If you have <u>advanced cancer</u>, you have no time to lose. You must accomplish three things with great haste to recover:

- stop the malignancy
- shrink your tumors
- remove the toxicity in your vital organs that leads to mortality.

If you have been given less than six months to live go directly to the 21 Day Cancer Curing Program on page 179. As soon as you are making progress, you can come back and read the explanations in the other chapters.

Also read the case histories; see how hopeless the situation <u>was</u> and how simple it is to stop the cancer, shrink the tumor, and feel safe from ever having cancer again.

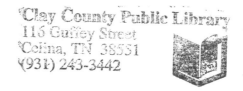

Is It Really A CURE?

The word **cure** in the title was chosen, rather than **treatment**, because it is scientifically accurate.

When the true <u>cause</u> of an illness has been found and, by removing it, the illness can be stopped or prevented, a true <u>cure</u> has also been found. When the cause is not found but the symptoms can be removed, helpful as this is, you have only found a <u>treatment</u>. My research was a search for the <u>causes</u> of cancer, how they might be removed, and whether their removal would lead to relief from the disease. I did not search merely for relief from the disease as most regular cancer research does. Even research into gene-replacement does not address the <u>cause</u> of numerous mutations in cancer. Nor does finding better ways to kill tumor cells. They are treatments.

Syncrometer® technology described in this book makes searching for causes and cures possible. Hopefully, there will also be a return to a search for the cure of diseases like diabetes, heart disease, multiple sclerosis, Parkinson's, and a lot of others that are now simply being treated.

The Cure For All *Advanced* Cancers

Published in the United States by New Century Press
1055 Bay Boulevard, Suite C, Chula Vista, CA 91911
(619) 476-7400, (800) 519-2465, www.newcenturypress.com
ISBN 1-890035-16-5

Other books by Dr. Clark available from New Century Press:
The Cure For All Cancers
Heilverfahren Aller Krebsarten (Cure For Cancers, German)
The Cure for All Cancers (Japanese Translation)
The Cure for All Diseases
Heilung ist möglich (Cure For All Diseases, German)
The Cure for All Diseases (Chinese Translation)
The Cure For HIV And AIDS

Reprinted 2004

RESEARCH ARTICLES AVAILABLE
In the interests of stimulating further research in these areas, the articles referred to in this book and other related articles are available from New Century Press at a nominal fee. By making these copies available the author wishes to eliminate the difficulties readers may have in gaining access to these materials. Send a SASE to New Century Press for an order form.

Notice to the Reader

The opinions and conclusions expressed in this book are mine alone. They are based on my scientific research and on specific case studies involving my patients. Be advised that every person is unique and may respond differently to the treatments described in this book. On occasion I have provided dosage recommendations where appropriate. Again, remember that we are all different and any new treatment should be applied in a cautious, common sense fashion.

The treatments outlined herein are not intended to be a replacement for other forms of conventional medical treatment. Please feel free to consult with your physician or other health care provider.

I have indicated throughout this book the existence of serious pollutants in food, dental materials and even medicine and intravenous supplies. These pollutants were identified using a testing device of my invention known as the Syncrometer.® Complete instructions for building and using this device are contained in my first book *The Cure For All Cancers*. Therefore anyone can repeat the tests described and verify the results.

The Syncrometer, an audio frequency oscillator is more accurate and versatile than the best existing testing methods. A way to determine the degree of precision is also presented. However at present it only yields positive or negative results, it does not quantify. The chance of a false positive or a false negative is about 5%, which can be lessened by test repetition.

It is in the public interest to know when a single bottle of a single product tests positive to a serious pollutant. If one does, the safest course is to avoid all bottles of that product entirely, which is what I repeatedly advise. These recommendations should be interpreted as an intent to warn and protect the public, not to provide a statistically significant market analysis. It is my fervent hope that manufacturers use the new electronic techniques in this book to make purer products than they ever have before.

It is also in the public interest to disseminate the information about cancer in this book, even before clinical evaluations of properly "blinded" treatment protocols are made, because the advice in this book does not interfere with existing treatment. Formal validations may take decades, during which time the suffering is great.

Since avoidance of certain foods and products is central to my method for pursuit of health, it is my hope that many persons train themselves in Syncrometer use. Others may elect to use testing laboratories. See *Sources* for some that use the latest technology and are willing to test supplements, foods, body products, and biological specimens (such as surgery and biopsy specimens) for the pollutants I discuss in this book.

Special Tribute

This work is dedicated to the unsung heroes of so-called "alternative" cancer therapies, both past and present. With their own money, and on their own time, they chose to do battle against humanity's most tragic mystery disease, cancer. Although this disease dates back to antiquity, its wild acceleration in the past 100 years has baffled us all. Facing the mythical monsters of the Greek literature in ancient times with mere rocks or swords could not have been more daunting than this disease. This challenge was often undertaken or continued even with the ridicule of peers, impending bankruptcy, and on-going lawsuits. Their compassion for cancer sufferers is immeasurable. If it were not for their writings, I could not have made my own discoveries. Knowledge is built upon knowledge. I am deeply grateful to all these persons for their sacrifice of life's comforts to further the cause of truth and to describe their work: Max Gerson, Virginia Livingston Wheeler, Harold W. Manner, Andrew C. Ivy, Robert R. Rife, William F. Koch, Ernst T. Krebs Jr. There are many more for whom this tribute is intended. Some had an MD, some had a Ph.D., some had both, and others none. No matter, they had the right stuff. Their hard work stands as a monument to the essential goodness of humanity.

Acknowledgments

The smallest coincidence can be the hinge on which future events turn. So it was for the microscope slide of *Fasciolopsis buskii*, made by Frank Jerome, DDS. It turned out to be the malignancy-causing parasite as described in *Cure For All Cancers*. Now, once again Dr. Jerome supplied a microscope slide he made in his parasitology class long ago. This time it was the rabbit fluke, *Hasstilesia tricolor*. The rabbit fluke turned out to be the true source of *Clostridium*, the tumor causing bacterium. My sincere Thank You!

In 1996, the collaboration with Patricia Connolly-Gorzen made possible our discovery of dental toxins and better dental practices.

Gratitude is also due to Elizabeth Sorrells, whose dedication was equally amazing. Thanks are due to the entire staff of the International Diagnostic Center, especially the pathologist, Dr. Miguel A. Ruiz, for their unique contributions.

I gratefully acknowledge the help of my son, Geoffrey Clark, as administrator of the International Diagnostic Center, provider of malonate-free food, environmentally safe lodging, and later as computer editor of this book. This project could not have been done without him.

The help of my sister, Edna R. Bernstein, was also indispensable, as literature researcher.

Gratitude is due to the Mexican dentist C.D. Joachin J. Zavala, and oral surgeon, C.D. Benjamin Arichega C.M.F. Without their expertise, none of our terminally ill cancer patients could have recovered.

And finally, Mexico itself is to be commended on its research-friendly climate. I am truly grateful to this forward-looking country that made this venture possible.

Contents

Figures

An Invitation

This book, *The Cure For All Advanced Cancers*, is about a completely self-sufficient cancer therapy that can be carried out by the patient at home at fairly low cost. It seldom requires medical care.

At one time **scurvy**, a vitamin C deficiency disease, was so life threatening it required medical care, but it no longer does. We all know what to do: eat fresh fruit and vegetables. It took 400 years from the discovery of its cure (1535) to utilization of the cure by the public in the early 1900's. Yet it had been published in <u>medical journals</u> many times![1] It took the unrelated <u>orange juice industry</u> to bring it to the public's attention in the early 1900's.

Why did it take so long to put into practice a simple truth, like the importance of eating fresh fruit and vegetables? Because ordinary people, not able to read the medical journals, had no way to learn of it. Unless the public has access to the great truths uncovered by scientists, they can not learn them even now.

Cancer as an epidemic is now 100 years old. Some of its true causes were already known 100 years ago, like parasites (in several animals),[2] coal tar,[3] synthetic dyes,[4] over-fried foods.[5] But these discoveries were ignored rather than treasured, as befell the scurvy cure.

---

[1] Davies, M.B., Austin, J., Partridge, D.A., *Vitamin C, Its Chemistry and Biochemistry*, Royal Society of Chemistry, 1991, chapter 2.

[2] A good discussion of this topic (more than just dogs) is by Bailey, W.S., *Parasites and Cancer: Sarcoma in Dogs Associated with Spirocerca lupi*, Annals Of the New York Academy of Sciences, v. 108, 1963, pp. 890-923.

[3] Greenstein, Jesse P., *Biochemistry of Cancer*, 2nd ed., Academic Press Inc., 1954, pp. 44-56.

[4] Ibid., pp. 88-96.

[5] Lane, A., Blickenstaff, D., and A.C. Ivy, *The Carcinogenicity of Fat "Browned" by Heating*, Cancer, v. 3, 1950, pp. 1044-51.

Hopefully the age of computers will set free the bird of truth as was never before possible. Patients now have easy access to information just like doctors and researchers do.

Yet this book is not a critique of current clinical management of cancer. No experiments were done on age-matched patients with similar cancers comparing my treatments to chemotherapy, radiation or surgery. Scientific/clinical evaluations await the future. The good news is that this new method is not incompatible with clinical treatments in most respects. But the use of certain vitamins may be considered undesirable by your oncologist if she/he is planning certain chemotherapies. There is a very large body of research literature that discusses the use of supplements in cancer.[6] Your oncologist may wish to peruse some of the references cited in this research report as well as throughout this book.

Most victims of cancer have been given an accurate diagnosis, meaning a label for their cancer. After this a **protocol** (procedure) for this particular cancer was applied, taken from a scientifically acquired bank of data. Here is a sample: MMM chemotherapy regimen for breast cancer, MOB chemotherapy regimen for cancer of the cervix, MOCCA chemotherapy regimen for myeloma, MOPP/ABVD chemotherapy regimen for Hodgkin's disease, and MOPLACE chemotherapy regimen for MOPP- and ABVD-resistant Hodgkin's disease.[7] Radiation and surgery protocols are also carefully described and prescribed. All this data and its efficacy is undoubtedly correct, taken within the boundaries of the varied assumptions made to get them.

A huge catalog of such data exists, with the precise protocol for each category and sub-category of cancer. Your doctor may still be creative and flexible <u>within</u> this protocol or use a <u>new</u>

---

[6] Jaakkola, K., et al., *Treatment with Antioxidant and other Nutrients in Combination with Chemotherapy and Irradiation in Patients with Small-Cell Lung Cancer*, Anticancer Research, v. 12, 1992, pp. 599-606.

[7] Haskell, Charles M., *Cancer Treatment*, 4th ed., W.B. Saunders Company, 1995. Taken from index, p. 1212.

experimental procedure, which is another statistically derived protocol[8].

Remember that oncologists are highly trained in the sciences; they do want the best for you. They must practice within the boundaries of conventional treatments or risk losing their license to practice. The result may be something that overtreats or undertreats. This is unavoidable. They too would like to know the cause and effect relationships that underlie cancer and do not try to cover up ignorance.

When you are first contemplating the options available to you, try to choose the best of both worlds for yourself. You will be torn in different directions.

A fictional example, about a painful toe, may help:

> One day, you tell your doctor your toe hurts and has been painful for several months. You are given a blood test, a physical examination, and some pain killers. You are asked to return in a few weeks. When you return and there has been no change, you are referred to a foot specialist.
>
> The new doctor scans, measures, palpates and Doppler-auscultates your foot and toe; details on posture, gait, health history, family foot problems are noted. All the results, put together after a complete workup, give you a label (diagnosis): *prosematis*. This label is now looked up in a huge catalog that is kept current by professional and government committees. There are very many entries of similar but slightly different conditions, like "pseudo prosematis," "atypical prosematis," "idiopathic prosematis." Success in treatment depends on the diagnosis being absolutely accurate. (A large part of the work and expense that goes into cancer treatment is in the accuracy of the diagnosis.) The catalog gives you the treatment protocol: ACP, IHO/W, PMT/GA in order of effectiveness for your prosematis.
>
> ACP means Amputation up to the exact Center of the Pain location. "When a circle is drawn according to pain intensity determined by artificially produced pain around that point and a pain intensity scale is used to determine the diameter of," and so forth. Exact details fill a page or more.

---

8 Warrel, R.P. Jr., Danieu, L., Coonley, C., Atkins, C., *Salvage Chemotherapy of Advanced Lymphoma with Investigational Drugs: Mitoguazone, Gallium Nitrate, and Etoposide*, Cancer Treatment Reports, v. 71, 1987, pp. 47-51.

IHO/W means Immersion in Hot Oil or hot Water for prescribed periods of time after immobilization in various ways and appropriate anesthesia, etc.

PMT/GA means Pressure is to be applied on top of (or from the bottom of) the center of the pain location to MT (maximum tolerated) with or without local anesthesia. The doctor can creatively decide whether GA (general anesthesia) may be used and the length of time to apply pressure in order to maximize treatment. It is explained to you that the treatment is effective for five years in 30% of cases but you will be carefully followed to catch the earliest recurrence.

You, the patient, may be shocked almost to tears, and ask the doctor how your toe pain could warrant such drastic measures, whether this really is prosematis.

Yet, this seems like a foolish question when your own educational training tells you the diagnosis was scientifically acquired, the measuring devices were all accurate, and a thousand scientific studies support the catalog of protocols for prosematis. Undoubtedly, the treatment is effective and will work for you. You tell yourself you must simply trust.

Only a modern human being could be so duped. These recommendations would be hilariously funny to a primitive person who would first of all throw away their shoes! But in your ignorance, walking to work each day in fashionable shoes, it is entirely serious.

Suppose you go home, too depressed to eat the rest of the day. You imagine how your toeless foot will look and wonder if a prosthesis exists. Will your spouse have more of an aversion to your toeless foot, or prosthesis? You take your shoes off and step into a hot shower. You tearfully watch TV. Then you notice the pain is temporarily gone. You keep out of those shoes, take more hot foot baths. Being scientifically oriented, you try more changes: a better diet, stopping bad habits, and resting your foot. Eventually, you clear it up yourself!

You can't help wondering how a clinical treatment could be so wrong, when all the data that went into it were so right. You wonder why ordinary things, not scientific in nature, like shoe fit, diet, and foot use did not come under scrutiny. The doctors were all kind and sympathetic, thoroughly believing in their treatment methods (and outlawing others for your protection). You may conclude, as I did, that a totally "scientific" system of belief and treatment can still be quite wrong, even though, admittedly, the treatments like amputation to cure prosematis would be 100% effective.

"Prosematis" is a fictional disease I made up to illustrate how more serious diseases, like cancer, are treated. Scientific data are a collection of accurately obtained, statistically sound measurements. Science is not the culprit. But its application requires wisdom—a human quality. It can be lacking in any individual or profession. Yet, we all have some of it.

An example of wisdom for an individual might be changing daily habits when cancer threatens, such as improving diet, stopping addictions, and stopping the use of recognized carcinogens. This book will elaborate on these.

An example of wisdom for the medical profession would be searching for carcinogens in the tumorous organ. Then searching for the same carcinogens in the patient's air, water, food, and body products.

For example the dye "butter yellow" is known to cause elevated alkaline phosphatase levels in animals. Many cancer patients show elevated alkaline phosphatase levels, too. Researchers should search for butter yellow in these cancer patients. To my knowledge such a study has not been done, nor do I see evidence of this whole approach! Here's another example. Scientists know that broken chromosomes are characteristic of nearly every cancer.[9,10] They also know that heavy metals, like copper, cadmium, and the lanthanides ("rare earths") cause chromo-

[9] Weiss, L.M., Warnke, R.A., Sklar, J., Cleary, M.L., *Molecular Analysis of the t(14;18) Chromosomal Translocation in Malignant Lymphomas*, N. Eng. Jour. Med., v. 317, no. 19, 1987, pp. 1185-89.

[10] Warrell, R.P., et. al., *Differentiation Therapy of Acute Promyelocytic Leukemia with Tretinoin (All-Trans-Retinoic Acid)*, N. Eng. Jour. Med., v. 324, no. 20, 1991, pp. 1385-93.

somes to break.[11] Yet doctors do not send biopsy specimens to a lab for heavy metal analysis!

Ordinary lay persons have a great deal of wisdom. This book will help you to practice and express your wisdom. You can build the same diagnostic and monitoring tool that I have used: instructions are in *The Cure for all Cancers*. Your wisdom, together with others', is much needed. When wisdom is accumulated, it can contribute to a <u>new</u> bank of information for persons in the future who face the same dilemma you faced. Wisdom can be gained by communicating and listening to others in similar predicaments. It is my cherished belief that you and others can solve human health problems with unprecedented speed and success.

I invite you to do so.

---

[11] Komiyama, Makoto, *Sequence-Specific and Hydrolytic Scission of DNA and RNA by Lanthanide Complex-OligoDNA Hybrids*, J. Biochem, v. 118, no. 4, 1995, pp. 665-70.

The Tumor

We have all believed that cancer is a <u>single</u> disease. That a malignant cell starts it all. This is not true. Cancer is <u>two</u> diseases. Malignancy is the second and last disease to set in. By curing this <u>last</u> disease, (malignancy), as we did in *The Cure For All Cancers*, the <u>earlier</u> disease becomes visible. This earlier, <u>first</u> disease is <u>tumor-growing</u>. It is a distinct and different disease from malignancy.

We have also believed that tumors, unless they are malignant, need not be feared, that they may be called <u>benign</u>, implying safety. This is like a zebra on the African plains believing that a lion who is standing very still, nearby, need not be feared. This is, again, <u>not true</u>.

In this book, I will show you the true nature of tumors, why they grow and even multiply. Why they are dangerous. By removing the <u>causes</u> of tumor growth, you will be able to <u>shrink</u> your tumors.

Even if you have a non-tumorous form of cancer, the same causes are at work. All cancers are alike.

Your body has built-in tumor shrinkers. Obviously, they are not working. Why? They are blocked. You only need to unblock them. It does not take months or years to unblock them. It only takes <u>days</u> to do this and begin the shrinking process.

You will <u>see</u> it happen, on X-rays or by blood test results. You may <u>feel</u> it happen when pressure and pain are reduced. But <u>how</u> the body shrinks your tumors, or gets rid of cells that have acquired numerous mutations, the exact mechanism involved, is still a mystery. Even the $p53$ mutations, the hallmark of cancers, disappear! Oncogenes, such as the myc family, stop reproducing. (We will talk about all these later.) The details must wait for future research. The good news is that it <u>does</u> happen, predictably, not by chance or "spontaneous remission."

Malignancy Review

Now that we can cure both the malignancy <u>and</u> the tumor growth, we may reflect: it makes good sense that malignancy and tumor growth <u>are</u> two distinct diseases. After all, the malignancy is simply the result of invasion of your tumors by a fluke parasite, *Fasciolopsis buskii*, and the presence of **isopropyl alcohol**.

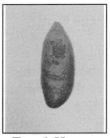

The common name for this parasite is **human intestinal fluke**. It goes through its

Fig. 1 Human intestinal fluke typical size

larval stages in your tumors, instead of in its usual secondary host, a snail. Your body serves the same purpose as the snail's—it provides food and shelter for the parasite. But at a huge cost! If isopropyl alcohol is present also, we will make abundant hCG and ortho-phospho-tyrosine (which I use

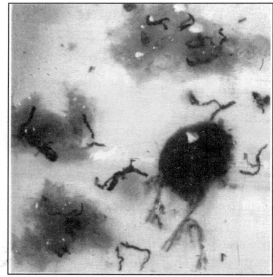

These were expelled from the bowel, they are in various stages of decay. They float. "Black hairy legs" are strings of eggs.
Fig. 2 Five flukes

as cancer markers[12]). Surprisingly there are <u>two</u> ways you can get isopropyl alcohol into your body. Some bacteria produce it, and it is used as an antiseptic in many of our body products and food!

Obviously, then, the most important thing to do first is eliminate these parasites, bacteria, and unnatural chemicals. This, in turn, eliminates the two dominant growth stimulators hCG and ortho-phospho-tyrosine.

Tumor Tour

hCG is **human Chorionic Gonadotropin**, the same hormone a mother produces in her placenta to protect the growing baby from attack by her own immune system. hCG will protect the tumor cells from attack, no doubt, by <u>your</u> immune system.[13] hCG is <u>only</u> present when isopropyl alcohol is present and organic germanium ("good" germanium) is absent, suggesting that it may result from a specific mutation (a mutation is a change in your genes). We will see evidence for this theory later.

Ortho-phospho-tyrosine is a powerful growth stimulant, perhaps made by the parasite larvae themselves, perhaps induced in our cells by the intestinal fluke parasite. Whatever the mechanism is, the explosive growth that results has disastrous consequences: metastasis to far flung places in the body. No amount of surgery, radiation, or chemotherapy and no amount of alternative therapy (vitamins, health potions, immune boosters) can keep up with such a *mitosis* (cell division) explosion.

But killing this parasite and all its tiny larval stages stops it in about a week, using the parasite-killing program discussed in *The Cure For All Cancers*. In <u>advanced</u> cancer we will use

---

[12] Sell, S., *Diagnostic Uses of Cancer Markers*, The Female Patient, v. 9, Aug 1984, p. 133-48. Tyrosine-Phosphorylated Proteins are discussed as markers for human tumors in these articles: Hunter, T., Cooper, J.A. Ann, Rev. Biochem., v. 54, 1985, p. 897. Yarden, Y. Ann. Rev. Biochem., v. 57, 1988, p. 443.

[13] *A Clue to Cancer*, Newsweek, Oct. 23, 1995, p. 92.

doses that kill all parasites and all their stages in the first twenty-four hours. Fortunately, the advanced cancer program is well tolerated by even the sickest person. We can then turn our attention to shrinking the tumors so you can get well. All this can be accomplished in three weeks so I call it **The 21 Day Program**.

Tumor Cell Handicaps

Tumor cells are a very special breed. They have become like drones, doing nothing, in a busy bee hive. Tumor cells do nothing to contribute to the organ they live in. Liver cells do liver work. Pancreas cells do pancreas work. Bone cells do bone work. But tumor cells do no work. It is not by choice, though.

Tumor cells have no tools to work with; this means they have no enzymes, nor RNA to make enzymes. RNA is *ribonucleic acid*, the blueprint for making proteins, and my Syncrometer never detects any in advanced tumors. RNA is necessary to make all proteins (enzymes are proteins).

A Syncrometer is a new electronic device which is described in *The Cure For All Cancers*. With it you can identify objects and chemicals in your tissues very accurately.

Tumor cells do not even have the raw materials to make proteins; this means they have no *amino acids*. Besides this, the tumor cells' energy-generators are mostly shut down, and the ones remaining are old and decrepit. The energy-generators in a living cell are the *mitochondria*. The mitochondria are shriveled, misshapen, and few in number.[14] It is the mitochondria's job to turn out energy which will be the cells' fuel. This is called adenosine triphosphate (ATP). We can hardly expect the

---

14 Ohe, K., Morris, H.P., and Weinhouse, S., *β-Hydroxybutyrate Dehydrogenase Activity in Liver and Liver Tumors*, Cancer Res., v. 27, 1967, pp. 1360-71.

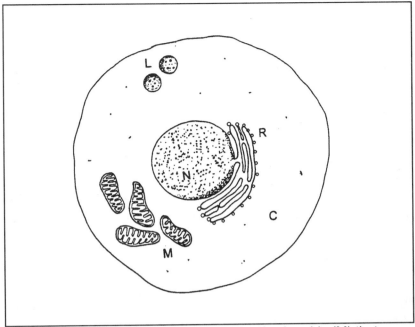

A healthy cell is a very busy place, with mitochondria (M) that use oxygen to turn out energy, the cytoplasm (C) where glycolysis takes place, the lysosomes (L) that tackle invading bacteria, the nucleus (N) where your genes make the RNA that will produce your proteins, the ribosomes (R) that stud the membranes attached to the nucleus, where proteins are actually made.

Fig. 4 A cell with nucleus, cytoplasm, mitochondria, etc.

tumor cells to do any work if neither the equipment (enzymes), nor the material (amino acids), nor the fuel (ATP) are available.

The mitochondria are in a broken down condition for two reasons: (1) constant interference by **malonic acid**, and (2) lack of thyroid hormones.

Malonic acid is constantly being eaten because it occurs in some common foods. It also trickles in from tapeworm larvae lodged in us and from a completely unnatural source, plastic teeth (we will discuss malonic acid later).

But the lack of *thyroxine*, a major thyroid hormone, is <u>not</u> due to a weak thyroid gland as in an ordinary low-thyroid condition. The thyroid gland makes its daily quota of thyroxine (five grains each day) and ships it out via the blood stream to each one of our 50 billion body cells! It must enter each cell to deliver its activating effect. But as the thyroxine enters the tumor cell, and approaches the mitochondria, it is attacked by *thiourea*. Thiourea destroys the thyroid hormone. This does not happen in the neighboring healthy tissue.

You might be asking yourself why we care if tumor cells are malnourished, have dysfunctional mitochondria, and other abnormalities. After all, aren't we trying to kill them? The answer is no, we are not. We are trying to heal them! Then tumors shrink and the tissue returns to normal.

Yet, thiourea is a normal chemical, made by each cell to facilitate cell division. It is only doing its job. Unfortunately it is being overproduced by the tumor cell, in its own effort to heal itself. Living things are supposed to heal themselves whenever they are wounded or injured in some way. Our cells instinctively know they must multiply themselves to heal. This provides healthy, young cells to fill the gaping hole or to replace the injured cells. The damaged cells are digested. Tumor cells are busily healing themselves by such multiplication. Why don't they stop? Are they never done healing? Why don't they stop dividing in two when they are done healing? What are they healing from?

Tumor Cell Division

They don't stop because the "brakes" on cell division are not being used. This allows the accelerator of cell division, thiourea, to be on continuously. The brakes are another chemical made by each cell for itself, called *pyruvic aldehyde*. (We will often call it the "brakes.") The brakes are gone. Pyruvic aldehyde can seldom be detected by the Syncrometer in the tumor-tissue. So, not only is there an accelerated multiplication of cells going on, but the brakes slowing them down are gone. At the same time the excess thiourea destroys the thyroid hormones, and without thyroxine the mitochondria can't do their work.

Why are the brakes gone? Pyruvic aldehyde is susceptible to *amines*, much as car brakes are susceptible to drops of oil. Amines react and combine with pyruvic aldehyde until it is all gone.

Our cells normally make thiourea for one minute, followed by pyruvic aldehyde for one minute, and so on, back and forth, like a pendulum, to keep a balance between the accelerator and the brakes on cell division. But when massive amounts of amines appear in the cell, there may be no brakes on cell division for fifteen minutes at a time, followed by just one minute of pyruvic aldehyde, typical of a fast growing tumor.

Why are there so many amines around? Some amines are produced naturally by our cells, perhaps to do exactly this— release the brakes by combining with pyruvic aldehyde on a tight schedule. But the excessive amount of amines in tumor cells is produced by <u>bacteria</u>. Simple bacteria! They have entered the cells as they always try to do. But for some reason the tumor cells can neither kill them, nor free themselves of them. The predator is living within! The cells' primitive solution to this impasse is to divide itself (release the brakes on cell division), so at least one of the two newly formed cells will escape and be free of the attacker, assuring survival. Like a fingernail you accidentally hit with a hammer, the nail will fall off eventually and reveal a new one growing underneath.

Tumor Cell Bacteria

It is understandable now, why tumor cells are not able to do any work. They are sick. Bacteria have attacked them. Their toxic amines have removed the brakes. Without brakes thiourea production is endless and thyroxine can't reach the mitochondria. Mitochondria are <u>dependent</u> on thyroxine.[15] Without it the generator-like enzymes cannot burn the food molecules that are waiting to be oxidized into ATP. This part of our metabolism is called *respiration*. Without enough energy, tumor cells only divide and contribute nothing. Unless you count making a cozy home for *Fasciolopsis* larval stages! That parasite then contributes ortho-phospho-tyrosine to accelerate them into malignancy.

Ordinarily when bacteria attack, either <u>your cells or the bacteria</u> win the battle. It is a life and death struggle. If the bacteria win, your cells die. They do not become tumor cells. They are dead and will be removed by your white blood cells. But if your cells win, the bacteria die and are digested by special little "fortresses" inside your cells called *lysosomes*. Unfortunately, thyroxine is needed to activate your lysosomes too! Because tumor cells are short on thyroxine an <u>impasse</u> is occurring. They neither die, nor can they kill their invaders. They are half alive and half dead. They are in a twilight zone, trying to solve the impasse by dividing.

If only we could help them heal, the impasse would be over. How to help them is the subject of this book.

Tumor-making bacteria are of a special kind, too: *Clostridium* species. They have the ability to make DNA in a special bacterial way.[16] They make huge amounts of DNA from RNA by the enzyme, *ribonucleotide reductase*. Their enzyme requires vitamin B_{12}, which <u>you</u> supply.

Clostridium species of bacteria are the constant companions of tumors, supplying the DNA, the toxic amines, and even the isopropyl alcohol which will eventually contribute to malignancy. The bacteria are thriving, while flooding your cells with excess DNA that can be used for cell division. Some of the

---

[15] Ingbar, Sidney H., Braverman, Lewis E., *Werner's The Thyroid A Fundamental and Clinical Text*, 5th Ed., 1986, p. 224-27, 949.

[16] Zubay, Geoffrey, *Biochemistry*, Addison-Wesley Pub. Co., 1984, pp. 706-07.

bacterial DNA will certainly get integrated (joined) with your own DNA. And most certainly, any viruses infecting the bacteria will seize their chance, too, to join and **transform** your DNA.

"Transformation" is a scientific term that describes what happens when your genes (DNA) have been joined by foreign DNA, such as from a virus. Your cells become changed (transformed), <u>stopping their normal</u> RNA and protein formation. The virus genes now hidden amongst your own can be triggered by <u>common chemicals</u> (as anyone with chronic *Herpes* infection knows) to reproduce. And <u>some</u> virus genes tell your cells to multiply! They have become *oncogenes*, genes that cause tumors.[17] Such an event is quite possible, even probable, when hordes of *Clostridium* bacteria have invaded your cells without killing them or being killed. This should not happen. It was not meant to happen.

Cell Defense Mechanisms

Cells that are struggling for their lives call out for help. They call for your immune system. They call for a temperature rise. They call for oxidizers. They call for reducers. Ultimately, they call for self-destruction in a self-sacrificing way to protect <u>you</u>. So that <u>you</u> could never develop an aggressive tumor. But what will go wrong?

- Your immune system will fail.
- Your temperature will not rise.
- Your oxidizers will vanish.
- Your reducing power will disappear.

---

17 Braude, Abraham, et. al., *Infectious Diseases and Medical Microbiology*, 2nd ed., W. B. Saunders Co., chapter 10. Pringle, C.R., *The Genetics of Viruses*, pp. 94-102.

How will your immune system fail? Perhaps the flood of hCG incapacitates it.[18] Perhaps the metals arriving on the site destroy your white blood cells' ability to find and "home-in" on the infected cells.[19] Perhaps the absence of germanium (the "good," organic kind) suppresses immunity and does not let interferon be made.[20] Perhaps our increasing exposure to benzene is crippling our immune system.[21] Perhaps our white blood cells are smothered with ferritin or immobilized due to lanthanides (discussed in detail later). We do not yet know. But lowered immunity is a hallmark of cancer. The most significant observation I make with the Syncrometer is that glutathione (GSH) is absent! Although I am not sure what the exact connection is, I observe that all healthy cells have glutathione, and all cells with bacteria, heavy metal, or malonic acid, do not. I conclude that your glutathione has been destroyed by trying to detoxify these. So for many reasons your cells cannot depend on your immune system to assist them.

Your body tries to raise its temperature. This will cook and fry many invaders. But a cancer patient's body does not respond. In fact, cancer sufferers are extra cold. Their body temperature is often more than one degree colder than normal! Is this the work of toxic amines? Is it a thyroid gland problem, beyond the local effect of thiourea? The answer still eludes us, but the

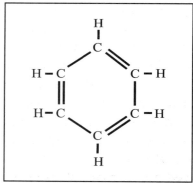

H is hydrogen, C is carbon.
Fig. 5 A benzene molecule

---

18 *A Clue to Cancer*, Newsweek, Oct. 23, 1995, p. 92.

19 Ward, P.A., Goldschmidt, P., Greene, N.D., *Suppressive Effects of Metal Salts on Leukocyte and Fibroblastic Function*, Journal of the Reticuloendothelial Society, v. 18, no. 5, Nov. 1975, pp. 313-21.

20 Suzuki, F., Pollard, R.B., *Prevention of Suppressed Interferon Gamma Production in Thermally Injured Mice by Administration of a Novel Organogermanium Compound, Ge-132*, Journal of Interferon Res., v. 4, no. 2, 1984, pp. 223-33.

21 Lucier, G.W., Hood, G.E.R. (eds), *Symposium on Benzene Metabolism, Toxicity and Carcinogenesis*, Environ. Health Perspect., v. 82, 1989, pp. 1-349.

result is that your struggling cells will not get the temperature rise they need.

Your body's oxidizers will vanish. *Oxidation* means burning up by adding an oxygen atom or by subtracting an electron. Here is an example of oxidizing benzene (which looks simple, but is very difficult to do in your body).

Each line between the carbon atoms represents two electrons being shared. Sharing creates a strong bond between them, like two people holding hands tightly.

Your body has the necessary enzyme to pry apart one of these strong bonds, and pull out an electron or insert an oxygen atom. The advantage gained is that the oxidized benzene atom is more soluble in water (namely urine) and can be excreted through the kidneys. Oxidation is used to detoxify substances as well as to burn food into energy. The detoxifying enzymes belong to a family called *cytochrome P450 enzymes*. But they must have **iron** to function. If you live in a home with copper water pipes, the excess copper in your water is competing with the iron in your food. It is well known that iron is lacking in cancer patients.[22] Other oxidizers like diamine oxidase, D-amino acid oxidase,[23] rhodizonic acid, and cytochrome C are also missing. We will discuss more on oxidation later.

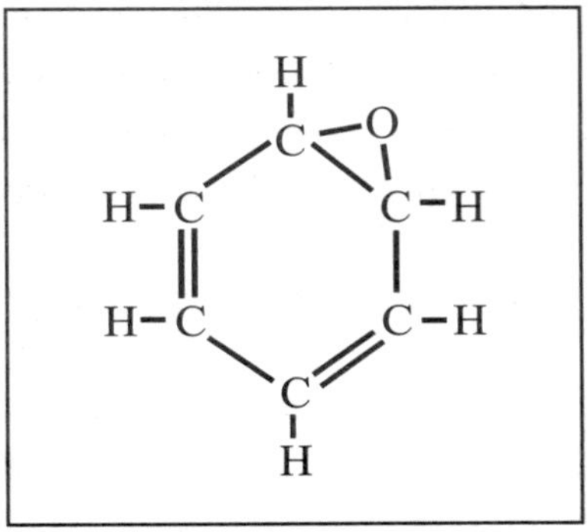

O is an oxygen atom.

Fig. 6 Benzene beginning to be oxidized

---

[22] Sigel, Helmut (ed), *Metal Ions In Biological Systems*, Carcinogenicity and Metal Ions, Marcel Dekker, Inc., v. 10, 1980, chapter 5. Foster, M., et. al., *Ceruloplasmin and Iron Transferrin in Human Malignant Disease*, pp. 129-66.

[23] The research states that the dye popularly called DAB can cause this enzyme depletion. Greenstein, Jesse P., *Biochemistry of Cancer*, 2nd ed., Academic Press Inc., 1954, p. 97.

Your body's reducers will disappear. When oxidizer-chemistry fails, the opposite can be tried, *reduction*. Now atoms of oxygen are removed or electrons are added. **Vitamin C** is a reducer. It gives away its own electrons to the chemical the body wishes to reduce. It gives away its hydrogen atoms too,

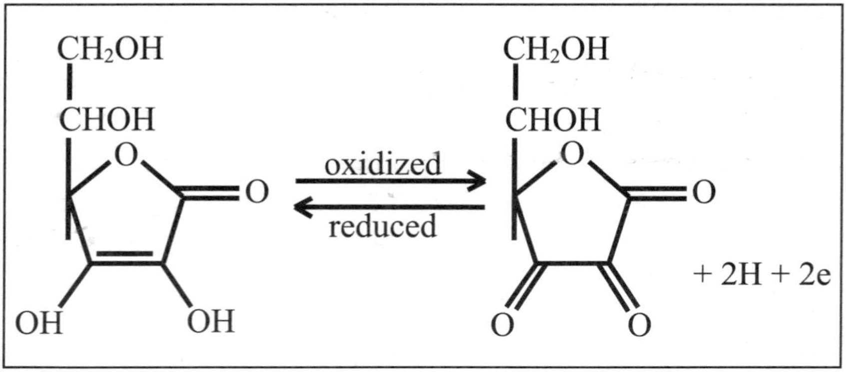

L-ascorbic acid   dehydroascorbic acid
Vitamin C can give up two electrons (two hydrogen atoms go also).
Fig. 7 Two states of vitamin C

and then is itself called *dehydroascorbate*. **Cysteine** and **glutathione** are two other reducers.[24] Reduction, like oxidation, is strong chemistry, but in a cancer patient this mechanism is very weak. There is very little reducing power in the blood.[25] Why someone loses their reducing power is not known, but I think it's largely due to exposure to heavy metals, like nickel and chromium from stainless steel cookware, or cadmium from galvanized water pipes, or mercury, thallium and germanium (the toxic kind) from amalgam tooth fillings.

Your beleaguered cells are reaching a crisis. They are losing their immunity, bacteria are attacking them, so they are trying to multiply themselves out of this predicament, and, of course, trying to self-destruct at a stepped up pace, too. We will discuss

---

[24] Black, M.M., *Sulfhydryl Reduction of Methylene Blue With Reference to Alterations in Malignant Neoplastic Disease*, Cancer Research, v. 7,1947, pp. 592-94.

[25] Schoenbach, E., Weissman, N., Armistead, E., *The Determination of Sulfhydryl Groups in Serum.II. Protein Alterations Associated with Disease*, J. Clin. Invest., v. 30, 1951, pp. 762-77.

self-destruction later, but obviously the end result for a person with tumors is that self-destruction did not keep up with cell division, and a small mass formed.

Cell Mutations

Meanwhile, as the cells are multiplying faster and faster, a sinister development takes place. The very act of mitosis (cell division) exposes the *chromosomes* to chemicals that might cause mutations. The protective nuclear membrane is temporarily gone, leaving the genes naked in the cell sap, called *cytoplasm*. Normally mitosis is done quickly and not very often, to reduce this risk. But in the *Clostridium*-infected cells, mitosis is going on much more frequently due to the overabundance of thiourea. A scientist, looking at a specimen of a very early tumor sees many more nuclei going into mitosis—they become densely stained when dyes are applied that color DNA, making it easy to spot and count the cells that are in mitosis. This gives scientists a measure of the rate of mitosis. The problem with constant mitosis is that it increases exposure of your genes to the hazards of *mutagens* (substances that cause mutations) in the cytoplasm.

Look at the drawing of intestinal cells.[26] They are piling up

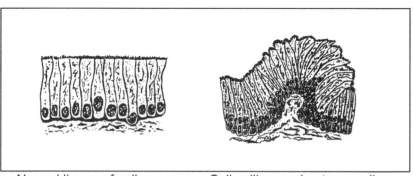

Normal lineup of cells   Cells piling up due to crowding.

Fig. 8 Beginning tumor formation

due to too much mitosis. It is a beginning "adenoma" typical of benign or pre-malignant tumors.

Soon mutations abound in this fast-multiplying tissue. But they will not be <u>random</u> mutations. They will be mostly **p53**, **LDH** and **alkaline phosphatase enzyme**, **vitamin A**, **bcl-2** and **bax** mutations. (We will discuss these soon.)

Metal In Cells

I do not understand why a tissue in distress or simply in accelerated mitosis <u>attracts</u> so many things. It attracts heavy metals. It attracts dyes. It attracts more bacteria and parasites. It attracts mutagens and carcinogens (these are chemicals specifically known to cause mutations or tumors). But it also attracts good things, like vitamins and immune boosters. This attractive force, which I call *morbitropism*, deserves intensive study.

If morbitropism attracts even minute quantities of toxins, is that significant? Yes. That peculiarity was noticed quite early in cancer research. Numerous <u>small</u> doses of a carcinogen, were more effective than fewer <u>large</u> doses.[27,28] In this respect, it was similar to the carcinogenic action of radiation: again, the <u>smaller</u> the dose, the more <u>effective</u> it was.[29] So that is why I advise people not to wear metal jewelry, to remove toxic tooth fillings, to change their metal water pipes to plastic, and avoid processed food (it has traces of dyes and antiseptic chemicals). Although the dose seems small, these particular toxins, over time, can be deadly.

Other attractive forces have already been studied: the liver attracts liver flukes, even if they are injected into a fish, far away from the liver near the tail; the flukes can somehow

---

[26] Koch, W.F., *Cancer and its Allied Diseases*, Pub. by author (Koch), 1933, pp. 40-41.

[27] Warburg, O., *On the Origin of Cancer Cells*, Science, v. 123, no. 3191, Feb. 24, 1956, pp. 309-14.

[28] Greenstein, pp. 104-05.

[29] Bain, J.A., Rusch, H.P., *Carcinogenesis with Ultraviolet Radiation of Wave Length 2,800-3,400 Å*, Cancer Res., v. 3, Jul. 1943, pp. 425-30.

"home in" to the liver. The attraction of certain metals, like thulium, gallium, technetium specifically to cancer sites has been the feature making bone scans possible. Cobalt is specially attracted to dividing cells.[30] The attractive force between bacteria and white blood cells can be "felt" for long distances; it is destroyed by heavy metals and fungus toxins.[31]

Perhaps some of these are not true forces—but just an accident of shape or chemistry, the way a kitchen sink drains and "attracts" water because of the hole in the base. Perhaps cell division itself makes cells act like a "sink."

Whatever the mechanism, heavy metals now arrive at the tiny site undergoing rapid mitosis: copper, cobalt, vanadium, germanium, lead, mercury, thallium, nickel, cadmium, and the lanthanides ("rare earth" elements). As well as arsenic, asbestos, freon, silicone, urethane, acrylic acid, and other non-metals. Copper, cobalt, and vanadium are always there, detected by the Syncrometer; the others are often there. Most of them are known mutagens.[32] Together, they begin using up all the sulfur that is available in the cells: all the cysteine, methionine, taurine, glutathione, SAM, pantothenic acid, coenzyme A, and vitamin B_1 (thiamin) because these all contain sulfur.

Metals (except the lanthanides) typically combine with sulfur to form sulfides. This also detoxifies them in the body, solubilizing them, so they can be excreted. Soon the cells are in sulfur bankruptcy. Cysteine and methionine are amino acids, glutathione is a reducer and immune-supporter, SAM and coenzyme A do other vital chemistry, and pantothenic acid and vitamin B_1 are essential parts (cofactors) that enzymes must have

---

[30] Liquier-Milward, J., *Tracer Studies on Cobalt Incorporation into Growing Tumors: Uptake of Radioactive Co^{60} by Normal and Malignant Cells*, Can. Res., 1957, pp. 841-44.

[31] Ward, P.A., Goldschmidt, P., Greene, N.D., *Suppressive Effects of Metal Salts on Leukocyte and Fibroblastic Function*, Journal of the Reticuloendothelial Society, v. 18, no. 5, Nov. 1975, pp. 313-21.

[32] Sigel, Helmut (ed), *Metal Ions In Biological Systems*, Carcinogenicity and Metal Ions, Marcel Dekker, Inc., v. 10, 1980, chapter 3. Issaq, H.J., *The Role of Metals in Tumor Development and Inhibition*, pp. 55-93, but this entire volume is devoted to various aspects of metal involvement in cancer.

to do their work. So metals cause depletion of some of your most vital compounds.

Metal sulfides can be escorted out of the body via the kidneys and intestines. After your sulfur is used up, the plain metals remain in circulation and are attracted to the tiny hyperactive tissue where cell division is accelerated.

Lanthanide metals cannot be detoxified this way. They belong to a special group of metals that are highly magnetic (paramagnetic), second only to iron.

They were once called "Rare Earths", though of course they are not rare. But they were so difficult to separate, one from another, that getting any one in pure form was rare indeed. There are 15 in all; although two other elements, yttrium and scandium, are often added to the group. The Syncrometer detects all the lanthanides in the metals used to restore teeth!

They are rarely found as pollutants in processed foods, nor in drinking water with two exceptions. One variety of water is loaded with yttrium and/or ytterbium. It is reverse-osmosis water. Evidently, the membrane used for treating such water has these lanthanides in it. And some varieties of vitamin C are contaminated with thulium.

The lanthanides do more sinister damage than regular heavy metals. They disturb your own DNA production; it begins too late (by 13 seconds)[33] but then runs overtime. The extra DNA is pushed into the lysosomes where the Syncrometer now detects the enzyme DNAse, which will happily destroy it. Yet, it represents danger.

The lanthanides seem to fill up your cells with iron deposits and calcium deposits. The link between lanthanum and calcium deposits has been studied[34], but the Syncrometer detects more. Cells "choked" with iron and calcium are not able to hoist a "flag" that begs your body to digest them. The flag is a cell

---

[33] Clark, H. R., *Syncrometer Biochemistry Laboratory Manual*, New Century Press, 1999.

[34] Smith, Bonita M., Gindhart, Thomas D., and Colburn, Nancy H., *Possible Involvement of a Lanthanide-Sensitive Protein Kinase C Substrate in Lanthanide Promotion of Neoplastic Transformation*, Carcinogenesis, v. 7, no. 12, 1986, pp. 1949-56.

chemical called **phosphatidylserine**; it can be forced to stick out of the cell membrane just like a real flag! In every normal tissue some worn out cells need to be digested, so healthy tissues are Positive for phosphatidylserine. But tumors test Negative for it, indicating this essential function is missing. "Raising" the "flag" attracts two common digestive enzymes, pancreatin and lipase, made by your pancreas in large amounts at mealtime. Children and healthy adults have these enzymes present in every organ at all times, but as you may guess, the Syncrometer detects neither of these in tumors.

So the lanthanides are preventing self-digestion—the very mechanism that lets tumors enlarge.

Uranium, a radioactive metal, is also found in the tumor. It, too, must come from metal tooth fillings since the Syncrometer finds uranium in about $2/3$ of all amalgam ordered fresh from the factory! If you have six amalgam fillings your chance of not having uranium in your mouth is one in 729.

PAHs In Cells

Non-metal mutagens also arrive at the threatening tumor site, apparently attracted in the same fashion. For instance, the Syncrometer detects polycyclic aromatic hydrocarbons (PAHs) at tumor sites. Some PAHs are extremely carcinogenic. Are they drawn by morbitropism? Or simply drawn by the "sink effect" of *purines* and *pyrimidines* that are present. Purines and pyrimidines are the *bases* that form part of all DNA. During cell division, DNA, with its purines and pyrimidines, are abundant in the cytoplasm, not hidden inside the nucleus. PAHs dissolve especially well in purines.[35] Carcinogenic PAHs, therefore, are particularly attracted to fast dividing cells.

---

[35] Weil-Malherbe, H., *The Solubilization of Polycyclic Aromatic Hydrocarbons by Purines*, Biochem. J., v. 40, 1946, pp. 351-63.

Decades ago, the common purine in coffee, called **caffeine**, was seen to easily dissolve PAHs.[36] And therefore attract them. The question then, was, is there anything in the human body to be attracted? Do we ever have PAHs, or things like PAHs, in our bodies? It was an intriguing question in the 1930's and 40's. All the more intriguing because of the resemblance between the PAHs and our own cholesterol molecules!

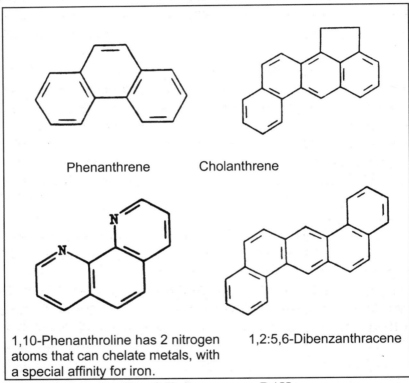

Phenanthrene   Cholanthrene

1,10-Phenanthroline has 2 nitrogen atoms that can chelate metals, with a special affinity for iron.

1,2:5,6-Dibenzanthracene

Fig. 9 Four common PAHs

Look at the sample PAHs pictured above. Hundreds of similar, though slightly different PAHs can be made in a lab and many of them will be carcinogenic.

---

36 Neish, W.J.P., *On the Solubilization of Aromatic Amines by Purines*, Recueil, v. 67, 1948, pp. 361-73.

Many PAHs are produced naturally in decaying organic matter such as coal tar[37] (from fossil vegetation) or crude oil (from ancient dinosaur bodies) or a grilled hamburger. Notice that they are combinations of benzene-like rings (look at the hexagonal shape of benzene, alone, on page 16). Benzene is a <u>flat</u> molecule, making the entire PAH flat. This will be an important feature.

Compare the PAH molecules with a cholesterol molecule. It, too, is very large, made up of benzene-like rings stuck together.

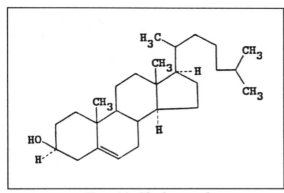

Fig. 10 Cholesterol

It too will be <u>flat</u>. But the rings do not have double bonds—not yet! So cholesterol is <u>not</u> carcinogenic—yet!

Heating cholesterol to a very high temperature, as in open fire grilling, <u>does</u> put double bonds into it and <u>does</u> make PAHs out of it.[38]

Yet, our own bodies never get that hot. Could there be enzymes that change our own cholesterol to PAHs? Yes. They were never found in the research studies of the 1930's and 40's. But the Syncrometer detects <u>numerous</u> PAHs that could be made from our own cholesterol (listed further on). But <u>only</u> when *Ascaris* is present! *Ascaris* is the common roundworm of cats and dogs. It parasitizes us, too, though it is less obvious.

Many of our hormones, including estrogen and testosterone, are <u>made</u> from cholesterol, and therefore have a similar structure, and therefore could be turned into PAHs as well.

---

[37] Greenstein, *The Carcinogenic Action Of Coal Tar* , pp. 44-88.

[38] Falk, H.L., Goldfien, S., Steiner, P.E., *The Products of Pyrolysis of Cholesterol at 360°C and Their Relation to Carcinogens*, Cancer Res., v. 9, 1949, pp. 438-47.

PAHs Invade DNA

Both cholesterol and PAH molecules are thin, flat, and shun water—just like the **bases** in our nucleic acids, our purines and pyrimidines. This similarity will lead to mutations!

Each of our chromosomes is made of a double thread of nucleic acid. Along the way are bases keeping them close together like thousands of hands clasped together. There are thousands of

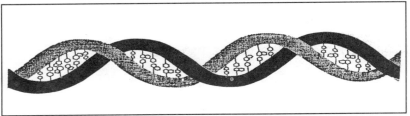

Two nucleic acid threads wound around each other.

Fig. 11 DNA

bases in each *gene* and over a thousand genes in each thread of nucleic acid. The double thread is wound around into a spring shape; this shortens it and makes it manageable. Only when a purine base is held by a pyrimidine base is the bond strong enough to hold the two threads close together. So while one thread has a purine base, the other has a pyrimidine and vice versa. But along a single thread, any assortment is possible. The neighboring thread will always provide the correct base to pair with it. **Obviously, the total number of purines must always equal the total number of pyrimidines.**

The spring-like shape allows the bases to be stacked like the steps of a spiral staircase, at the same time keeping the threads close together in a tight fit. Yet, <u>cholesterol-like</u> molecules <u>can</u> break into this careful arrangement when the chromosomes are lying unprotected in cytoplasm during mitosis. Cholesterol-like molecules are very thin and flat and are perfectly suited to slide between the bases and get stuck there. In this way they cause mutations. It is called *intercalation*. It is probably quite accidental, happening when cholesterol-like molecules are plentiful nearby.

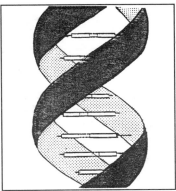

The double threads of nucleic acid are twisted like a spiral staircase. The "rungs" are made of a <u>purine</u> base from one thread and a <u>pyrimidine</u> base from the other thread. The bases attract each other with a force. The spaces between the "steps" can be invaded by PAHs or cholesterol derivatives.

Fig. 12 DNA and bases

Our bodies have developed elaborate systems of getting rid of old cholesterol and hormones safely by detoxifying them. But the detoxification products themselves have molecular shapes dangerously similar to the mutagens of the PAH family. Could cholesterol occasionally and erroneously be turned into a carcinogenic PAH? My evidence shows that it does,[39] and other researchers have also considered the possibility.[40]

The Syncrometer detects a <u>host</u> of carcinogenic chemicals of the polycyclic hydrocarbon class in <u>every</u> tumor, even in <u>warts</u>. These were called "carcinogenic" originally because a minute quantity of a PAH could be injected into a mouse or other animal, or rubbed onto the skin, and sometime later—often many months—tumors would appear, predictably. These tumors could be removed and planted in a

[39] Clark, H.R., *Syncrometer Biochemistry Laboratory Manual*, New Century Press, 1999.
[40] Greenstein, p. 49.

27

different animal, causing new tumors[41]—they had developed a life of their own! So they were called "cancerous."

Here are some PAH-like carcinogens detected by the Syncrometer in every tumor, whether benign or malignant:

- 20-methylcholanthrene. This was deemed to be the <u>most</u> carcinogenic of all chemicals when it was discovered; $^1/_{10}$ of a mg ($^1/_{10}$ of a flyspeck) placed under the skin of a mouse , would induce tumors many months later and would kill the mouse.
- 1,10-phenanthroline, somewhat similar to phenanthrene, and always accompanied by its iron-derivative *ferroin.*
- Phorbol (phorbol-12-myristate-13-acetate, or "PMA") one of a family of naturally occurring tumor promoters.[42]
- 1, 2:5, 6- dibenzanthracene, a very potent tumor inducer.
- 3,5 cholestadiene, a tumor inducer and oxidation product of cholesterol.
- Chrysene, an oxidation product of cholesterol and tumor inducer.

Some carcinogens, studied by early scientists, were so long lasting after a single minute dose that they could still be seen by a fluorescence-meter seven or eight months later! This explained why it might take so very long (a long "latency") for cancer induction. The carcinogen was tightly intercalated, could not be detoxified or pulled out, and was causing mutations all that time.

PAHs From Parasites

How can these powerful mutation-causing chemicals be produced in our own bodies and allowed to intercalate them-

---

[41] Greenstein, p 22.

[42] Birnboim, H.C., *DNA Strand Breakage in Human Leukocytes Exposed to a Tumor Promoter, Phorbol Myristate Acetate*, Science, v. 215, Mar. 5, 1982, pp. 1247-49.

selves between the bases of our nucleic acids? Is our body manufacturing its own demise? It is actually not our own doing at all! It is the foreign biochemistry of our parasites! (I will sometimes call it mis-biochemistry.)

Ascaris worms are responsible for the 1,10 phenanthroline, 20-methylcholanthrene, and dozens of related carcinogens! Tapeworm stages contribute phorbol and dibenzanthracene!

Ascaris worms also bring two harmful bacteria: *Rhizobium leguminosarum* and *Mycobacterium avium/cellulare*. More research is needed to determine whether these are really responsible for our mis-biochemistry.

Tapeworm stages bring *Streptomyces* bacteria which spread through the body. It could be these that are actually responsible for the tapeworm mis-biochemistry. *Streptomyces* are also known for their production of mycins, some of which are potent inhibitors of RNA and protein formation. The Syncrometer detects an assortment of these mycins in tumorous organs.[43]

So although PAHs are one of the biggest abnormalities in a tumor, they are caused by parasites, one of the easiest problems to eliminate!

Once parasites and bacteria, including *Clostridium*, are gone, PAHs and their mutations are gone! Excess DNA for mitosis is gone, the amines coming from bacteria are gone, so pyruvic aldehyde (brakes) can return the cells to slow mitosis. Next thiourea levels decrease, allowing thyroxine to replenish, and a whole host of cell functions begin to normalize!

Fungus And Benzene

Fungus, too, plays a significant role. Fungus species produce special chemicals called **mycotoxins** to fight the bacteria that are constantly trying to take away their feeding grounds. That is why our most popular antibiotics are mycotoxins.

---

[43] Clark, H.R., *Syncrometer Biochemistry Laboratory Manual*, New Century Press, 1999.

Three mycotoxins which are especially bad for a cancer patient are **aflatoxin** (on peanuts), **patulin** (on apples), and **zearalenone** (on Russet potatoes). Actually, the molds that make these mycotoxins grow everywhere in such abundance that we have government agencies to monitor them, even in animal feed. But the presence of zearalenone in Russet potatoes is not controlled by an agency (because it is my own recent discovery). That is why I recommend only red and white potatoes.

All tumors have these three mycotoxins within them. Aflatoxin and patulin were studied decades ago by scientists. Aflatoxin is a large flat molecule that intercalates between the bases of our nucleic acids. Patulin combines directly with our nucleic acids, also causing them to mutate.

Aflatoxin seeks out the liver. Patulin seeks out the parathyroid gland, according to the Syncrometer. But zearalenone seeks out fat. It can be found in our skin-fat when we are well and in our organ-fat when we are ill. While it is in our fat tissue, it very slowly detoxifies into benzene![44] To my knowledge this is the first and only incidence of benzene formed by a plant or animal. It is, of course, quite abnormal to have zearalenone in our fat. Mother Nature depended on our parents to teach us not to eat moldy food!

Benzene destroys our "good" (organic) germanium, changing it into "bad" (inorganic) germanium.

Germanium and Asbestos

Good germanium (called carboxyethylgermanium sesquioxide) brings us special immunity; it induces **interferon**[45] and

---

[44] Ibid., Clark, H.R.

[45] Suzuki, F., Brutkiewicz, R.R., Pollard, R.B., *Ability Of Sera From Mice Treated With Ge-132, An Organic Germanium Compound, To Inhibit Experimental Murine Ascites Tumours*, Br. J. Cancer, v. 52, 1985, pp. 757-63.

raises the helper-to-suppresser ratio of our **T-cells**.[46] Good germanium protects our chromosomes from virus invasion.[47]

Another way that good germanium is turned into bad germanium is by asbestos. The Syncrometer detects asbestos everywhere in our environment. For instance on apples and plums, undoubtedly picked up from conveyer belts that contain asbestos, because when the fruit is washed and the stem and blossom removed, the Syncrometer finds the asbestos gone. Sugar also tests positive to asbestos, possibly from also being transported on belts, and you can not wash sugar! So many of our sweetened foods are polluted with small amounts of asbestos.

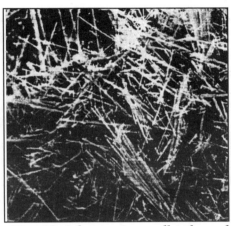

As soon as it is swallowed, your white blood cells try to remove it by "eating" the sharp asbestos needles. Unfortunately, the asbestos wins the battle and is soon free

Fig. 13 Asbestos is needle-shaped

again, but your white blood cells will continue to fight. Your body tries another plan: cover the tips with a protein that will act like gum, keeping the needles together and blunted.[48] The protein chosen is *ferritin*, whose neatly shaped molecule is now torn by the asbestos spears, exposing its iron core. Exposed iron is highly oxidizing—it over-oxidizes everything in the vicinity, including good germanium, making it bad.

---

[46] Ikemoto, K., Kobayashi, M., Fukumoto, T., Morimatsu, M., Pollard, R.B., Suzuki, F., *2-Carboxyethylgermanium Sesquioxide, a Synthetic Organogermanium Compound, As An Inducer of Contrasuppressor T Cells*, Experientia, v. 52, 1996, pp. 159-66.

[47] Clark, H.R., *Syncrometer Biochemistry Laboratory Manual*, New Century Press, 1999.

[48] Fubini, B., Barceló, F., Areán, C.O., *Ferritin Adsorption on Amosite [asbestos] Fibers: Possible Implications in the Formation and Toxicity of Asbestos Bodies*, Jour. Tox. Env. Health, v. 52, 1997, pp. 343-52.

How bad is "bad"? Oxidized germanium may be responsible for attacking the spleen somehow and causing the anemia that is a common cause of death for cancer sufferers, because the Syncrometer always detects bad germanium at the spleen. More research is needed here. But certainly depleting good germanium reduces our immunity. More importantly, **when the Syncrometer does not detect good germanium it always detects mutations in the form of p53 and excess hCG.** This implies good germanium is <u>necessary</u> to prevent cancer, and other research suggests this also.[49]

Unfortunately, it does little good to take organic germanium supplements! There are two reasons for this. Commercially, the organic forms are made in a laboratory so traces of inorganic germanium, such as germanium dioxide, are still present; and secondly, unless you get rid of asbestos (and benzene), your body will inevitably change the good germanium to bad.

Fortunately, asbestos can be removed in days from your vital organs by avoiding asbestos contaminated foods and drinking <u>lots</u> of fluids. So that, too, gets top priority along with parasite killing in the 21 Day Program.

More Mutagens and Tumor Formers

I detect many other mutagens, besides PAHs, in tumors. Here are a few:

- **Betapropiolactone** (not a PAH) also associated with *Ascaris*; a tumor inducer.
- **Ortho-amino-azotoluene** (the active portion of Sudan IV), **Sudan Black B**, and **4-diaminoazobenzene** (DAB), three of numerous *azo* dyes, pervasively present in foods, clothing, as well as hair dyes. They cause mutations that raise the blood LDH and alkaline phosphatase while

---

[49] Gerber, G.B., Léonard, A., *Mutagenicity, carcinogenicity and teratogenicity of germanium compounds*, Mutation Research, v. 387, 1997, pp. 141-46.

causing disappearance of vitamin A-related body chemicals. Vitamin A is a growth regulator!

- **Fast Green, also called Food Green 3**, a dye that is legitimately used to <u>color</u> fruits; it penetrates the entire fruit. The dye is evidently contaminated with lanthanide metals since these accompany the dye and are eaten with bananas, grapefruit, eggplant, cucumbers, etc.

- **Urethane**, a pollutant from the plastics industry (commonly seeping from plastic teeth); it is a potent tumor former.[50]

- **Hydroxyurea**, associated with *Ascaris*. It kills white blood cells. (Used for this purpose as treatment for some leukemias!) It combines with ribonucleotide reductase.

- **Cycloheximide**, associated with tapeworm larvae; it inhibits protein formation in you, but assists viruses.

- **Acrolein and acrylic acid**, made by overheating oils or seeping from plastic teeth, but large amounts produced by *Ascaris* larvae. Induces DNA overproduction.

- No doubt all the **environmental carcinogens** we have been told about, like tobacco smoke, pesticides, and saccharine, are now headed toward the handicapped organ too. There is no detoxifying ability there and no immunity; they must simply pile up there.

So, instead of getting help from the rest of the body in response to its cries, the tiny mass, trying desperately to throw off its bacteria and heal, is getting malicious metals and merciless mutagens sent its way. Yet, it must struggle on, whipped by thiourea, choked by malonic acid and dyes, constantly tripped by mutations. It will not grow into an uncontrolled tumor, though, as long as it can still self-destruct (*apoptose*) as fast as it multiplies. This is the state of a wart.

---

[50] Mirvish, S.S., *The Carcinogenic Action and Metabolism of Urethan and N-Hydroxyurethan*, Advan. Cancer Res., v. 11, 1968, pp. 1-42.

Warts, First Cousins To Tumors

A wart, too, has an assortment of heavy metals detected by the Syncrometer. It has the mutagens made by mis-biochemistry of *Ascaris* and tapeworm stages. It even has p53 mutations and myc oncogenes.

But it <u>can</u> keep up its self-destruction, its apoptosis. Its *bcl-2* gene is working properly. The bcl-2 gene produces bcl-2 for thirty seconds, followed by *bax* for thirty seconds, in endless continuity. Bax, in turn, is produced by your bax gene.

The ratio of these two gene products determines the rate of apoptosis. A wart has started to multiply abnormally, but its genes that govern killing off excess cells still work, so a wart's growth reaches a limit.

A true tumor is also multiplying abnormally, but its apoptosis mechanism is broken, so it grows limitlessly. If we could keep from mutating our bcl-2 and bax genes, our small, helpless masses would stay that way.

Cell Problems Intensify

But by now, our small mass has a large quantity of metals and dye accumulated. Besides, these toxins are spreading to our vital organs: the spleen, bone marrow, liver, and parathyroids. The effects of mis-biochemistry (parasite induced mutagens, like 1,10-phenanthroline) are spreading, too.

Sulfur levels are getting too low to let metal sulfides be formed for safe excretion. Inorganic copper, cobalt, germanium, thulium (a lanthanide), vanadium, and azo dyes will become the "ultimate toxins", the deadly reapers for the entire body.

I find cancer sufferers are usually not dying of cancer (tumor formation), as such, but of metal and dye toxicity! And of mis-biochemistry. This means that as glad as you will be to see your tumors shrink, you must not become complacent! You must also remove the toxins!

Copper combines with 1,10-phenanthroline, as well as iron. Copper-phenanthroline complexes cause wholesale chromosome breaks[51]. Cobalt activates the clostridial enzyme that makes DNA out of RNA,[52] and it activates *arginase,*[53] an enzyme that supplies polyamines, necessary for growing tissues. Toxic germanium stops protecting us from p53 and hCG mutations. Even the normally beneficial iron can join the harmful metals when it produces oxygen radicals.[54] Vanadium combines with abnormally exposed nucleic acids. Normally phosphate combines with nucleic acids to form "nucleoside phosphate complexes" called nucleotides. But the chemistry of vanadium is rather similar to phosphate. So it forms "nucleoside vanadyl complexes." Vanadyl complexes are well known to molecular biologists as *synthetic RNAse inhibitors*, which I observe displace your natural ones.

I have discovered that vanadyl complexes do one more thing: they cause *p53* mutations. p53 is the gene that makes our "policeman" protein.[55] It stands guard over our nucleic acid threads. It can recognize mutations, like intercalation, and stop those cells from multiplying. It allows no further gene duplication until the mutation has been "fixed." The PAH or other mutagen must be pulled or snipped out from between the bases

---

[51] Pope, L.M, Reich, K.A., Graham, D.R., Sigman, D.S., *Products of DNA Cleavage by the 1,10-Phenanthroline-Copper Complex*, Journal Of Biological Chemistry, v. 257, no. 20, Oct. 25, 1982, pp. 12121-28.

[52] Zubay, p. 231, discusses how cobalt activates ribonucleotide reductase.

[53] Liquier-Milward, J., *Tracer Studies on Cobalt Incorporation into Growing Tumors: Uptake of Radioactive Co^{60} by Normal and Malignant Cells*, Can. Res., 1957, p. 843.

[54] Weinberg, E.D., *The Role of Iron in Cancer*, European Jour. of Cancer Prevention, v. 5, 1996, pp. 19-36.

[55] *The Cancer Killer*, Newsweek, Dec. 23, 1996, pp. 42-47.

and any missing bases replaced correctly before p53 will release its hold.

I find p53 mutations also occur when tapeworm larvae are present, even without vanadium. (Conversely I find p53 mutations <u>don't</u> occur in the presence of vanadium or tapeworm larvae <u>if</u> good germanium is present!)

When the p53 <u>gene</u> has become mutated, multiplication is allowed to go on and on, <u>in spite of</u> the gross mutations that are now occurring and being passed along. If p53, also called the "tumor suppresser gene", is incapacitated, how long can the hyperactive little mass be controlled so a tumor does not develop? Everything now depends on bcl-2 and bax. If this last mechanism fails, you will have a tumor.

The Final Defense

More and more mutations, many of them translocations (misplacement) of chromosome parts, are occurring now that p53 is gone (mutated). Bits of chromosomes litter the cytoplasm making it look like a war zone. The cells are completely disabled as productive members of their community due to these mutations. Yet they must multiply, because *Clostridium* is filling the cells with toxic amines, the brakes (pyruvic aldehyde) are out, and the accelerator (thiourea) given full reign.

It is only a matter of time before the bcl-2 gene will also mutate.[56] Its characteristic mutation is yet another translocation. After this, the cells cannot self-destruct.

The Syncrometer detects overproduction of bcl-2 protein in all growing tumors, whether benign or malignant. It should be produced for thirty seconds only, out of each minute. Now it is produced for forty seconds, leaving only twenty seconds for bax.

---

[56] Tsujimoto, Y., Bashir, M., Givol, I., Cossman, J., Jaffe, E., Croce., C., *DNA Rearrangements in Human Follicular Lymphoma Can Involve The 5' or the 3' region of the bcl-2 Gene*, Proc. Natl. Acad. Sci. USA, v. 84, Mar. 1987, pp. 1329-31.

bax, a protein bit from another gene, should be detectable for its share of time, the remaining thirty seconds out of each minute. Healthy tissues, right beside the tumor-growing organ are producing bax at the proper rate. In a growing tumor, bax is always underproduced. Gradually the ratio worsens, until it appears as if bcl-2 is always present and bax is not. bcl-2 and bax decide whether a cell will self-destruct by starting to digest itself internally.

Recall that cells filled with lanthanides, and therefore, calcium and iron deposits cannot be digested externally by pancreatin and lipase.

The Conspiracy Gains Control

We have now seen a dozen contributors to the tumor-growing process. They interact like the pieces of a puzzle. Is it possible to determine which piece comes first? And which comes next? Is there an orderly sequence? A jigsaw puzzle can be put together starting with any piece. Perhaps the pieces that go into making a tumor can all combine independently, too. Or perhaps there is a specific sequence. Only more scientific research can answer this question correctly. Meanwhile, we can imagine various ways. Here is one:

1. Tapeworm larvae infect our tissues, releasing malonic acid, which interferes with respiration (the making of ATP in mitochondria). We also get malonic acid from food and plastic teeth.
2. Invading *Clostridium* bacteria supply DNA, isopropyl alcohol, and toxic amines in the vicinity of larvae.
3. These amines can shift the balance between pyruvic aldehyde and thiourea production in favor of thiourea, speeding up cell division, mitosis.
4. Excess thiourea consumes thyroid hormones (like thyroxine), which in turn disables lysosomes, your cells' bacteria killers, and mitochondria.

5. Metal and non-metal toxins are attracted to the sick cells by forces not completely understood, but commonly observed, which I call morbitropism.
6. Heavy metals consume our sulfur and sulfur compounds; reducing power declines.
7. Oxidizing defenses decline, too, as p450 enzymes decline, due to insufficient iron, a combined effect of nonorganic copper and germanium, asbestos, and 1,10-phenanthroline.
8. Lanthanides get stuck in cells, causing calcium and iron deposits. These block the "flag" for external digestion, phosphatidylserine. (Calcium also causes extra cell division.) Without the flag, pancreatin and lipase don't digest these failing cells while they do others.
9. Major carcinogens (PAHs and others) are produced by two very common parasites, *Ascaris* and tapeworms. These carcinogens are now absorbed preferentially by the fast dividing cells.
10. Parasite-related bacteria (*Streptomyces, Mycobacterium avium/cellulare, Rhizobium leguminosarum* species, and the c-myc related virus) contribute in ways that are not yet clear and cause symptoms of illness such as night sweats.
11. Mutations occur.
12. Azo dyes from food, clothing, and body products can no longer be detoxified and are attracted to our vital organs as well as locations of rapid cell division. Azo dyes cause further mutations.
13. Enough mutations occur to disable the cells' oxidizing and reducing powers. Some enzymes are overproduced while vitamin A receptors are underproduced. The cell can still divide, however.
14. Good germanium is gone, so vanadium causes p53 mutations by forming ribonucleoside vanadyl complexes. Tapeworm stages or their bacteria also can induce p53 mutations.

15. bcl-2 and bax genes become disregulated so that self-destruction of disabled cells (apoptosis) does not occur quickly enough.
16. The small mass becomes an aggressively growing tumor. If it were transplanted into a different healthy animal, it would take its immortality, its *Clostridium* and other parasites, and its mutations with it. It would grow and consume its new host.
17. If the human intestinal fluke (*Fasciolopsis buskii*) finds the tumor, and isopropyl alcohol is present (*Clostridium* makes it), then ortho-phospho-tyrosine is produced, and I consider the tumor to be malignant.

It makes good sense that part of a tissue can become a runaway tumor, unable to stop its endless cell multiplication when a dozen or so common factors are present.

The prevailing concept is that tumors have become "uncontrollable." My observations point the finger of guilt at the rest of the body, not the tumor itself. It is the rest of the body that has supplied the metals, dyes, malonates, parasites, and bacteria. It will do no good to remove the tumors although it helps temporarily; the disease is systemic; they will simply grow again.

It is tempting to think that the dozen tumor-causers discussed here are the only ones of any significance. This may not be true. They may merely be the prevalent factors in our society. There may be other ways a tissue can become tumorous. Much more research is needed.

But for the present, removing these returns over 95% of cancer patients to health, while tumors shrink and disappear! How can this be accomplished most speedily and efficiently?

Cancer Diagram

Here is a picture for review.

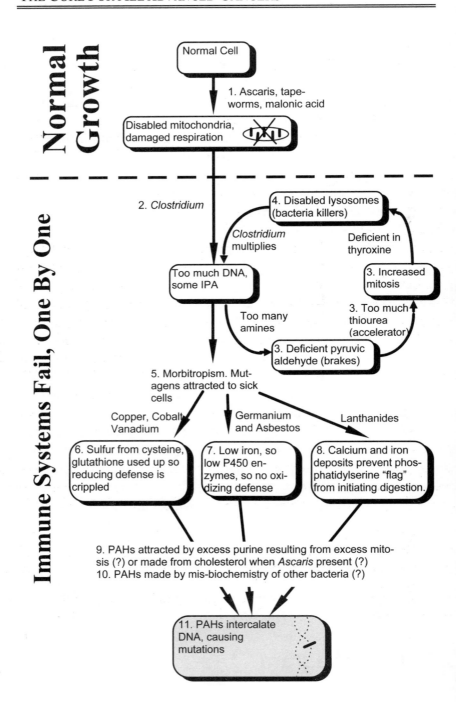

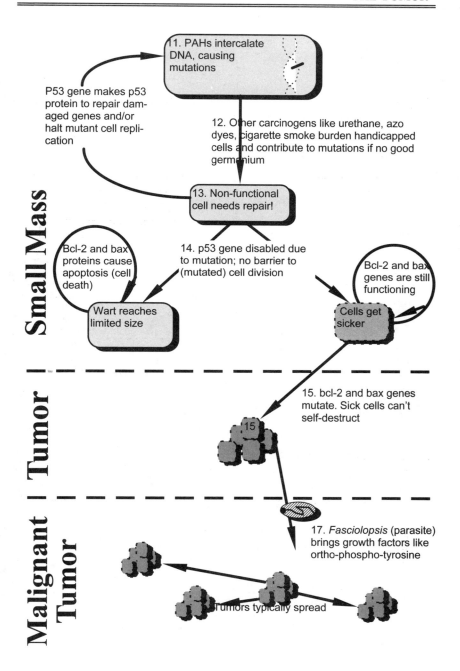

11. PAHs intercalate DNA, causing mutations

P53 gene makes p53 protein to repair damaged genes and/or halt mutant cell replication

12. Other carcinogens like urethane, azo dyes, cigarette smoke burden handicapped cells and contribute to mutations if no good germanium

13. Non-functional cell needs repair!

Bcl-2 and bax proteins cause apoptosis (cell death)

14. p53 gene disabled due to mutation; no barrier to (mutated) cell division

Bcl-2 and bax genes are still functioning

Wart reaches limited size

Cells get sicker

Small Mass

15. bcl-2 and bax genes mutate. Sick cells can't self-destruct

Tumor

17. *Fasciolopsis* (parasite) brings growth factors like ortho-phospho-tyrosine

Malignant Tumor

Tumors typically spread

41

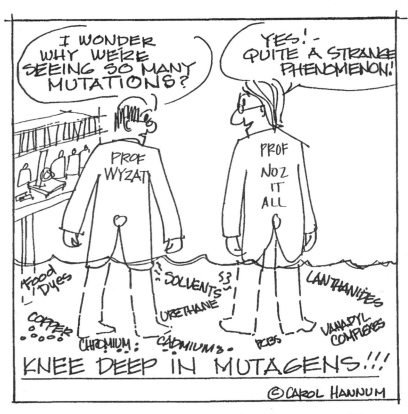

Fig. 14 Parts per trillion analysis is now possible

Use the earlier book, *The Cure For All Cancers*, as a <u>reference</u> guide for your life-style and environmental changes.

The Tasks

In spite of a myriad of problems that beset an advanced cancer patient, there are still only two causes for all of them: parasites (including bacteria) and toxins. Specifically, there are three tasks:

- Kill clostridium bacteria.
- Kill all other parasites.
- Remove metals, malonic acid, and several other carcinogens from your body.

Killing *Clostridium* will be the most challenging because it involves dental work. Killing other parasites will be the easiest, and if you have already read *The Cure For All Cancers*, you may have already begun using the herbal parasite killing program and the zapper. We will review this with special emphasis on preventing reinfection.

Removing heavy metals (including the lanthanide elements), malonic acid, and carcinogens like urethane, asbestos, acrylic acid and azo dye, is also easy because it is part of the same dental solution, together with diet changes.

Killing *Clostridium*

Clostridium bacteria are *anaerobes*. This means they are very primitive, not even tolerating oxygen. Their origin goes back to the time when the earth had no oxygen. To survive, they have found clever ways to avoid oxygen. They may live with bacteria that use up the oxygen around them. They may live <u>inside</u> parasites that shelter them from oxygen. They may live in canned food, oxygen free if they have been allowed to enter during canning (botulism is caused by *Clostridium botulinum*). They may live at the bottom of deep wounds, like punctures, where oxygen does not enter because circulation is bad (tetanus is caused by *Clostridium tetani*). If oxygen suddenly appears, they quickly make capsules around themselves, like heavy armor, to survive until it becomes anaerobic again.

Clostridium Colonies

We are *aerobic* beings. All of our cells need and use oxygen. We do not have an organ or a location that is naturally oxygen-free. But we do have a location—in the colon—that is low in oxygen and could be made oxygen-free artificially. Other bacteria, in very large numbers, could use up the oxygen so *Clostridium* species could live there, too. But it would be a precarious existence. The colon would frequently need new supplies of *Clostridium* to reinforce the colony there. That is what actually happens.

The presence of clostridium bacteria in our intestines has been considered normal by scientists. Yet, I did not detect them in young children.[57] Instead they had bifidus bacteria, which adults did not have. Evidently at some time while growing up, the *Bifidus* disappear and *Clostridium* takes over. Several Mexican persons who were tested also did not harbor *Clostridium*. Yet, all American persons, even when well, harbored *Clostridium* in the intestinal tract. But only in the colon, not higher up.

Cancer patients, though, harbor *Clostridium* throughout the intestine, reaching all the way to the stomach! They harbor a seething mass of *Clostridium* bacteria.

The cancerous organ, even as far away as the brain or eye, has been invaded by *Clostridium*, too. In very advanced cancer, the entire body is invaded. The Syncrometer detects *Clostridium* (and extra DNA) in dozens of tissues. They are probably able to circulate freely, now, even in the blood stream.

It would probably be advantageous for the patient to receive hyperbaric oxygen therapy for an hour each day for a week; this would reoxygenate the tissues the fastest, and kill most of the

---

57 This is based on four children, ages nine, six, four, and two. Two samples of intestinal contents were tested by Syncrometer for each child.

Clostridium. Our clinic did not have the use of a hyperbaric oxygen chamber. Yet, they can be vanquished in other ways, too. They can be pushed back down the tract, all the way to the colon, and even eliminated from there. But then, mysteriously, the colon is promptly re-inoculated! From where?

The only truly anaerobic location in our bodies is artificial—a prosthesis! We have unknowingly built one into our teeth during tooth repair! If our teeth become colonized with *Clostridium*, they become a source of distribution to the colon and tumors.

Tooth fillings, if imperfectly applied, create a crevice between tooth and filling that is suitable for anaerobes to live in. Dead teeth also invite *Clostridium*. If your teeth have gray or bluish-black discoloration, you probably have *Clostridium* infection. It is fairly easy to spot, visually, in a dead or filled tooth. But of course it is hidden from view under a cap or crown or simply under a filling. Usually, many species of Clostridium grow together. I test for six species. They are usually all present when there are large plastic fillings, and when crowns, root canals, or dead teeth are present.

The next time you have a tooth extracted, ask the dentist to give it to you, so you can search for the thin, black lines of clostridium invasion yourself.

Clostridia are not necessarily present under small fillings, such as those in front teeth. It is probably easier to get a small filling to stick perfectly to the tooth than a large one, so no crevice develops.

Evicting The Colonies

Once the teeth and colon have been colonized by *Clostridium*, they can not be easily eradicated. No immune power can reach the colony in the teeth; there is no circulation to the fillings! So all immune support fails.

Are there other ways? Can an antibiotic be used to counter-act the *Clostridium* continually? Can the rest of the body be sufficiently oxygenated to prevent invasion by *Clostridium*? Can the tooth crevice, causing **microleakage**, be sealed off so bacteria couldn't escape into the body? Could the bacteria in the crevice and tooth be killed by zapping? Some of these ideas are promising, but I

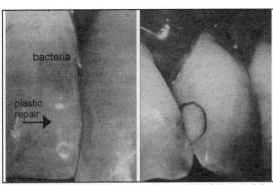

The left tooth has a plastic repair. Above this is discoloration due to bacterial invasion. The plastic filling in the tooth on the right has a black outline of bacteria.

Fig. 15 Teeth with visible bacteria

find the best way to kill Clostridia is brushing with oregano oil (see page 548), a natural penetrant and antiseptic.

But if you have advanced cancer, you can not risk a temporary solution—don't delay. Extract all your decayed teeth—teeth with caps, crowns, root canals, and large fillings of any kind. You will be accomplishing more than just eliminating clostridium bacteria, as you will soon see.

While you are waiting for your first dental appointment, you can begin to clear clostridium bacteria

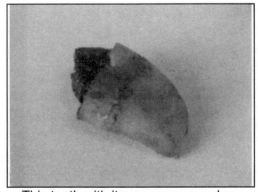

This tooth with its crown removed reveals a black surface underneath and fine gray lines of further invasion of the tooth. It is invariably *Clostridium* at work.

Fig. 16 Black tooth under crown

from the <u>intestinal tract</u>. No antibiotics, no change in diet, no extra lactobacillus or bifidus bacteria taken as a supplement can clear them. Only one substance, normally found in your stomach, can banish them. It is *betaine*, together with *hydrochloric acid* (HCl). Neither alone is completely effective.

- Betaine or betaine hydrochloride (betaine HCl), about 300 mg (see *Sources*), take three, three times a day with food.
- Hydrochloric acid (USP) 15 drops of a 5% solution stirred into food and put into your beverages at mealtime. Total: 45 drops a day. **Do not put drops directly into your mouth!** It will dissolve your teeth.

All clostridium species (as represented by my set of six slides) will be gone from the colon, all the way up to the stomach in three days, but <u>not gone</u> above the stomach nor in your tumors. They are trickling down from your infected teeth. This is waiting for the dental work to be completed. Meanwhile, you should be brushing with oregano oil, just ½ drop on your toothbrush. Increasing the betaine or hydrochloric acid does not help.

Your body will feel an incredible relief when the clostridium-infected teeth are gone. People describe this as the lifting of a weight. The effect is similar to removing a thorn that is deeply imbedded in you. No antibiotics and no bandaging can control the blood poisoning that will develop if you do not extract the thorn. There is no alternative to pulling it out, and the relief is immediate. After extracting your decaying toxic teeth you still must do careful Dental Aftercare (discussed later), but the big step has been taken and you may now feel secure you <u>can</u> recover from your tumor-disease.

Clostridium Carriers

Although the earth is teeming with clostridia of all varieties we do not get infected from eating them with dirt accidentally. But that doesn't mean you don't have to be very careful when preparing food. Because in dirt is a more sinister parasite, the **rabbit fluke**.

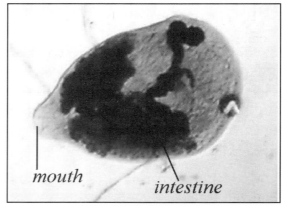

The rabbit fluke, *Hasstilesia tricolor*, brings *Clostridium* into

Fig. 17 Rabbit fluke

our bodies indirectly, the way the Trojan horse brought its soldiers. *Hasstilesia* goes directly to the esophagus after it is eaten. Here the clostridia emerge and while attempting to travel through our bodies, may find a tooth crevice to survive in, as well as the colon.

The colon will be more anaerobic as we age, perhaps because it usually becomes more sluggish in later years. In this way *Clostridium* becomes a permanent member of the "flora."

As if *Clostridium* isn't bad enough, I find *Hasstilesia* also brings *Streptococcus* bacteria, c-myc (an oncogene that could cause cells to divide), *Plasmodium malariae* (a protozoon), and *Besnoitia* (another protozoon)! Everywhere the rabbit fluke goes, these five "friends" go too. Fortunately, they are all killed by the herbal parasite program and zapping.

To kill *Clostridium*, you need to:

1. Get rid of the source. Use the Parasite Killing Program in the next section to eradicate the rabbit fluke.
2. Get rid of colonies in the colon. Take betaine and hydrochloric acid.
3. Get rid of colonies in the teeth. We discuss this in the Dental Work chapter.

Kill All Parasites

We will fight parasites in many ways. With herbs, with electricity, with ozonated oil, with cysteine (an amino acid), and with hydrochloric acid. Getting rid of parasites would be absolutely impossible using clinical medicines that can kill only one or two parasites each. Such medicines also tend to make you quite ill. Flagyl is used for amoebas and Giardia; when the correct dosage is used, it can cause extreme nausea and vomiting. Imagine taking ten such drugs to kill a dozen of your parasites! Good news, perhaps, for the drug makers but not for you.

Herbal Parasite Program

Three herbs can rid you of over 100 types of parasites! And without so much as a headache! Without any interference with any drug that you are already on! Does this sound too fantastic? Just too good to be true? They are nature's gift to us. The herbs are:

- Black Walnut Hulls (only when they are <u>green</u>)
- Wormwood
- Cloves (only <u>freshly</u> ground)

In *The Cure For All Cancers* I give instructions for making your own (green) black walnut hull tincture extra strength, and grinding your own cloves. But in this book I expect you do not have time to do that. Reliable sources for ordering these (and other) products are given in the *Sources* chapter, page 589.

How much to take, and how often is summarized in the *21 Day Cancer Curing Program* chapter. But here are some important points.

We have seen persons who were bedridden get out of bed within a week after taking <u>ten</u> teaspoons <u>daily</u>. Perhaps in these cases the tumors themselves were releasing the parasites in large numbers.

If you are incapacitated or bedridden, pencil in a higher dose for yourself in the 21 Day Program on page 179.

The tincture can be diluted in water and sweetened or spiced.

Don't spread the dose out longer than one half hour.

If swallowing is difficult or even repulsive, spoon it down carefully; do not gulp it, to avoid nausea. You may also add two drops of peppermint oil (see *Sources*) to block nausea. Stay seated, to avoid dizziness. Do not drive a car afterward in case you do feel dizzy or nauseated. Eating 10 minutes afterwards can help. So can going straight to bed.

You should help your liver detoxify the alcohol in the tincture by taking niacinamide, 500 mg, each time you take a dose of tincture.

Take the wormwood and clove capsules one at a time, carefully. Have bread within reach in case a capsule sticks or nausea is felt. Eat bread if there is any discomfort afterward. Allergic reactions are very, very rare, but if you are susceptible to allergies, keep your medicine nearby.

How often should you repeat the parasite program? Daily, until your tumors are gone. This is because your tumors shelter parasites (along with *Clostridium*, dyes, and other toxins). As your tumors drain, parasites emerge, and must be killed. If you have liver disease, making the alcohol prohibitive, or if there is stomach cancer where bleeding is a risk, use the non-alcoholic varieties (see *Sources*).

If you are the caregiver, how often should you do the parasite killing program to protect your patient? Although the answer is somewhat arbitrary, repeating it once a week is recommended.

Zapping Parasites

Zapping is a way of killing bacteria and parasites electrically. You can make a zapping device yourself; the instructions are given in *The Cure For All Cancers*; total cost is around $35.00.

It runs off an ordinary 9 volt transistor battery, and is harmless to you. I find it kills parasites and bacteria wherever the electricity reaches. But some locations that are not reachable are tooth crevices, the intestinal tract, gallstones, and the inside of tumors. In spite of these limitations, the benefits can often be felt with each use! In addition, the benefits accumulate with each use, whether felt or not. In fact, I have preliminary evidence that zapping can raise immunity by removing the abnormal coating of ferritin on the outside of white blood cells. We will discuss ferritin coating later.

In the 21 Day Program you are instructed to zap every day. A "zap" consists of seven minutes of electrical current, a rest of about 20 minutes, another seven minutes of current, another 20 minute rest, and a final seven minutes of current.

The reason for doing three seven minute sessions is that bacteria typically emerge from parasites that are killed. After these bacteria are killed, viruses emerge. So it takes three sessions to kill them all.

You can zap more than once a day or continually if you wish, but be sure to zap at least once a day. Do this until you are completely well.

Cysteine

After taking the herbal parasite program, later in the same day, begin the **mop-up** program. This is to kill escaped viruses and the eggs still trapped inside dead parasites.

The mop-up program consists of cysteine and ozonated oil. The dosages are given in Day 1 of the 21 Day Program. Because your own tumors will be reinfecting you, you need to mop up daily as well as kill parasites until tumors have shrunk.

Because cysteine is a reducer and ozonated oil an oxidizer, they must <u>not be taken together</u> to retain effectiveness.

The cysteine and ozonated oil will be very good for you in other ways, too. Cysteine gives you reducing power and precious sulfur. Ozonated oil gives you oxidizing power that reaches into distant places like bile ducts. Since they have opposite actions, they must be kept apart for <u>at least five hours</u>.

You may sometimes experience minor side effects from taking cysteine. Fatigue and nausea are the most common. Tearing eyes and dripping nose are common too. Dizziness may occur. All this is avoided, though, just by eating. Have bread handy or wait till mealtime to take your dose of cysteine. Side effects lessen with each dose taken and wear off in an hour.

A strong and beneficial diuretic effect may also be noticed.

The cysteine should be the L variety, like "l-cysteine", not "d-cysteine" which is unnatural. It may be "cysteine hydrochloride" or simply free "cysteine." But <u>not</u> "cystine"; that is a different amino acid.

Ozonated Oil

Ozone has molecules made of three atoms of oxygen stuck together. Oxygen in the air consists of just two atoms stuck together. The extra oxygen atom is easily released, making ozone a good oxidizer.

Ozonated oil gives you no noticeable side effects, but it should not be taken more than necessary. One could expect the extra oxygen to jump across from oil molecules to your fat molecules, aging them too soon. In my experiments ozonated oil did not oxidize vitamin C, nor cysteine or glutathione, nor ferrous iron. Fortunately the dose is small (one tablespoon), so unknown risks are small. Yet it is advisable to take vitamin E (see *Sources*), a known anti-oxidant, after taking ozonated oil. Give the oil five hours to do its work, first.

Ozonated oil is not generally available in health food stores, and even if it were, it may have a short shelf life. I have not researched the effectiveness of ozonated olive oil kept at room temperature for more than a day, or refrigerated for longer than a week, or in the freezer for more than a month. So it's best to make your own, and make it fresh.

You can easily make your own ozonated oil. Purchase an ozonator (see *Sources*) and a bottle of olive oil. Add a pinch of vitamin B_2 and 4 drops HCl (5%) per cup to the oil and shake to destroy any benzene and to kill *Ascaris* eggs. Attach an aerator to the end of your ozonator hose and drop it to the bottom of the olive oil. Aerators are available at any pet store; if possible choose ceramic or wood. If the bubbles make the oil flow over the top, pour more of it off. Turn the ozonator on before dropping the hose in the bottle. Ozonate for 25 minutes (not longer). When done, cap the bottle and store in freezer till you are ready to use it. It melts quickly when needed. If it has aged more than a month, make a fresh supply.

Ozonators can cost from $200.00 to $700.00. So you may be tempted to skip the one tablespoon of ozonated olive oil that is required. Don't! It is an essential part of your recovery! You may need more ozonated oil in the future, and also ozonated water. An ozonator is a good investment.

Ozonated oil can be mixed with vegetables or a casserole dish. Remember, it should be taken at least five hours after cysteine to avoid clashing with it.

Now parasites, particularly *Fasciolopsis*, *Ascaris*, tapeworm larvae, and rabbit fluke, are gone!

> . . . except the ones marooned in your tumors, and soon those will be eliminated, too.

Reap The Benefits

Killing *Ascaris* means you have gotten rid of 1,10-phenanthroline. Without phenanthroline in your vital organs, you are no longer attracting and chelating your precious iron and copper; more will be left for you instead. Without this interference, your bone marrow, liver, and spleen can begin to regulate your most vital functions again. It begins immediately. So *Ascaris* annihilation is supremely important in a life-saving venture. Without the mutagens made by *Ascaris*, your list of mutations is shortened. Without *Mycobacterium* and *Rhizobium* you will feel much better.

Killing tapeworm larvae means you have gotten rid of phorbol and dibenzanthracene from your vital organs, two other powerful mutagens. And without streptomyces bacteria, RNA and protein formation can start again. Without both parasites, p53 mutations are all but gone, only waiting for vanadium (dental) to be removed.

Killing rabbit flukes means you are no longer bringing *Clostridium* nor *Streptococcus* into your body for distribution to teeth, colon, or tumors. Nor the c-myc oncogene.

While clostridia are our tumor-causing bacteria, streptococci are our pain-producers. Streptococci produce *phenol* which not only causes pains of many kinds, but also ages us. Phenol, although considered a reducer in regular chemistry, oxidizes our vitamin C into toxic "oxidation products" that cause wrinkling of skin, cataract formation and other aspects of aging! Perhaps health and youth would stay much longer in humans if we didn't regard *Clostridium* and *Streptococcus* as being "normal" colon flora!

> ## Most important now is not reinfecting.

Stay Clean

In <u>all</u> cases, where I have seen that a cancer victim did not get good results after using the parasite program and zapper described in *The Cure For All Cancers*, I found remaining parasites! Was the program ineffective? Or did the person get reinfected? I find when the program is administered again, it is effective. So I conclude that the biggest problem for a cancer sufferer is the ease with which they can become reinfected from food and their own tumors!

The sources of reinfection with *Ascaris*, tapeworm, and rabbit fluke eggs are <u>so pervasive</u>, you may reinfect faster than you can <u>eliminate</u> them! A glass of milk, a cheese sandwich or a green salad will reinfect you in <u>five minutes</u> if they are not sterilized first. Cancer victims have no ability to kill these parasites—their immune powers are gone!

A person <u>without</u> cancer <u>can</u> eliminate them. There are no "safety islands" in them, namely tumors. And stomach acid kills them or the immune system takes over for them.

For a cancer patient, swallowing a few *Ascaris* eggs is equivalent to swallowing a few cholera bacteria or the ebola virus. Even <u>a few</u> will be disastrous unless killed.

Where would you find *Ascaris*, tapeworm and rabbit fluke eggs? <u>On your vegetables</u>! And <u>in your dairy products</u>!

Agribusiness uses, and <u>must</u> use fertilizer. Fertilizer is cow, pig, and horse manure. All animals have parasites. The eggs pass with the manure. Manure does not simply wash off lettuce and strawberries as you "clean" them under the kitchen faucet. They <u>stick</u> tightly to the cabbage (even inner leaves), beans, and spinach that have been splashed with manure or are simply dusty with dirt that has manure in it![58]

The other source of reinfection with *Ascaris* is a pet. All pets have *Ascaris*. The carpet has *Ascaris* eggs trapped between the fibers. They fly up with the dust that settles everyday on the table and dishes. In the bedroom you inhale them all night.

Remove the bedroom carpet, get a new mattress, dry clean the blankets and small rugs (laundering does not kill *Ascaris* eggs). Sterilize other carpets with a special stain-free iodine solution added to the carpet shampoo mixture (see *Recipes*). Give away your pet until you have recovered.

Cleaner Cooking

You can not change the way milk and produce are handled or grown. But you can protect yourself. You must kill parasites yourself, or peel the produce, or refrain from eating it.

There are two ways to kill rabbit fluke: chemicals or heat.

Sanitizing your unpeeled **vegetables and fruit** is quite easy. You can use Lugol's iodine or hydrochloric acid (HCl). Do not use chlorine bleach. It is a good disinfectant, but supermarket bleach is itself polluted with heavy metals, solvents and dyes; besides, you would get too much chlorine.

A one minute dip in very dilute Lugol's solution or hydrochloric acid kills everything it reaches. But they do not reach into crevices without a lot of agitation. Sanitized foods keep much longer. Specific instructions are in *Recipes*, on page 533.

Our traditional methods of food preparation have never tried to make food sterile. Even cooked and baked food is not sterile. Some pathogens require higher temperatures to be killed. That is why hospitals heat surgical instruments to 250°F in a special pressurized oven called an *autoclave* instead of simply boiling at 212°F.

---

[58] For an interesting report by the FDA, see Rude, R.A., et. al., *Survey of Fresh Vegetables for Nematodes, Amoebae, and Salmonella*, J. Assoc. Off. Anal. Chem., v. 67, no. 3, 1984, pp. 613-15. Nematodes include *Ascaris*.

Dairy food is fairly easy to sterilize (page 543) but often contains traces of azo dyes. For that reason, dairy products are omitted from the 21 Day Program.

Meat is best sterilized by heat, but a higher heat than you are used to using. Rabbit fluke stages and *Ascaris* eggs survive boiling temperature (212°F/100°C). Even baking seldom raises the internal temperature of meats or other foods higher than 180°F even if the temperature is set to 400°! (Meat pop-up temperature devices go to 160°F.) This is far from the boiling point. So to cook your meat safely, I recommend microwaving or "cooking twice." Microwaving has other disadvantages, such as destroying good germanium. The details on food sterilization are given in the chapter *Food Rules*, page 517.

If you neglect sterilizing your fruits and vegetables, you can assume you have *Ascaris*, tapeworm eggs, and rabbit fluke eggs again—immediately repeat the parasite program.

Kosher Foods to the Rescue

During my testing foods labeled with a Kosher symbol were found to be far superior in cleanliness and purity. Canned foods did not have rabbit fluke. Sweetened foods did not have asbestos. Processed foods did not have azo dye pollution. Even meats did not have rabbit fluke or *Ascaris* eggs. But dairy foods, while free of parasite eggs, often had azo dyes. For this reason, the ban on dairy foods for the 21 Day Program must stand. Read more about Kosher foods in *Recipes*.

Clearing Toxins

The third task is to remove inorganic copper, cobalt, vanadium, lanthanide metals, germanium, malonic acid, azo dye, asbestos, urethane, silicone, acrylic acid, and acrolein from your body.

These come from three places. The first, your dentalware, will be cleaned up with the same dentalwork used to eliminate

Clostridium. The second, your food, will be discussed in more detail in the Tumor Shrinking Diet chapter. The third, your environment, is the subject of the Safe Surroundings chapter.

After your body has been cleared of pathogens and toxins, your tumors <u>must</u> shrink. They always do, in case after case after case. In fact, we must be careful not to shrink them too fast! The contents must be detoxified and cleared <u>slowly</u>, in order not to overburden your vital organs. But before going on to the detailed instructions, we must pay attention to *pain.*

Pain Killing

Reducing pain is the first and most important need for any cancer sufferer. It is a patient's <u>right</u> to have pain relief. You may be in excruciating pain, and on morphine because no other painkiller "touches it." Or you may be stoically "putting up" with it, not sleeping, barely able to get up from your chair to get to the bathroom. Pain is the true master of us all. It even takes away our initiative to get well. If a cancer sufferer has decided to give up the battle, this wish should be understood and respected. But removing pain can change all that! And initiative and determination to conquer this disease can return.

We have been told that pain in cancer is <u>due</u> to the cancer. This is <u>not true</u>. The pain is caused mainly by bacteria. There is very little contribution from other causes. The simple act of pulling infected teeth can reduce the pain to half within hours even though the pain is at the hip or abdomen, far away from the teeth. The Dental Aftercare program reduces it further.

<u>Streptococcus bacteria play the major role in producing pain</u>. They reside in numerous little pockets all over our bodies, even if we consider ourselves "well," making *phenol*. When the phenol can no longer be detoxified at some location, it builds up to produce pain. All our painful locations have streptococcus bacteria living there!

Streptococcus bacteria killers include **cayenne pepper, inositol, ozonated water,** and **oregano oil** (*Oreganum vulgare*), and zapping. None of these work decisively in the body. Yet in a week you could be in a lot less pain by taking inositol and oregano oil before meals plus cayenne capsules with meals.

Take ½ tsp. inositol in ¼ cup water; it is sweetish. Oregano oil may be taken as 3 drops placed in an empty capsule for moderate pain; 20 drops for severe pain, followed by bread. Repeat 3 times a day if on morphine. The cayenne dose must be worked up gradually to get to a dosage of six capsules three times a day for three days in a row.

Once you make progress killing streptococcus, you must hold onto those gains. The underlying reason for having streptococcus colonies must be found. It is often due to the presence of <u>asbestos</u> or <u>lanthanide metals</u>, namely, <u>local</u> lack of immune power.

I believe our major source of asbestos is food that has rolled along old asbestos-containing conveyor belts. Sticky foods like sugar pick it up and spread it to all sweetened foods in the marketplace. Wherever a minuscule tuft of asbestos lands in your body, there is a location of low immunity because the local white blood cells (our immune "soldiers") become coated with ferritin. (See page 30.) *Streptococcus* can then grow unchallenged.

Lanthanide metals ride along with fruit and vegetable dyes used to intensify their color, and with pesticide. The most polluted dye, Fast Green (also called Food Green 3), penetrates entire bananas, grapefruit, eggplants, etc., bringing you thulium, lanthanum, gadolinium in large quantities.

Streptococcus infects us by riding along with the common parasite, rabbit fluke, in the same way as *Clostridium*. This fluke is smaller than a pinhead and the eggs are everywhere in dirt. We have been taught since primeval times to wash our food for the very purpose of removing dirt—even dust. We wash our hands for the same reason. And plain washing does get off most of it. But tiny amounts remain. The small amount that is stuck in crevices or remains glued to the food we eat is important to us now, although it does not make ordinary people sick or feel pain. Unfortunately as we age, we lose the very hydrochloric acid that can kill this parasite and its bacteria in our stomachs. In this way our immunity sinks and we acquire more and more colonies of streptococcus—and more and more aches and pains. A new-born baby is very susceptible too, due to immature immunity and is fed only sterilized food for its safety. The cancer patient is most susceptible of all, and with every mouthful of non-sterile food, receives another dose of rabbit fluke.

Streptococcus does not have special needs, such as *Clostridium* does—it colonizes wherever there is the slightest opportunity: in traumatized joints, in organs with asbestos lodged in them, in ears after infections, in hearts that are parasitized, and in tumorous organs.

As soon as you stop reinfecting with rabbit fluke, and zap your streptococcus, or kill them with the items mentioned, pain will stop, whether it is in the bones, abdomen, chest or head, or any other location. Soon your body is cleared of them except for those that are marooned in your tumors. After the tumors are drained and shrunk, all pain stays away until you reinfect. If you are in pain, this is the most compelling reason to sterilize your food as you would for a baby. (See *Food Rules*, page 520.)

Who Comes To Dinner?

The Syncrometer detects many other varieties of bacteria, too, at a tumor site or a location of pain, but these are more easily banished. Many are common food bacteria:

Shigella sonnei, food origin
Shigella flexneri, food origin
Shigella dysenteriae, food origin
Salmonella paratyphi, food origin
Salmonella typhimurium, food origin
Salmonella enteriditis, food origin
E. coli, food origin
Staphylococcus aureus, dental origin
Rhizobium meliloti, food origin
Rhizobium leguminosarum, only with *Ascaris*
Lactobacillus casei, food origin
Lactobacillus acidophilus, food origin
Streptomyces griseus, only with tapeworm larvae
Streptomyces albus, only with tapeworm larvae
Streptomyces venezuelae, only with tapeworm larvae
Mycobacterium avium/cellulare, only with *Ascaris*

A glance at the list shows that common food bacteria eaten at mealtime can find their way to your tumors and to your joints or muscles, wherever you have pain! Immune protection by your white blood cells is lacking there.

Normally, even harmful food bacteria simply pass along and out of the digestive tract. Yet, for a cancer patient they can escape from the digestive tract and enter the body. The protective lymph nodes and white blood cells in the lining of the intestinal tract have lost their immune power. You will get it back as you recover.

Until then the bacteria, besides the parasites, found in common dirt must not be allowed to enter with food and invade you. They make amines that remove the "brakes" on cell division. They also make ammonia. Ammonia is extremely toxic to living cells, giving you fatigue and illness besides. Some bacteria make growth factors and "cancer antigens" as seen by Syncrometer. For a list see *The Cure For All Cancers*.

If you have extreme pain, or even moderate pain, this is your clue that bacteria are still arriving. You can assume you are eating them! Fight back with a two pronged approach:

> 1. Eat sterilized food to stop reinfection.
> 2. Kill those bacteria already present with a daily regimen, as follows:

Divide And Conquer

- *Salmonellas* are eradicated with Lugol's' iodine solution, three times a day. In severe pain, a fourth dose is given at bedtime. It clears up in a day—unless your food is contaminated with it (throw out all leftovers immediately).
- *E. coli* and *Shigellas* will be eradicated by a combination of turmeric and fennel herbs.
- *Streptococcus* will be eradicated with oregano oil and by killing the rabbit fluke and zapping. You should, of

course, stop eating asbestos and lanthanide metals. You must remove the ferritin coating from your white blood cells and any lanthanide metals coming from metal teeth, as well, to restore your immunity. We will discuss them later.

- *Staphylococcus* varieties will be eradicated as dental work is completed. Extraction sites must be kept free of food particles, of course, so they can heal. This is accomplished in the Dental Aftercare program.

How do you know which bacteria you have? You can assume that you have all of them. That is why the parasite program, Lugol's solution, turmeric, fennel, and oregano oil are part of the 21 Day Program. Food sterilization, and dental work take care of the rest. Ferritin plus lanthanide removal, the mainstay of immune recovery, is also easily accomplished.

Fight Phenol Too

Although *Streptococcus* and rabbit flukes are instantly killed by the parasite program, the pain causing part, the phenol, is not instantly gone. There are several ways to destroy phenol:

1. Inositol, 1-3 tsp. before each meal.
2. Raw beet juice, 2 tbs. with added vinegar, 1 teaspoon to 1 tablespoon before meals.
3. Rhodizonate, 133 mg (available in Mexico).
4. Magnesium oxide, 300 mg with each meal.

A single dose of any of these treatments destroys all phenol quickly, but you may still not feel pain relief for several reasons. You may already be reinfected because your tumors themselves release bacteria. Also, we find it takes about a week of practice to learn to make sterile food. Another reason is that you may still have benzene accumulations in your tumors or fatty tissues. Benzene is detoxified into phenol. It takes three to five days before benzene can be cleared with vitamin B_2 doses (these are part of the 21 Day Program). So, although pain reduction will <u>begin</u> immediately, it typically takes the first week of the 21 Day Program dosages for substantial relief.

Minimize Morphine

Try to switch from morphine to codeine and then to non-prescription pain killers—even if you must quadruple the number of tablets. It is often difficult to move from the addictive drugs (morphine and codeine) to the non-addictive varieties. Morphine and codeine are more powerful. But remind yourself why you were put on them—your "case" was considered hopeless. The side effect of morphine, <u>inability to thrive</u>, was not considered important anymore. Doctors routinely do <u>not</u> tell the patient or family when they have given up on them. A prescription of morphine is your clue! Switch as soon as you can to regular pain killers. Try to <u>mix</u> several pain killers so less of any <u>one</u> is required. Also, try these alternative pain killers:

- Castor oil packs (see *Recipes*).
- One aspirin plus 50 mg niacin (not when bleeding or very low RBC are problems).
- Benzoquinone, 1-2 mcg by injection (provided clinically only; available in Mexico).
- Colloidal silver, homemade (commercial varieties were polluted with lanthanides). Try one tablespoon first. After 10 minutes take another tablespoon. Increase this way till you get pain relief. Stop at ½ cup. Repeat as needed.
- Coffee enemas, one to four a day (see page 558).

Safer Painkillers

Both nonprescription and prescription painkillers are heavily polluted with antiseptic (isopropyl alcohol), petroleum residue (benzene), and traces of azo dyes. These will go straight to your tumors; some will be stored in your body fat.

If you cannot test your pills for these, try to make them safer. First, wash off any color coating under the cold water faucet. Then roll in a bit of B_2 powder. Then allow to dry. Pills that are white and capsules containing powders need the same treatment because dyes contaminate them also.

What If Pain Comes Back

Pain can come back with a vengeance even after it has left. If it does, you already know the causes—the same bacteria as before! Since you cleared it up once before, repeat everything, being very meticulous. Just assume that you picked up *Ascaris,* tapeworm stages, the rabbit fluke, or dental and food bacteria. Kill them all again. Take black walnut tincture extra strength, cloves, wormwood, Lugol's, turmeric, fennel, and oregano drops all at 10 minute intervals and finally wash it down with 10 drops hydrochloric acid (5%) in water. You may need to repeat everything later in the day. Reinfection is so easy and immunity so low.

Coincidental Pain

Another contributor to pain is spasms from the gallbladder and bile ducts. Although this has nothing to do with cancer, it is often a part of the total pain picture.

Gallstone pain may be directly over the gallbladder (right side, lower chest) or radiating through to your upper back! It may be especially intense in shoulders, upper arms, behind or between shoulder blades. The only solution is to do a liver cleanse (see *Recipes*). Fortunately, this serves extra purposes: it will make your digestion stronger, you will be able to gain weight, and you will feel better. And fortunately, sick people, even terminally ill people, tolerate it very well. In about one thousand cases there have been no emergencies resulting from a liver cleanse. Follow it exactly including the suggestion to use ozonated olive oil. The ozonation will reach into the bile ducts, penetrating many stones and killing bacteria and viruses there. Four to six liver cleanses with ozonated oil will make a big difference to your health. Follow each cleanse with vitamin E (100 u, see *Sources*) the following day to minimize over-oxidation. Also take the usual parasite killing dosage the following day. Of course, if you are in great pain and your ozonator has not arrived, do the liver cleanse anyway, with plain olive oil.

How can you know for sure, whether some or all of your pain is due to gallstones, which is easy to correct? You can do a simple test: the Epsom salts test. Spasms from the bile ducts (the excruciating pain) are relieved by Epsom salts. If you have not taken any food or beverage (besides water) for four hours you may try this test. If you <u>have</u> eaten, this test will make you sick because Epsom salts mixed with food will cause nausea. Wait until your stomach has not had food for four hours. If the pain level allows you to wait until six PM, it will be a better test.

Give yourself a rounded tablespoon of Epsom salts in ¾ cup water. If you sense <u>some</u> relief—it need not be total relief— spasms from the bile ducts <u>are</u> contributors to your pain. At this point, you could decide to continue with the liver cleanse since you have already done part of it. Even if you had food containing fat in the morning, even if you had pain killers in the morning (both of which are normally not allowed), there is little to lose, except gallstones, or an *Ascaris* worm, and burgeoning bacteria that are somehow causing spasms.

In advanced cancer the rule of waiting two weeks between liver cleanses can be set aside. The time interval can be decided by how you feel. Especially if you are in <u>great</u> pain, you can repeat the liver cleanse every third or fourth day. You may get slightly more pain relief each time. As soon as pain is tolerable, rest your body; delay the next liver cleanse until pain is intolerable again or for two weeks.

Another coincidental pain could be from a fracture in hip, vertebra, or rib. Such pain can be excruciating, and a fracture should be searched for by x-ray. Nevertheless, it is extremely painful only if infected with bacteria. Do your dental work as soon as you are able to sit in the dentist's chair. Start the Dental Aftercare program the same day.

Wearing a supportive brace may help with pain, but gives you the risk of "overdoing" by sitting up too much or walking too much. There could be sudden collapse of vertebrae or a perforation of pelvis by leg bone. These "accidents" will keep you flat on your back for six months while healing occurs! So I don't recommend wearing a brace; you should stay fully aware of your limitations, real improvement, or worsening.

To heal a fracture, you need lots of calcium, magnesium, and the bone hardeners: manganese and boron. We also use a special herbal tea (see Bone Healer recipe and Bone Herb tea in *Recipes*).

Pain from friction of a lung sac (pleura) against the chest can be excruciating, too. Purchase a rib brace to immobilize your chest as you heal; a rib brace is not conducive to over exertion.

Headache can also be severe, especially in brain cancer. If it returns after clearing up, suspect a new tooth infection. Go back to the dentist and be extra meticulous with your dental aftercare (page 83). Repeat the parasite program. Be extra careful to sterilize your food.

Remember, your body is eager to heal and be pain-free.

Be sure to zap daily. Keep bowel functioning well (do a daily enema, see *Recipes*).

Finally, if things don't go exactly as planned, and you must use stronger pain killers, don't punish yourself with remorseful thoughts. It is not a moral issue. When pain is lessened, you will automatically be able to reduce them. Not sooner.

Dental Work

There are two purposes for doing the dental clean-up:

---

1. to clear up *Clostridium* infection
2. to remove mutagens and carcinogens from your mouth.

Clearing up *Clostridium* infection requires removing abscessed teeth, teeth with microleakage (infections in crevices under fillings), and eliminating infections in the jawbone itself where teeth once were, called **cavitations**.

Removing mutagens and carcinogens means all metals and plastic materials in your mouth. You may believe you have only "gold" or "silver" in your teeth. But these are really gold or silver alloys, containing many metals, including carcinogenic ones[59].

The Syncrometer® detects about 30 metals in any "gold" or "silver" filling. These include nickel, copper, cobalt, vanadium, thallium, germanium, cadmium, mercury, platinum, titanium, and even uranium! In my Syncrometer studies, I have found copper, cobalt, and vanadium to be present in every tumor. Seeping from both metal and plastic teeth, these metals are common denominators in advanced cancer cases. I have also found inorganic "bad" germanium in enough cases to consider it another common denominator. These begin to build up in your tissues in the early, tumor-forming stage. I am not sure whether these toxins play a role in actual tumor growth, but eventually they cause the anemia, liver failure, kidney failure, mutations, hypercalcemia, and immunity failure that causes death. So I want to emphasize again, that even if a magic wand shrank your tumors, you are still in mortal danger unless you get your dental work done!

---

[59] Phillips, R.W., *Skinner's Science of Dental Materials* 9*th* Ed., W.B. Saunders Co., 1991, ch. 20, Dental Casting Alloys, pp. 359-84.

If you have plastic materials in your dentalware, I find they will seep urethane, maleic acid, malonic acid, and various azo dyes. Methacrylate dentures even seep acrylic acid. Urethane and azo dyes have had decades of research in the past; they were found to be highly carcinogenic. Maleic and malonic acids were found to be respiratory inhibitors which, in turn, cause tumors to form. And acrylic acid, another carcinogen, is the same chemical that is made by frying foods in unsaturated fats. With so many well-studied carcinogens in dental materials, we should ask a child's question: Have they ever been tested for carcinogenicity? If so, what were the results?

Is it impossible to make plastics that don't have all these carcinogens? Not at all. The Syncrometer detected more dental ingredients that were free of them than those that had them. But if each dental material (such as composite, ceramic, glass ionomer) requires the use of ten ingredients, then the chance of finding the final restoration free of carcinogens is essentially zero. Using a Syncrometer, each ingredient could be tested separately for one dozen of the most harmful chemicals–not impossible–but quite impractical.

So to accomplish the two purposes of eliminating *Clostridium* infection and seeping carcinogens, you must extract teeth with large metal or plastic fillings, root canals, crowns or caps. They once were infected—before you had them "repaired". Now they are infected again and must be removed.

Why Is There Metal In Plastic?

Metal is not an essential ingredient of plastic manufacture. How can plastic material become polluted with it? I can speculate on several ways, but the fact is I am not the only one finding it.[60]

---

[60] Benjamin, M., Jenne, E., *Trace Element Contamination, Copper From Plastic Microlitre Pipet Tips*, Atomic Abs. Newsletter, v. 15, no. 2, Mar-Apr 1976, p. 53. Sommerfeld, M., et al., *Trace Metal Contamination Of Disposable Pipet Tips*, Atomic Abs. Newsletter, v. 14, no. 1, Jan-Feb 1975, p. 31.

Perhaps the use of inferior "practical" grade chemicals to make plastics with, or recycled ingredients, causes wholesale pollution of dental materials with toxic metals, dyes, or solvents.

I also find insufficient hardening of plastic in your mouth allows seepage of plasticizers, dyes, and other ingredients from the soft tooth.

A method for hardening (curing) your own dentures and partials is given in Recipes, page 574. Unfortunately, no way of hardening fillings and glues has yet been found.

Another possibility involves the chemical <u>antiseptics</u> used in manufacturing plastics. Although important, they are <u>themselves</u> polluted with metals, solvents and dyes. Pollution that stems from antiseptics spreads further and further. It is like having a wet kitchen sponge that drops to the ground; after that, dirt will be spread wherever the sponge is used to "clean" a surface. Ultimately, there is nothing left unpolluted with the antiseptics themselves and the toxins found in them. Look at the assortment of antiseptics legal for use in manufacturing processes, including the dental and plastic industries.[61]

---

[61] A complete list of allowable solutions for food-contact articles is in the (U.S.) Code of Federal Regulations (21 CFR Ch. 1, 4/1/95 ed., §178.1010 *Sanitizing solutions*).

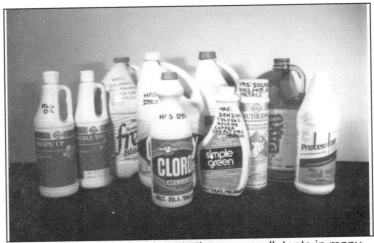

The Syncrometer detects the same pollutants in many manufactured products as in these antiseptics. Coincidence?
Fig. 18 Only two of these antiseptics had no pollutants

Learning to manufacture pure and safe dentalware should not be difficult for an industry with a research budget. Hopefully, it will soon develop. Learning to harden it adequately should be the second goal.

Be Your Own Dentist

Meanwhile, you must try to be your own dentist. Your teeth are too important not to understand the issues. If your dentist is willing to assist you, you are most fortunate. You may otherwise learn the basics from the following sample X-rays. Use this diagram to orient yourself.

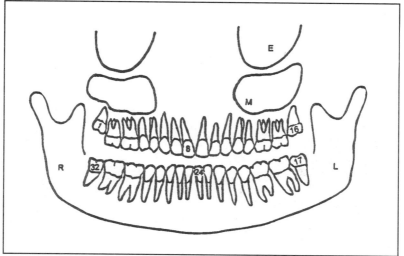

R is right side; L is left side; M is maxillary sinus; E is ethmoid sinus; and the teeth are numbered from 1 to 32, with 1 being the upper right wisdom tooth

Fig. 19 Diagram of a panoramic X-ray

First, obtain a good quality *panoramic* X-ray of your mouth, in duplicate if possible. A panoramic views the entire mouth, including jaw and sinuses, allowing you to see much more than single teeth. Take one negative home to study.

On your panoramic you can identify metal, plastic, root canals, crowns, abscesses along roots, cavitations (hollow spaces or mushy bone at old extraction sites), and other suspicious things. Circle whatever your dentist or radiologist identifies as suspect for future reference. Make notes.

Here is a sample of a panoramic X-ray that has been printed. Remember that a print of an X-ray negative reverses the light and dark areas. Since you will be comparing this print with your own X-ray, you must compare light areas on the print shown here to dark areas on your X-ray.

To read your panoramic X-ray, tape it up on a window. First find the angles of your jawbone, noting top and bottom view, left and right side, with the right side (R) on <u>your</u> left, as if facing yourself. Use a hand magnifying glass to study it.

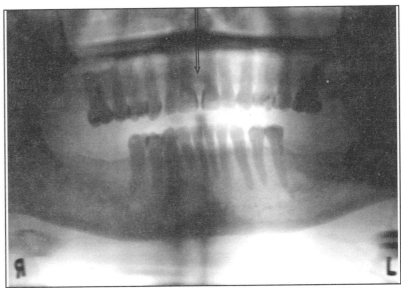

Fig. 20 A print of a medium quality panoramic X-ray

You Be The Judge

It doesn't take an advanced degree in dentistry to judge whether it is a good or bad X-ray. Are all the root tips visible? If not, you wasted your money; you got the panoramic so you could see the root tips and beyond! Since the X-ray can be viewed right at the time it is made you can request a retake (it costs very little extra and supplies the duplicate you wanted anyway).

This particular X-ray should have been done over, because, looking at the upper teeth, no root tips are visible. The mouth was not correctly positioned for the X-ray. Also, the teeth at the ends are a solid black, so nothing can be deduced about them.

The intensity setting on the X-ray machine was not correct for them.

Next, look at the lower teeth. The root tips are on the print, but not very clear. The X-ray machine produced two dark vertical lines at the centers, obscuring the roots further (a good reason to get it redone on the spot). Under each end-tooth is a roundish white spot. On the X-ray film, which you would be examining, these would be dark spots. These are the holes in the jawbone that allow the nerve and blood vessels to pass through.

A tooth was pulled three months ago on the lower left side. Note that the bone has already filled in almost to the top, so that a nearly flat line is seen to mark the ridge of the jaw bone from one side to the other. This shows good healing.

Locate the center. You have four small flat teeth in front on the lower side. The center is between them so two are on the left side and two on the right. The center on the upper side is easier to find; see the arrow.

The fifth tooth from the center at upper left (L) has a black cloud emerging upward from the root tip like a swarm of gnats above it. This is an infection, the bacteria are parading up towards the brain. Brain tumors are made of such events. Trying to save such a tooth would be a bad mistake, even though it "looks good and was giving no trouble." Plastic (black edges) can be seen on the inner edge of the top center teeth; this was done for cosmetic purposes. A few more bits of plastic are seen here and there. No cavitations (dark areas) are seen in the bottom half where the visibility is good.

A large tattoo (spattered amalgam) did not show up on this X-ray although the dentist spotted it easily just by searching, visually, some time later, while working on the mouth. Tattoos can be notoriously difficult to find, either way.

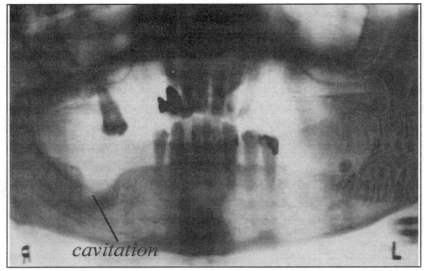

Fig. 21 Panoramic showing large cavitation at lower right.

The second panoramic, although poor quality, shows a large cavitation at the lower right. One or two teeth extracted there long ago left a large hole with infection (dark area) along the sides. Thorough cleaning will allow it to fill in with bone again and stop the chronic illnesses this patient suffered from.

At the upper right, a solitary tooth is sitting in a bed of infection. The dark black areas are metal. Syncrometer tests of this patient showed that the tooth bacteria, *Staphylococcus* and *Clostridium,* were both traveling to the breast. Staph was producing growth factors and *Clostridium* was turning RNA into DNA to spur the tumor there.

If you notice a suspicious tooth or location, but can't quite make a determination, repeat the x-ray at the tooth location; it is called a *periapical* X-ray. **But not the regular kind.** Newer digital X-ray equipment is much superior. Compare these digital X-ray frames with your panoramic.

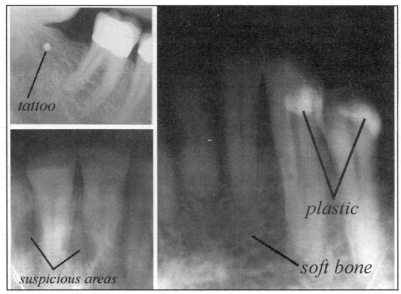

Fig. 22 Digital X-rays give superior view

Two or three "takes" of each location may still be needed to find your hidden cavitations, "surprise" plastic leftovers, tattoos, and simply, infected bone.

After examining your X-rays, make your decisions—do not ask the dentist to make them for you—and mark the teeth for extraction. The dentist may not agree with you because his/her job is to <u>save teeth</u>. Your job is to <u>save your life</u>. Your dentist can't be expected to know that your life depends on this.

Another option is to go to a foreign country to find a sympathetic dentist (see *Sources*).

What You Can Salvage

How can you decide what is a large and not-so-large filling? Since this is to some extent a subjective decision, you should consider the options. If you mark for extraction a number of bad teeth, but leave single teeth behind that are marginally good, you will get a partial denture that must fit around the single stragglers. These will constantly get food clogged around them, giving you discomfort. You will need to take out the partial for cleaning much more often than if you had a simpler partial that included all the molars and premolars in any one quarter (quadrant) of your mouth.

The same thinking applies to front teeth. If you have only two or three good front teeth, you should consider the need to remove partials for cleaning more frequently than you would need to remove a full denture.

Fillings that could be replaced with an inlay or onlay may simply be removed, leaving the hole open. Later, when your tumors are gone you may have them filled using zinc oxide and phosphate paste as the glue. But this does leave you with a grave risk—the risk that the dentist "didn't get it all." And this could hardly be considered the dentist's fault, since he/she must work blindly. Plastic is almost invisible and undetectable by any means. Even a digital X-ray could not detect a tiny bit left behind. A reliable plastic identifier has not yet been found. If you are terminally ill, the tiniest remnant of plastic could tip the scales to failure. Your spleen, bone marrow and liver are already full of plastic toxins, as a cup of water is "full" to the brim. Your spare storage tissue, fat, is full, too. Even a tiny plastic remnant is too much. Extraction is safer.

When the open tooth is brushed daily with oregano oil and colloidal silver, and occasionally with bleach (USP, more on this below), it does not decay further. I have not seen these teeth undergo further decay in one year's time. Remember that the purpose of the original filling was to stop decay. You can now do that without the filling so no harm is done for about one year, enough time for you to get well first. You will be able to monitor your teeth yourself by watching for discoloration. Any beginning infection can be quickly eliminated by yourself. (See *Home Dentistry*, page 91.)

The Visit To The Dentist

Find an <u>oral surgeon</u> willing to clean up your mouth for you. It is more than "just pulling teeth." They must be willing to let you examine your own X-ray, participate in decisions, and use your homemade antiseptics.

Make two appointments (if you have time), one for X-rays and one for dental work. That way you will be able to study the X-ray. Dentists often want to get started right away, but you may need more time than that for these important decisions.

Arrange for a friend to accompany you to the dental office. All professional persons pay more attention to a party of two than a single person. Ask for permission to have your friend nearby. Your friend can hand you your antiseptics. Your friend should sit quietly near you, not wasting the dentist's time with talk or questions.

Treat yourself to a good meal before going for dental work. You will be on liquids for a while afterward.

If you have "dentist-phobia", take a strong dose of pain killer (not aspirin) one half hour before your appointment time.

Your Antiseptic Is Best

Make and bring your own antiseptic. Even though the surgeon and dental assistant wear gloves, a cancer patient <u>can't help</u> picking up bacteria. This is not the dentist's or surgeon's fault. They are coming from your own mouth. Sterility for the mouth is impossible. While blood vessels are broken (bleeding), bacteria can enter your circulation.

By far the best antiseptic to use during dentalwork is plain bleach.

Bunyan [in *The Use of Hypochlorite For The Control of Bleeding*, Oral Surgery, v. 13, 1960, pp. 1026-1032] reported that rinsing with 0.2% hypochlorite solution stops postoperative bleeding within 1 minute after a tooth extraction or other oral operation. The hypochlorite solution functions also to contract and harden the blood clots and make them more resistant to infection.

In addition to the effective hemostasis and the change in the character of the clot, the author reported a reduction of swelling of traumatized gingival tissues and diminution of the postoperative pain.[62]

Don't use <u>household</u> bleach because it is not safe for internal use! Obtain food grade (USP) bleach from *Sources*. Purchase the same strength (5%, not stronger) as regular household bleach so you can handle it safely. If bleach is not available bring Lugol's iodine solution or a colloidal silver solution with you to the office.

Bleach (5%) is very caustic.
You must not use it at full strength.

You must dilute it. Follow the recipe on page 547 <u>exactly</u>.

We will name your new, diluted bleach, Dental Bleach. Take a half cup of Dental Bleach with you in a convenient jar. Rinse your mouth with it before you sit down in the dental chair. <u>Never swallow it!</u> Hold the jar in your lap. Later, when the dentist signals you to rinse your mouth, use your solution again. Also rinse one last time before leaving the office. The dentist will appreciate this extra care because she/he is less likely to see post-dental infection in you.

Second best would be Lugol's iodine solution (six drops of actual Lugol's iodine in a half cup of water). Use up the entire amount before leaving the dental office.

Third best is colloidal silver. Make your own colloidal silver solution since the commercially available ones I tested had the familiar pollutants associated with antiseptics. The same instructions apply to colloidal silver; use ½ cup.

As soon as the extractions are completed the sockets left behind must be cleaned by the surgeon to remove bits of adhering

---

[62] Block, Seymour S., *Disinfection, Sterilization, and Preservation*, 3rd Ed., Lea & Febiger, 1983, p. 178.

tissue together with a few millimeters of bone. This will prevent leaving a residue for bacteria to thrive on later. Then it is squirted with a dropperful of diluted Lugol's iodine solution, or straight white iodine (see *Recipes*). If you are allergic to iodine use colloidal silver instead. You must supply these.

Commercial antiseptic made for the dental profession is not satisfactory. It invariably contains isopropyl alcohol besides other chemicals. On the positive side, though, is that they are not trapped in your teeth, they do dissipate and get detoxified.

Save The Pieces

Tell the dentist before sitting down in the chair that you would like to keep the extracted teeth, root canals, and fillings, but they can all be tossed into a bag together. If the dentist tells you this is not allowed due to Public Health regulations, agree to fill out the appropriate application forms. They may need to be sterilized first (in 50% bleach water—don't autoclave because that would put mercury vapor into the air). It is amazing that your own teeth may be considered too dangerous—too bacteria-laden and full of mercury (a hazardous waste!)—to be handled, even by you, the owner! (Were they safer in your mouth?) But they do belong to you. You may be curious in the future about what they contain, and could have been leaching.

You can preserve them in a few days, when you are up to it. Cover them with Dental Bleach or Lugol's to sterilize them again. If the strong odor does not leave, you may understand how the internal infection of these teeth was poisoning your body! Finally, you may wish to look for the *Clostridium* infection, which would be a darkened area under fillings or in crevices. After drying, store them in a paper bag (plastic traps moisture).

Save loose pieces of metal and plastic because you may wish to have them analyzed at a later date, too. Or you may simply wish to gloat over the retrieved "treasure" as you identify corrosion and gross infection.

When extractions are done, congratulate yourself for the achievement. Start the Dental Aftercare program at once. Do not eat or drink, (besides water) for the rest of the day after an extraction.

All root canals and dead teeth must be extracted, as well as teeth with large fillings. Teeth with implants have not been studied sufficiently to know which metals they shed or if *Clostridium* infections start in their vicinity. For this reason, you must use your own judgment on implants.

After extracting rotten or filled teeth, the dentist or surgeon needs to do <u>two things</u> before stitching up the wound: cavitation cleansing and amalgam cleanup.

Huggins Cavitation Cleaning

The tooth was held in the socket by soft tissues like tiny ligaments. Unless these are removed, too, they will decay and provide opportunity for bacteria to reside there. The sockets left behind should be carefully cleaned with special tools for this purpose.

This procedure has been taught in the past by Dr. Hal Huggins and many dentists are familiar with it. It is called cavitation cleaning. It prevents future infection and inability to heal at that site. In spite of such superior treatment of the socket, you may occasionally expect a bone fragment to reveal itself later. As it loosens and works its way out, infection and pain accompany it. Go back to the dentist. This could be a source of your pain elsewhere in your body if it is not removed.

<u>While the new sockets are being cleaned, any old infected sockets (cavitations) should be cleaned out as well</u>. The dentist can spot the obvious cavitations on the panoramic X-ray. Afterwards, each cavitation site also gets squirted with diluted Lugol's solution or straight white iodine or straight colloidal silver. Hidden cavitations (those that don't show up on the X-ray) can be cleared without surgery; we will discuss this soon.

Arichega Gum Cleaning

The second task after extracting your teeth, and cleaning cavitations is to <u>remove imbedded amalgam</u>. This procedure has been developed by Dr. Benjamin Arichega of Mexico. Each quadrant of your mouth needs an amalgam cleanup. The top of the gum line will be gray from absorbed mercury. It is easiest for you to have this done while extractions are being done. The dentist begins by cutting a straight line on top of the bony ridge of the jaw where teeth once were.

Next, he/she snips away $\frac{1}{8}$ inch (3 mm) of the gum on each side of the incision. A ribbon, $\frac{1}{8}$ inch wide and extending from the wisdom teeth to the closest front tooth is discarded. The remaining gum tissue stretches over the top easily and is sutured over. Surprisingly, the new gum tissue heals <u>much faster</u> than the old, mercury-saturated gums. You can count on your gums being healed in two to three days. The new gum tissue produces a strong even union, without small holes where food can get trapped. We call it the Arichega technique, after the oral surgeon who invented it. While the dentist is cutting out mercury-drenched gum tissue, the exposed bone can be cleaned of amalgam bits that are easy to spot now.

Dental Aftercare

One of the purposes of doing this dental clean-up is to kill all *Clostridium* bacteria that have invaded the deeper regions of the jaw bone after being spawned in the decaying teeth and crevices under tooth fillings. From here they colonize your tumors as well as the bowel.

Antibiotics are not to be relied upon by a cancer patient undergoing dental work because antibiotics only <u>inhibit</u> the bacteria until they die or your immune system takes over. In a cancer patient, this immune response may never happen. And as soon as the antibiotic is stopped a new, more serious, bacterium can surface to bewilder and defy everybody.

Antibiotics cannot stop tooth decay. They do not reach the crevices in teeth because there is no blood circulation there. For the same reason, antibiotics do not reach cavitations.

Antibiotics are merely an adjunct to good Dental Aftercare. So a very vigorous program is needed to clear up infection even after the infected teeth are pulled because deep wounds such as the base of the socket where the bacteria used to be is precisely the preferred location for more *Clostridia*. They refuse to leave. Just removing the tooth does not automatically clear up an abscess that was at the tip of a root. Other bacteria may leave but not *Clostridium*. Even cleaning the socket thoroughly may remove *Staphylococcus* but does not remove *Clostridium* bacteria.

This Dental Aftercare program is successful in killing *Clostridium*. You will need:

- a water pick
- hot water, towels
- empty syringe (barrel only, purchase at pharmacy)
- pure salt or sterilized salt water
- Dental Bleach

Acquire these before your dental appointment. Practice using the water pick. Practice using the syringe to squirt water (do not attach needle).

The immune power of your arterial blood is much greater than in your veins. How can you bring arterial blood into the jaw area to heal it faster after dental work? Simply by hot-packing it from the start!

The first day of dental work is critical.

If you miss this, a massive spread of infection can occur because the mouth is always a "den of bacteria", and your own tooth infection is itself the source.

Remember, even before leaving the dentist's office, just as soon as you are out of the chair, rinse with Dental Bleach. Then, again, as soon as you get home from the dentist. Next, swish your mouth gently with a cup of warm water. The heat brings in arterial blood. Keep the cotton plug in place for you to bite down on and reduce bleeding, even while swishing. Don't <u>suction</u> the water forcefully around your mouth, you could dislodge the blood clot that needs to form in the socket. Slowly move the warm water about your mouth.

At the same time apply a hot towel to the outside of your face where the dental work was done. Wring a wash cloth out of the hottest water you can endure, trying it out on an unanesthetized location first. Or fill a plastic baggie halfway with hot water, zipping it shut securely. Do this for thirty minutes, four times a day, for a few days. Then three times a day for a week— even when there is no pain.

Don't suck liquids through a straw for twenty-four hours; the sucking force is too risky. Don't allow your tongue to suck the wound site, either; and <u>don't put fingers in your mouth</u>.

As the anesthetic wears off there will be very little pain <u>if</u> the bacteria in the tooth sites have been killed. But you could introduce the bacteria yourself, <u>by eating</u>, or by putting fingers into your mouth. Consider your mouth a surgery site. Anywhere else on your body, the surgery site would have been scrubbed first, then painted with iodine or other strong bacteria killers, and later sprayed again with antiseptic and bandaged to keep <u>everything</u> out—certainly food particles and fingers!

But the mouth cannot be bandaged and you must eat! To be successful, <u>eat a big meal just before your dental appointment</u>. Then eat nothing with particles in it that could lodge in your wound sites for two days! In fact, on the day of surgery, drink only water afterward. You may need a pain killer on the first night; choose a non-aspirin variety to minimize bleeding.

Bleeding should have reduced considerably by bedtime. The cotton plug put in your mouth by the dentist may be thrown away. Rinse with Dental Bleach once more before bed.

Dental Day Two

The next day you need to be well-fed, yet eat <u>no solids</u>, <u>nor liquids with particles in them</u>. The particles easily lodge in your wound. Your choices are:

1. Chicken broth, filtered.
2. Herb teas, sweetened, filtered.
3. Fruit juice, using undyed, pesticide-free fruit, filtered.
4. Vegetable juice, filtered (including raw beet juice).
5. Puddings made of cornstarch or flour.
6. Complete "feed" (see page 535).

Filter through a coffee filter placed in a strainer. These liquid foods must also be sterilized before drinking (see *Recipes*).

Immediately after eating, rinse your mouth with a cup of very hot water to which you have added ¼ tsp. salt. Fill syringe with hot salt water and squirt each extraction site several times. Do not be afraid to start some bleeding; this could be expected and is even <u>desirable</u> if an infection has already started; bleeding washes bacteria <u>outward</u>. Water squirting and swishing <u>never</u> dislodges the healing clot. Only strong suction or infection dislodges it. If pain increases instead of decreases on the second day, you are already infected. Continue swishing and hot packing for one hour. Devote the whole day to fighting infection. If the pain subsides, the infection has been cleared. If not, you will need a more forceful stream of water. Begin using the water pick at its lowest speed setting. Water pick repeatedly until it clears. (It could take four hours!)

Hot pack the outside of your face just as on the first day. If pain is subsiding on the second day, you are being successful. But the gums are <u>not</u> healed; you cannot take chances yet on eating food. Nearly all infections come from eating solid food on the second day.

Floss the front teeth with homemade floss being extra gentle. For floss, cut strips of plastic shopping bags ½ inch by 4 inches. Regular floss and toothbrush are too harsh for the nearby sensitive tissues. After flossing, clean these teeth by hand-rubbing, using paper towel dampened with water and oregano oil.

Also rinse your mouth with Dental Bleach several times during the day and bedtime.

Dental Day Three

On the third day, you may <u>drink</u> blended solid food; do not try to <u>chew</u> solids.

Use your water pick now after each meal. Fill the tank with hot water to which you have added a few drops of Lugol's iodine, or 1 tsp. colloidal silver, or salt. Set it at the gentlest level, at first, squirting each site carefully. Floss the front teeth and brush them with Dental Bleach (other antiseptics are not strong enough).

Notice how difficult it is to squirt out any trapped food. Swishing is <u>not</u> sufficient! Continue hot packing the face. If pain returns and water picking has not succeeded in clearing it, you must <u>hurry</u> back to the dentist to search for the food particle. The wound will be opened and cleaned out for you.

Bleeding

A moderate amount of bleeding is normal, even days later. Bleeding caused by water picking is not too serious. But if you sense an emergency, apply ice cubes wrapped in a paper towel or cheesecloth. Bite down on them till bleeding stops. Continue ice-packing for 4 hours. As soon as it is safe, return to hot-packing. If ice packing does not stop the bleeding, go back to the dentist or emergency room.

Cancer sufferers may have a low platelet count or be on a large amount of "blood thinners" which promote bleeding. Yet, oral surgery is a very skilled profession. Dental work is safe in the surgeon's hands. Platelets can be given just beforehand; blood thinners can be temporarily stopped; and a transfusion can be given before or immediately afterward. These same patients often state that they feel better, immediately after the dental extraction, than they can remember in months! It was the dental problem that was poisoning their platelets and their blood! It may be the last transfusion that will be needed even though there is some unavoidable blood loss with dental extractions.

Stitches should be removed earlier for cancer patients than others because they will get infected by the third day! Do not use self-digesting sutures; you need the extra dental visit to let the dentist observe your mouth.

Be Vigilant The Next Week

Continue water picking, hot packing, and rinsing your mouth with Dental Bleach after each meal until the gums are healed over. This may take five to seven days, longer for some sites. Floss and brush your front teeth once a day. If pain stays away you can take credit for killing your mouth-bacteria. You may reduce the treatments to three times a day, then twice.

Clostridium can return even after a week of steady recovery. Remember that its true source is the rabbit fluke, a tiny parasite that we eat accidentally with filth on unsterilized food. If you detect an odor from your mouth, at any time, it is *Clostridium* making a comeback, even without pain. A crumb has lodged in the wound and is decaying. Try bleaching, squirting, swishing, and water picking for half a day; then hurry back to the dentist if the odor persists.

If you got through the whole ordeal without needing more than one nights' pain killer and without needing to return to the dentist for extra clean-up, give yourself excellent grades. And if you got through, in any way, still give yourself very good grades!

It is common for dentists to recommend cold packing to reduce swelling after dental work. I recommend hot packing because I consider swelling less important than infection or pain. It is also common for dentists to rely on antibiotics to clear up infection. I find this is not sufficient.

Small Fillings

Again, you must search for a special dentist. The dentist must let you bring your own sealer. All sealers and desensitizers that are available from dental supply sources are typically polluted with the customary tumorigens and solvents: copper, cobalt, vanadium, malonates, urethane, azo dyes, germanium, isopropyl alcohol, and benzene. Do not risk any brand. But a sealer made of only calcium hydroxide (lime water) is safe and pure, if prepared by a pharmacist, yourself, or the dentist. A saturated solution is easily made and applied from a small dropper bottle. Purchase from a chemical supply company (see *Sources*).

Small fillings of plastic can be spotted on the digital X-ray that could not be seen on the panoramic. They must be drilled out meticulously.

The dentist should be very careful to notice any left over amalgam at the edges or the bottom of the plastic fillings left over from previous amalgam. Amalgams are routinely not cleaned out carefully when they are replaced by plastic. Furthermore, crevices may be found to be filled with amalgam that simply cannot be cleaned out. The dentist cannot go into a discussion of this while your mouth is stuck in open position! You should be familiar with this possibility. The dentist with a video system can show you the deep-seated metal bits. If the old amalgam cannot be removed without reaching the nerve, extract the tooth instead. Arrange for this with the dentist or surgeon beforehand.

Removing small amalgam fillings should be done very carefully, using a rubber dam, in order not to produce "dust" that spatters the entire mouth. Drilling out amalgam is a special skill. Find an experienced dentist. Only after your tumors are gone should you refill these cavities.

The cavity is then filled with a paste of zinc phosphate or zinc oxide and eugenol. These compounds will be pure if purchased from a chemical supply company or if purchased separately from a dental supply company. (No premixed variety has ever tested pure by the Syncrometer.)

The cavity may also be filled with an <u>inlay</u> of *Sculpture* or *Targis*. Inlays are already hardened in the dental lab and did not seep in my experiments. A glue of zinc phosphate paste, purchased as two separate bottles, will be safe. If removing a filling kills the tooth so it can now feel nothing, extract it. If filling removal got so close to the nerve that you are now in pain, extract it also. Only shallow fillings are candidates for salvaging.

Jerome Tattoo Removal

While the amalgam was being put into your teeth or taken out—tiny bits got away or flew away with great force into your cheek folds, into neighboring gums, into exposed bone nearby and down to the bottom of newly made sockets. Nobody will ever see these again, or so it was thought. (And guilt can never be laid.)

Larger bits of amalgam, called tattoos, can be seen on the panoramic or digital X-ray. Your dentist has already spotted them no doubt. But smaller particles do not show up. You must ask the dentist to search visually, with a magnifier and remove them <u>all</u> regardless how painstaking the job is. This and many more facts of dentistry are discussed by Frank Jerome, DDS in his book, Tooth Truth (see *Sources*). Each quadrant of your mouth needs a careful examination for mercury, and treatment by prying out tiny pieces stuck in your cheek folds, plus any pieces buried in your jaw bone. In addition, the ¼ inch ribbon of mercury-soaked gum on top of the jaw ridge must be removed as previously discussed.

Hidden Cavitations

These are more than the customary infected bone sites. They are primarily <u>bioaccumulation</u> sites. The Syncrometer detects them easily by searching for mercury and other amalgam-related metals <u>in the jawbone</u> (meaning a bone slide is in the circuit). Here the Syncrometer also finds plastic-related chemicals from fillings and silicones from toothpaste! *Streptococcus* is also there. The real reason for this bioaccumulation site is probably the presence of lanthanide elements. Wherever the lanthanides occur, the white blood cells become "choked" with iron and calcium deposits. After this they stop "eating" any more toxins destroying your immunity at this location. Hidden cavitations still contain their mercury even 20 years after amalgam was changed to plastic!

Only digital X-rays can picture these hidden bioaccumulation sites, and even here their identification can be difficult. Fortunately, they can be cleared without surgery. A magnet of about 100 gauss can attract the iron and lanthanide deposits in them (see page 170). It takes about one week. After these have left, remaining metals, plastics, and bacteria leave also, and are seen in the white blood cells for a few days, showing that immunity has returned suddenly and swiftly. Thereafter, the jaw bone is cleared.

Another way to clean out these hidden cavitations is with a DMSO mouthwash (see *Recipes*), although less reliable. In three to five days the entire toxic team of carcinogens (and *Streptococcus*) are seen to leave the jawbone.

Home Dentistry

Although dentists and dental surgeons alike have done their utmost to clean metal, plastic and infection from your mouth, there are still minute traces left behind. They continue to arrive in your tumors and fat reservoirs. Syncrometer testing reveals that half of the remaining teeth may still have traces of plastic. Only a final tooth-polishing can make them truly safe. On this hangs your fate if the LDH, liver enzymes, or alkaline phosphatase are much too high.

Ask the dentist for several "finishing strips." If these are not available you may use the finest grade emery cloth (such as 400 grit), by cutting strips out of it (approximately four inches long and one eighth inch wide). Put a few drops of Lugol's into a large glass of water, big enough to dip your hands into to sterilize them before the final polishing and "finishing" of your teeth.

First, you must brush your teeth very thoroughly with Dental Bleach. The easiest way is to be seated in a recliner chair facing into a bright light or sunshine and have a friend do the polishing. Otherwise you must do it yourself, standing in front of a mirror. Individually sterilize each of your hands and a finishing strip. Notice the clear plastic in the middle of a finishing strip. Slide it between the first two teeth. Saw back and forth as much as the teeth allow. Repeat between all other teeth. The heaviest work is at the ends—the sides of the last tooth in the row. Saw with a long sweep of the strip. Saw at least 20 times. Use the strip as ingeniously as you can to polish the top surface, too. Keep dipping your hands in Lugol's before each time you work in the mouth. When the polishing is complete, brush teeth again, and rinse with Dental Bleach.

Ideally, each newly polished tooth is now tested with the Syncrometer for remaining plastic, amalgam, or clostridium bacteria. Resonance with urethane and DAB dye or bisphenol implicates leftover plastic. Resonance with platinum, palladium, thallium, or nickel implicates amalgam. After finding which teeth are still contaminated, test the tooth surfaces individually to identify its exact location. Then repeat the polishing on that surface. Test each tooth for *Clostridium*, too. Note that even the tiniest brown spot tests Positive for *Clostridium*. Try to polish it away. If you can't, go back to your dentist for assistance. Do not have these tiny cavities filled afterward. But brush with oregano oil and colloidal silver in turns after meals, and Dental Bleach at bedtime.

This beginning Home Dentistry is a creative innovation of huge significance. Being able to do simple dentistry using the Syncrometer to guide you may pave the way to caries prevention that has eluded us so long. You can find a tooth infection long before it becomes a cavity.

You are finally metal-free, plastic-free, dye-free, and *Clostridium*-free. All that will be needed is to draw these out of your storage sites—fat tissue and tumors themselves—to begin tumor shrinkage.

Making Your Dentures and Partials

There are different opinions among dentists about <u>when</u> to make an impression of your mouth: <u>before</u> tooth extraction or later <u>after</u> your mouth has healed. There are advantages and disadvantages to either choice. The life-saving process is extraction—so don't delay a single day with this, even if the denture-making schedule is postponed.

For "instant teeth" the impressions are made before extraction. Ideally, the fitting is done immediately after extraction while still under anesthesia, so a very good fit can be made. But, of course, the mouth often changes its shape as it heals. Major adjustments will be necessary a month or so later.

Methylmethacrylate and **polyurethane** can be hardened by yourself at home and are therefore safe from seeping, even if a pink color is chosen for your dentures or partials. Other materials hold promise but need more research. See *Hardening Dentures* in *Recipes*.

Congratulations

You have completed the hardest task required to shrink your tumors: you have evicted *Clostridium* from its fortress.

A glance in the mirror shows you a beautiful set of teeth, sweet-smelling breath at all times and chewing better than before. You have enabled your body to survive.

On The Road To Recovery

Of course you have done a lot more than just eradicated *Clostridium*! You have also removed heavy metals, mutagens, dyes, and other toxins that were seeping from your fillings. Before this you killed *Ascaris*, tapeworm larvae, and rabbit fluke. The next step is to remove these same pathogens and pollutants from your diet and environment. And the final step is to drain them from your tumors so the tumors collapse and dissolve.

You might be wondering how much it will cost for this very specialized dental clean-up. Although the dental work may seem straightforward (extractions and filling removal being very common procedures) the way you need them done is not at all common. Using homemade antiseptics, requesting cavitation cleaning and tattoo removal, and finding a dentist with digital X-ray equipment are all non-traditional. In Mexico, in 1999 the rate, including the cleanups, was about $80.00 per extracted tooth.

How To Make A Million Dollars In Your Spare Time, At Home: Sue!

Pollution problems should be solved by people themselves, not industry or government; the responsibility is too great. Family health is at stake. Only people's groups would not be influenced by other priorities. What I am suggesting is that people form their own groups, find labs willing to do analysis of dental supplies, form collaborations with dentists willing to use tested materials, and follow-up on the job done with analysis of saliva (also by lab testing).

I was joking about making a million dollars, but maybe suing the American Dental Association is the last resort solution it takes to bring the problem to the attention of the American People, and provoke change.

That is another reason for saving what was removed from your mouth (besides curiosity). Any extracted teeth with fillings could be analyzed. They could be set to soak in water overnight and the water analyzed for seeped ingredients. These ingredients were seeping into you. The real object is not to point out guilt but to find a developing problem <u>before</u> your entire family has been damaged, generation after generation. Before your family must spend half its generated income on health restoration.

Bad health underlies mental illness, addictions, and criminal behavior besides the customary diseases. Even reproductive disturbance is a state of bad health. It makes no sense to place a piece of estrogen (as in bisphenol-A, used in dental plastic) in the mouths of children, to be sucked on day and night. Both girls and boys are likely to be affected, especially before puberty. Again, a people's group would not let this happen, if it were known, whereas a professional or governmental group is bound by laws to have other priorities even when they know it is happening.

A list of labs doing analyses for metals, solvents, and other chemicals is given in *Sources*. Many others can be found in the yellow pages of telephone directories. Be sure you understand the <u>sensitivity</u> of the testing each lab can do. Obviously, the ability to test to parts per <u>trillion</u> is better (more sensitive) than parts per <u>billion</u>.

Despite what I feel is the uninformed state of the dental profession, the average dentist is devoted to human welfare, besides just his or her own. This is apparent in the movements, <u>within the dental profession</u>, to outlaw mercury, to outlaw all metal, and to advocate better nutrition. Not all agree. But that is my point. Progress is made from discussion, and trying to achieve higher standards. If you find a dentist knowledgeable about microleakage and cavitations, willing to support your strange, new agenda, then you have truly found a treasure.

Tumor Shrinking Diet

To shrink your tumors your diet should be:

1. free of malonic acid
2. free of carcinogenic dyes and metals, isopropyl alcohol and benzene, asbestos and acrylic acid
3. free of parasite eggs and harmful bacteria
4. free of mold

because these are the things that made your tumors grow and drastically lowered your immunity.

This means that <u>safe</u> food is more important than <u>nutritious</u> food for you at this time.

Avoiding malonic acid in your food is the first rule in curing tumor disease. Malonic acid accumulates in tumors. No tumor has been found without it in over 1000 cases. This shows that malonic acid is a <u>common denominator</u> of tumors. What is it doing there?

Cancer researchers for one hundred years or more have been searching for the <u>direct cause</u> of our tumor growths. They suspected a chemical. They used mice and other animals to test chemicals by injecting them, putting them in the feed, or rubbing them into the skin. Chemicals were tested one by one, in the belief that there was <u>one</u>, and only one, responsible for it all. Many chemicals looked promising at first, but one by one, they were discarded—because they failed to <u>always</u> produce a tumor at the same place, in the same time, in all animals tested. It could not be imagined that a combination of chemicals was responsible. And that some might be supplied by the body itself. This degree of complexity could not be researched with traditional chemistry; even now it cannot be realistically pursued.

Only *Syncrometer biochemistry*, which is electronic, has the speed and accuracy to allow a return to the fundamental questions that were already asked one hundred years ago: What is different about tumors? What is unique about them? What do they have in common? Is the problem chemical, biological, or a matter of physics? The answers to these questions would surely lead to tumor prevention and cure. Now that Syncrometer technology has arrived, the involvement of malonic acid is clearly seen. To understand the role of malonic acid and the harm that it does, we must understand the basics of metabolism.

Your Metabolism

We get energy from food we eat by **oxidizing** it. This is the same way we get energy from fuel; we call it "burning." Burning fuel uses up oxygen and releases energy in the form of heat; it happens quickly, in a burst; we try to slow it down by controlling the draft in order to be less wasteful. Living cells burn food very, very slowly, controlled by enzymes, so that heat trickles out very slowly too (to keep us warm) and most of the energy can be saved as standby fuel—called *ATP*.

Getting energy from a food molecule means that an electron has been taken away from it; a nearby oxygen atom will soon grab it up. Intense heat causes this to happen in the case of burning fuel. But in a living cell enzymes cause electrons to be pulled away.

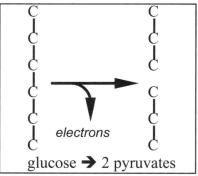

glucose ➔ 2 pyruvates

Fig. 23 Glycolysis, the first part of food metabolism

The first part of food metabolism in our cells is called *glycolysis*. Several enzymes approach a molecule of food, such as glucose (sugar), removing its electrons and finally snipping it in half. Removing electrons is called oxidation, even when no oxygen atoms are involved. **Pyruvic acid** (pyruvate) is produced.

In this way the food has been prepared for the second part of metabolism, called the **Krebs cycle**. Note that acetyl CoA is the hub that links glycolysis to the Krebs cycle.

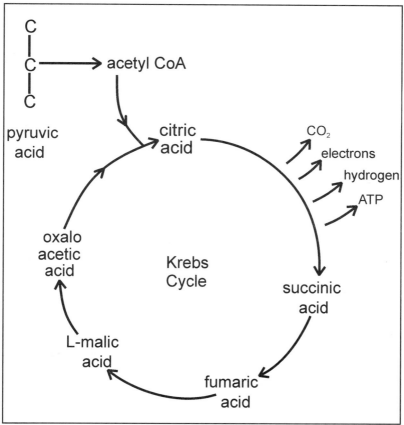

Fig. 24 The Krebs cycle, the second part of food metabolism

Now pyruvate (after turning into acetyl CoA) is joined by oxaloacetate to make citric acid (the same as in lemon juice). This gets oxidized to succinic acid, then to fumaric, then L-malic (as in apple juice) and back to oxaloacetate. Throughout the Krebs cycle oxygen is being used, electrons and hydrogen are being freed, and carbon dioxide (CO_2) and ATP are being formed. In addition each electron, along with its partner hydrogen, will combine with oxygen to make water, H_2O.

Meanwhile the path taken by electrons will be carefully supervised. It is called the "electron chain," the links of which operate with familiar molecules known as vitamins much like a hot-potato game. More on this later.

Very tiny chemical steps must be taken to get the most energy out of the food. That is the secret of energy conservation and that is why the Krebs cycle has so many "intermediates" and corresponding links to the electron chain.

Now the pyruvate molecule is completely oxidized to CO_2 and H_2O and a great deal of energy is produced in the form of ATP to be used later; although a tiny bit is let out now for immediate use. The second part of our food metabolism, the Krebs cycle, produces much more energy than the first part, glycolysis. It provides the "lion's share" of our energy.

The primitive part, glycolysis, may date back to the time before the earth had oxygen. Lots of bacteria, such as *Clostridium*, and some lower animals can survive quite well on glycolysis alone. Yeast is another example; when we want it to grow we give it sugar and cover it, to keep out oxygen.

The primitive and advanced parts of food metabolism together are called *respiration*. It is the reason we breath (respire); we must take in the necessary oxygen for the Krebs cycle. Many of the enzymes involved in respiration need to be attached—not loose in the cytoplasm (water portion) of our cells. These stationary enzymes are housed in special factories, the mitochondria, which have many shelf-like surfaces inside for enzyme attachment.

Malonic Acid

When our cells are accidentally fed the respiration inhibitor (poison) **malonic acid**, they mistake it for succinic acid because the molecules are "look-alikes." But, of course, the enzyme that is trying to pull away one of its electrons is rudely surprised.

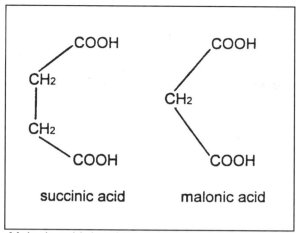

Malonic acid deceives our enzymes who think it
is succinic acid
Fig. 25 Malonate and succinate

The electrons are not in the right place. The Krebs cycle stalls. And because every step is dependent on the previous step the entire chain of metabolism, called respiration, stalls. It was known by 1909 that malonic acid is a severe respiratory inhibitor.[63]

By 1920, Otto Warburg, a scientist in Germany, had invented a new device that could measure how much oxygen was actually used by a bit of living tissue, the "Warburg apparatus". It was fun to measure the oxygen consumption of leaves, seeds, insects, frogs, pieces of different tissues, embryos, young and old tissues, and calculate their respiration rates. But Warburg measured the respiration of a <u>tumor</u> and found it hardly used oxygen at all,[64] that respiration was somehow inhibited! He devoted his scientific career to exploring this phenomenon. <u>Never was it guessed</u> that our tumors—human tumors—actually contained malonic acid! That we were eating it! It could not be guessed because malonic acid was known as an industrial chemical. It would not be logical to suspect it in foods or in the animal body.

---

[63] Webb, J.L., *Enzyme And Metabolic Inhibitors, Vol. II*, Academic Press, 1966, p. 2.
[64] Warburg, O., *The Metabolism of Tumours*, Constable & Co., Ltd., 1930.

After a lifetime of work Warburg finally concluded that **any substance that damaged respiration would cause tumors**; he had proved it many times, in many animals, with many respiratory inhibitors (including urethane, which seeps from plastic teeth). But exceptions could be found, showing there were additional "common denominators" he could not guess at that time. After giving his life to this work, he grew disappointed that damaged respiration was not <u>the one and only</u> cause of tumors. He, too, believed that a single cause must somehow be the only and sufficient cause of tumors. We now know that nothing is that simple in biology. His legacy, the discovery that tumor cells have inadequate respiration, is monumental. His book, *The Metabolism of Tumours*, can be found at university libraries.

When the Krebs cycle is blocked by a respiratory inhibitor, cells are immediately in a crisis, like when computers crash. The cells can still do glycolysis to make energy, but, of course, must do it many times faster than before. Like a car that has slipped out of high gear into first gear, but must still keep up the 55 mph speed—much more fuel will be used for the miles traveled. The tumor cell consumes everything in its vicinity for fuel: the blood sugar drops, blood fat level drops, muscle protein is used up. The patient becomes emaciated. And, in spite of all this activity, there is no energy and little enough body heat.

Numerous other respiratory inhibitors besides malonic acid and urethane were found in the next decades. Exotic things, like antimycin A, made by *Streptomyces griseus*, a most unlikely bacterium as it seemed then! Rotenone was found (a fish poison and now a common pesticide) and maleic acid, another non-biological substance. It could not be guessed—only the Syncrometer technology has revealed—that we are <u>inundated</u> in malonic and maleic acids, urethane, rotenone, and antimycin A, not one, but all of them!

Inundated in malonic acid because it is in our food, besides other sources. We are probably eating much more malonic acid now than we did in the past. Tomatoes are now a year round food. Orange juice is consumed in units of three or four oranges at a time, not one, as would have been the practice long ago.

Perhaps the malonic acid content of foods has even increased due to agricultural practices, such as the use of certain pesticides, time of harvesting, and method of artificial ripening. I have preliminary evidence that <u>organic</u> carrots and broccoli (sold in plastic bags, thereby avoiding spray treatment) do not contain malonic acid, whereas the ordinary varieties do. Nor do oranges grown on your back yard tree. This needs more research.

Scientists studied malonic acid, also called *malonate*, intensely for decades though never suspecting its true significance for humans. A lengthy and excellent review of malonate research has been published in *Enzyme And Metabolic Inhibitors Vol. II* (see previous footnote). Here is a <u>partial</u> list of topics reviewed.

◊ Malonate inhibits uptake of glycine and alanine.
◊ Malonate may chelate iron so it can't be incorporated into hemoglobin.
◊ Malonate inhibits healing.
◊ Motility of sperm is reduced by malonate.
◊ Bacterial phagocytosis by human neutrophils is depressed by malonate.
◊ Malonate chelates calcium.
◊ Malonate drops the resting potential of muscle.
◊ Malonate causes air hunger (dyspnea).
◊ Methyl malonate is toxic to the kidney.
◊ Acetoacetyl Co A can transfer its Co A to malonic acid to make malonyl Co A. This could lead to acetoacetate buildup, namely ketonuria and possibly a block in fat utilization of even numbered carbon atoms, leaving odd numbered carbons to predominate.
◊ Malonic acid reacts with aldehydes.
◊ Thallium is chelated by malonic acid into a stable compound. (This could explain accumulation effect in a tumor.)
◊ A color test for malonates is tetra hydroquinoline-N-propinal to form blue-violet compounds. It is sensitive to 0.01 mg malonate.
◊ Malonate complexes with zinc and magnesium.
◊ A fall in malate concentration due to malonate causes depletion of NADP.

◊ Malonate induces ketonemia.

◊ Malonate reduces oxygen uptake. Coenzyme Q10 is required to make ATP.

◊ Malonate raises cholesterol.

◊ D-malic acid complexes with malic dehydrogenase and NADH, but is enzymatically inactive.

◊ Maleic acid is competitive inhibitor of succinic dehydrogenase.

◊ Synergism between rotenone and malonate occurs in mitochondria.

◊ Malonate causes oxidation of NADH and cytochromes.

◊ Rats can convert malonate to acetate in the presence of malonyl Co A.

◊ Malonate reduces survival of infected animals.

◊ Malonate fed to dogs is recovered as methyl malonate in urine.

◊ Malonate can pick up an amino group from glutamine.

◊ Hemolysis of red blood cells may be caused by malonyl dialdehyde (MDA), a derivative of malonic acid.

◊ Malonate catalyses renal glutaminase; with less glutamine uric acid levels fall.

◊ Malic acid (apple juice) is the best antidote to malonic acid. (But commercial sources contain patulin which depletes cellular glutathione.)

◊ Malonic acid is present in urine.

◊ Malonate depresses the reduction of GSSG to glutathione.

◊ Malonate inhibits protoporphyrin formation 32%.

◊ Malonate inhibits insulin stimulation of muscle respiration.

◊ Malonate inhibits acetylcholine synthesis.

◊ *Mycobacterium phlei* respiration is stimulated by malonate. (All schizophrenia cases I see test positive to this bacterium in the brain!)

◊ Malonate is put into soy sauce in Japan.

◊ Malonate stimulates *Entamoeba histolytica* growth.

◊ Malonate inhibits phosphate entry into cells.

◊ Potassium transport into cells is inhibited by malonate.

◊ Malonate causes systemic acidosis.

◊ Calcium and iron transport by rat duodenum is severely reduced by malonate.

◊ Malonate inhibits pyruvate oxidation.

◊ Malonate causes increased utilization of glucose due to the Pasteur effect of a blocked Krebs cycle.

◊ Lactic acid formation is increased with malonate inhibition of respiration.

◊ Glycolysis is stimulated by malonate.

◊ Malonate has different effects on different tissues.

◊ Much less glucose goes to form amino acids and proteins in the presence of malonate.

◊ Malonate induces the appearance of the pentose phosphate shunt.

◊ Malonate diverts fatty acid metabolism to acetoacetate.

◊ Malonate increases the formation of fatty acids up to 10-fold.

◊ Maleic acid is a potent inhibitor of urinary acidification.

◊ Malonate inhibits oxidation of fatty acids.

◊ Malonate fed to dogs produces acetoacetate, acetone and alcohol.

◊ Malonate can reduce the concentration of magnesium and calcium to 25% or 50%.

◊ The methyl derivative of malonate depresses renal function.

◊ Malonic acid can form malonyl coenzyme A, which is very stable, thereby depleting the system of coenzyme A. (Coenzyme A has a nucleic acid base, adenine, plus pantothenic acid and sulfur in its makeup. You will have an increased need for these nutrients.)

◊ Malonate inhibits urea formation by reducing the supply of oxaloacetate.

◊ Malonate inhibits cell cleavage (the formation of a wall between 2 dividing cells).

◊ Benzaldehyde reacts with malonic acid.

With this much harm coming from malonic acid, why have we not noticed this as we eat malonate-containing food? Shouldn't we drop dead or at least get sick? Perhaps native American Indians <u>did</u> notice and get sick. They considered tomatoes toxic. Perhaps their superior physical condition—enabling them to run ten miles a day!—also enabled them to detect the toxic effect of a food. Perhaps we don't detect it because we are already so debilitated.

105

Obviously, the cancer patient must stop consuming any malonic acid-containing food; it inhibits respiration, the very stuff that Warburg found would cause tumors to grow.

Fortunately, the list of malonate-free foods is much longer than malonate-containing foods. The cancer patient may eat only malonate-free foods.

Malonate-Free Foods

Here is the malonate-free food list; stick to it; do not eat foods that are not listed. The fastest way to recover the health of your sick organ, is to stop poisoning it with malonic acid. You may notice the difference in a few days.

There is an extra benefit for persons who switch to a malonate-free diet. You may notice less sleepiness after eating and a higher body temperature after a few weeks, which brings with it a rosier complexion. This is just what is needed now.

Eat Only These

Remember, that a food may be malonate-free and still not be good for you for other reasons. Remember, too, that this is a plant list, since animals do not make it. But milk from the supermarket (not including goat milk) is an exception; it has traces. Yet, cows' milk (based on 2 samples) directly from the cow did not have malonic acid, either. Nor did several human milk samples. Evidently, malonic acid is part of processing pollution. So dairy foods are listed as safe, but only with special treatment. Your 21 Day Program does not allow any dairy foods, though, not even with treatment.

Acorn squash (with peel)
allspice
almonds (including brown skin)
aloe vera
amaranth
apples (red delicious, golden delicious, green)
apricot kernels
artichokes
avocados
bananas
banana squash (without peel)
bean sprouts
beans, adzuki
beans, pinto
bee pollen
beet tops
beets, red
bell peppers (red, green)
black pepper
black-eyed peas
blueberries
bok choy
brazil nuts
broccoli (organic, in plastic bag)
brewers' yeast
Brussels sprouts
buckwheat
butter (soften, add HCl and vit. C)
butternut squash (without peel)
cabbage (purple, white)
cactus (nopalitos)
cantaloupe (and seeds)
carrots (organic in plastic bag)
capers
cardamom
carob powder
cauliflower
cayenne pepper
chayote squash (with peel)
cheese (melt, add HCl and vit. C)
cherries (Bing)
chili peppers (California, jalapeno, pasilla, serrano, yellow)
chili peppers - red (dried)
cilantro
cinnamon
coconut (without the milk)

collards
corn (yellow & white)
cornmeal
cranberries
cream (add HCl and vitamin C)
cucumbers
cumin
currants
dairy products (add HCl and vit. C)
dandelion (greens)
dill (fresh)
dulse (sea vegetable)
eggplant
eggs
extract of wintergreen
eyebright herb (dried)
fenugreek
figs (dried)
flax seed
flour (unbleached white)
garbanzo beans
garlic cloves
ginger capsules
ginger root (inside only)
goldenseal
grains and legumes from India (see Sources), chana dal, split urad chilka, split moong chilka, whole urad, moth, whole moong USA green with skins, masoor, chori, kabu fee chana, whole val, moong zib, whole moong dal, toor dal, yellow peas, split val, oily toor (the dals are legume-like)
grapefruits (and seeds)
grapes (green, red & purple)
green bean thread
green beans
green olives (in jar)
grits
hazel nuts
Helleborushominy (white canned)
hydrangea root
jicama
kale
Kamut (grain)
kiwi
kumquats

leeks
lemon grass tea
lemons (also sweet lemon)
lentils
lettuce (iceberg, green leaf and red leaf)
lingon berries
loquats
maple flavoring
maple syrup
masala (spice)
millet
mint leaves
miso (sweet)
mullein flowers
macadamia nuts
mushrooms (common white)
nectarines
nutmeg
oats
olive leaves (for tea, see *Sources*)
onions (white, yellow, green)
paprika
parsley
Pau d'Arco
peaches
peanut butter
peanuts (without red skin)
pears (Bartlett, Bosc)
peas (green)
peas (split green)
peas, black-eyed
peas, green (in shell)
peas, snow
peppermint
pimentos
pineapple
plums (red and blue)
pomegranate

potatoes (russet, red, sweet)
psyllium seed husks
pumpkin
pumpkin seeds quassia
quince with seeds
quinoa
radishes (red)
raspberries
rhubarb
rice (white, cooked in pressure cooker)
salsa picante hot sauce
sesame seed
shave grass
soy lecithin
soybean (whole)
spearmint (dried)
spinach
strawberries
sunflower seeds
sweet basil
sweet lemon
Swiss chard
tahini
tapioca (pearl)
thyme
tomatillo turnip greens
Uva Ursi capsules
Viscum album
walnuts
watermelon (ripe inside portion only, excluding seed)
wheat berries, flour
yellow split peas
zucchini squash (yellow, pale green, mottled, with peel)
zucchini squash blossoms

The presence of malonic acid in plants was reported as early as 1925.[65] Yet, it has never been suspected that we are eating it daily in significant amounts! Here are some popular foods that contain it.

---

[65] Turner, W.A. and Hartman, A.M., *J. Amer. Chem. Soc.*, v. 47, 1925, p. 2044.

Foods That Contain Malonic Acid

Be aware that in <u>packaged</u> foods, the processing could contribute the malonic acid. Pesticide absorption by plants could also be responsible.

alfalfa sprouts	limes
apricots	mangos (large, small yellow)
araica (dried)	Nori sea weed, packaged
beans (black, great northern, lima	onions (purple)
mung, navy, red kidney)	oranges, all kinds
black olives (canned)	papaya (Mexican)
broccoli	parsnips
butternut squash peel	passion fruit
carrots	persimmons (Fuji, regular)
chaparral (dried)	radish (Daikon)
chocolate	red skin of peanuts
ginger root skin	Tamari soy sauce
grape jam, commercial	tomatoes
green zucchini (dark)	turnips, rutabaga
Kombo (seaweed)	wheat grass

Why is malonic acid always found in the tumor and not in other organs? Does the tumor attract it the way a rapidly dividing tissue attracts metal or carcinogens? Or does the metal already piled up in the tumor cells attract the malonate because of its chelating nature? Perhaps malonate accumulates in tumor cells simply because it cannot be detoxified there.

I believe there is a normal route for your body to metabolize malonic acid, because when malonic acid-containing foods are eaten, I observe the immediate appearance of *malonyl-Coenzyme A* ("malonyl CoA").

Malonyl CoA has been well studied by scientists and found to be the beginning of fat formation. So my conclusion is that the body can use up <u>some</u> malonic acid by making fat. But most malonyl CoA is produced from other food components besides malonic acid. So this alternate fat-making mechanism that uses up malonic acid seems to me like a "favor" evolution is trying to do for us.

It is not a perfect solution. In the process of making fat with malonate, <u>biotin</u> and <u>coenzyme A</u> are quickly used up, too, so this route doesn't work very long. A tumorous organ never has biotin or coenzyme A in detectable amounts. Its normal ability to metabolize malonic acid is lost, so it must try the next route, detoxification.

Detoxifying Malonate

A popular detoxification method used by the body is to pin a *methyl* group onto the offending molecule. In this case that means:

malonic acid + methyl group ⇨ methyl malonate

But transferring methyl groups requires **vitamin B$_{12}$, folic acid,** and **SAM** (S̲-a̲denosyl m̲ethionine). That uses up the organ's supply of vitamin B$_{12}$ and folic acid, but at least the malonic acid is gone. Of course we must still get rid of the methyl malonate, which is toxic, but that's another story. Another drawback of pinning a methyl group is that it uses up your methyl supply, which means methionine, choline and betaine. This, in turn, depletes other metabolites, including glycine, taurine, cysteine, lecithin, hormones, and neurotransmitters. Keeping SAM supplied also means keeping S (sulfur) and A (adenosyl) supplied, which depends on adenosine triphosphate (A̲TP), which is exactly what is not being made when respiration is inhibited.

The organ under siege is becoming vitamin deficient and malnourished, and so is the rest of your body that is trying to support it by sending more supplies to it.

Your tumorous organ will be free of malonic acid as soon as you dose it with vitamin B$_{12}$, folic acid, methyl groups (methionine, betaine), sulfur (cysteine), and vitamin C. But not the tumor itself. If it has a tough, thick wall around it, these supplements cannot enter, so we must wait for the second week of the 21 Day Program.

Now that we can detoxify malonic acid into methyl malonate, what's next? There are three more steps:

malonic acid ⇨ **methyl malonate** ⇨ **maleic acid**
⇩
D-malic acid ⇦ **maleic anhydride**

Fig. 26 Detoxification route of malonic acid as seen by the Syncrometer

Because these compounds all begin with <u>M</u>, I call them the "M-family." Fortunately just vitamin C is needed to detoxify the remainder.

Tumor cells have lost the ability to do the detoxifying chemistry on their own, but if you supply the ingredients, they can still carry out the detoxification routine.

Couldn't we simply stay on these supplements and not be deprived of the malonate-containing foods? Unfortunately, we would have to stay drenched in supplements, even taking them in the night.

Other Malonic Acid Sources

Once I identified malonic acid as a common denominator in all tumors I searched everywhere for it. First, I found malonic acid to be present wherever a tapeworm stage was located. Then it was found in food. Then I found malonic acid was seeping from the plastic of dental restorations. (All varieties seeped: the composites, ceramics, glass ionomers, and porcelain. Possibly because they all contained some acrylate[66]). Then most recently I learned that acrylic acid that we eat with heated oils gets changed into malonic acid by our metabolism. And a final source was simply as a pollutant. Malonate is so ubiquitous a pollutant, present in processed food, medicines, antiseptics, and body products, it is detected constantly by the Syncrometer.

---

[66] Riihimäki, V., Kivelä-Ikonen, P., Ruuth-Rautalahti, K., Louekari, K. *Acrylic Resins*, Occupational Medicine Third Edition, 1994, ch. 51, p. 754.

As pervasive as malonate is, you may have already removed it all. You have killed tapeworms, removed dental plastic, and are in the process of excluding it from your diet.

Some Expected Benefits

The most surprising benefit from the malonate-free diet and malonate-free mouth is stopping the production of *effusates*. Effusates are caused by seepage of body fluid into places where it does not belong. The lung is a favorite tissue for "water accumulation" of this type, but the abdomen is another common site. Legs, groin, lower abdomen are less common sites.

The actual culprit is <u>maleic anhydride</u> a substance that is formed from malonic acid in your body. It could also be formed from maleic acid trickling from plastic teeth! This may seem to be a small source, but when <u>all</u> of it travels to your tumor, and <u>none</u> gets excreted, it amounts to a great deal of damage, similar to a water drip—just one drop—dripping on your floor day and night, on the same spot.

Maleic anhydride as a cause of tissue edema has been known a very long time, but only when inhaled.[67] It was never guessed that cancer sufferers with effusions actually had this chemical in them. Effusates are life-threatening for a cancer patient. The effusion stops the day after all malonate-related chemicals are gone. Small effusates can often be reabsorbed but large ones must be drained. It may be your last drainage! When an effusate is not drained bacteria find these fluids. And the pressure of this fluid against heart and lungs, against liver and intestine, or against lymph nodes in the groin can produce severe pain and breathlessness. If you "fill up" again, you are still getting malonic acid!

Another surprising benefit of removing all malonate from your body is improved kidney function. Methyl malonate is a serious kidney toxin. Stopping use of malonic acid foods and getting every vestige of plastic out of your mouth can start your

---

[67] *The Merck Index, 10th Ed.*, Merck & Co., Inc., p. 814.

creatinine level (indicative of kidney health) dropping to more normal levels in a few days. *Polycystic* kidneys are greatly benefited. But eating the tiniest bit of an ordinary malonate-containing dairy product (not allowed in this program) can ruin your progress in days! You must have <u>no</u> methyl malonate. Methyl malonate is detoxified with vitamin C.

No amount of the detoxifiers, vitamins B_{12}, C and folic acid could stop effusates from occurring or creatinine levels from rising when malonates were still arriving in the body from any source. We were forced to conclude that detoxifying malonic acid <u>after</u> consuming it did not prevent the damage done by it. It should not be consumed at all.

The supplements needed to detoxify all the malonates in your body are included in the 21 Day Program.

In a few days, with your new malonate-free diet and reinforcing supplements, your tumor cells will no longer have to put up with Krebs cycle blockage. And a daily dose of thyroid will help your mitochondria to divide so fresh young mitochondria are born to handle the improved Krebs cycle activity. They will soon be larger, more numerous, more capable. The tumor cells will begin to do their own work. Soon they will look like neighboring healthy tissue on the scan.

Damaging Dyes

Your anti-tumor (tumor-shrinking) diet should also be free of carcinogenic dyes.

This is as logical as coming out of the rain if you wish to stay dry. Of course, we have believed that our diet <u>is</u> free of cancer-causing dyes, since laws were passed outlawing them decades ago. Actually, the Syncrometer detects the most <u>notorious of all</u> carcinogenic dyes, 4-dimethylaminoazobenzene (**DAB**) in foods as varied as jello, cool-aid, candy, and milk. **Sudan Black B**, **Fast Green**, and **Sudan IV** are also common pollutant dyes. The Syncrometer finds them in many hair dyes, too; dyes penetrate the scalp to load up the body, especially the spleen and body fat. Cheese, butter, cream, which state that annatto seed or riboflavin (natural dyes) have been added, also have traces of these dyes! Not only these, but a host of *azo* dyes, a finding as unbelievable as it is revealing. Azo dyes have a special chemical structure that involves two nitrogen atoms (–N=N–). They have been implicated in cancer induction for decades.[68]

How can this be? Is it the result of an error in identifying it to the manufacturer using other food dyes? Is it the result of cross-contamination? A manufacturer using unsafe dye for some legitimate purpose and safe food dye nearby cannot keep them totally apart? One cannot expect the work force in a factory to understand the issues—the terrible seriousness of keeping them apart—the system must be made fool proof. Or is it due to confusion in naming of dyes? (Both Sudan IV and DAB have over 40 names each![69] Their popular names are "Scarlet Red" and "Butter Yellow.") Could there be a loophole in the legislation banning carcinogenic dyes to be used in food? Have hair dyes completely escaped legislative attention? Why is it legal to use carcinogenic ingredients in them?[70] Just because you are not eating them? With over 20,000,000 people (mostly women) dying their hair in the United States alone, should it not be made safe? Could there be simple negligence, in spite of safeguards such as required testing of each batch of synthetic dye to be used? There is one glaring defect in this "safeguard." The testing done is for the presence of the stated dye, a legitimate one, to make sure it comes up to the percentage (usually 85%) on the label. Testing is not for possible illegal contaminants in the remaining 15%. The components and quality of this remainder is left up to GMP (good manufacturing practice)!

---

[68] Greenstein, J.P., *Biochemistry of Cancer, 2nd Ed.*, Academic Press, NY, 1954, p. 88.

[69] Howard, P.A., Neal, M., *Dictionary of Chemical Names and Synonyms*, Lewis Publishers, 1994, pp. I-144, I-193.

[70] Ames, B.N., Kammen, H.O., Yamasaki, E., *Hair Dyes are Mutagenic: Identification of a Variety of Mutagenic Ingredients*, Proc. Nat. Acad. Sci. USA, v. 72, no. 6, June 1975, pp. 2423-27.

Neither the FDA nor private laboratories do testing for illegal azo dyes.

Certainly, this is a loophole in the regulation of dyed foods. Dyed food should be spot-tested constantly. This would probably uncover the mysterious "transmissible factor" that pollutes nearly all (over 90%) of the processed food in the U.S. marketplace.

Sudan IV

The dye industry of Germany was an early industrial development—already thriving in the 1880s. During WWI, surgeons used Sudan IV to rub into soldiers' wounds because it had been seen to speed wound-healing. Soon these boys grew tumors from within and around the wound site. It did not take long to make the connection. Use of Sudan IV to heal wounds was stopped by the war's end. It was a cruel hoax to perpetrate on young war heroes and their families, but incredibly, researchers are still experimenting with its use![71]

Just how carcinogenic is Sudan IV? The Syncrometer detects it as soon as you have eaten dyed food, in the lung, tongue, salivary glands, esophagus and stomach. It is also seen in the bone marrow, liver and spleen. The next day, Sudan IV lines the whole intestinal tract including the colon, and is present in adrenals and kidneys, too. It is not easily detoxified by your body and therefore, cannot be quickly eliminated. It accumulates in the body's fat—both organ fat and skin fat.

Scientists had done the necessary research on Sudan IV and many other carcinogenic dyes by the 1960s. They had taken the molecule apart. The left hand portion of the molecule is responsible for the carcinogenic action. By itself, this portion is called o-aminoazotoluene or **AAT**, not easy to recognize or pronounce. It forms the heart of numerous azo dyes. When a single dose of AAT is given to mice or rats, it combines with both

---

[71] Tan, S.T., Robers, R.H., Blake, G.B, *Comparing DuoDERM E^R With Scarlet Red In The Treatment Of Split Skin Graft Donor Sites*, British Jour. Of Plastic Surgery, v. 46, 1993, pp. 79-81. (Scarlet red is Sudan IV.)

DNA and RNA and stays stuck for 84 days.[72] It produces mainly tumors of the liver, gallbladder, lung, and urinary bladder (particularly papillomas here). A single dose causes cancer in newborn mice.[73] Most azo dyes were taken out of the food market because of their carcinogenicity but now are present everywhere in trace amounts, detected by the Syncrometer.

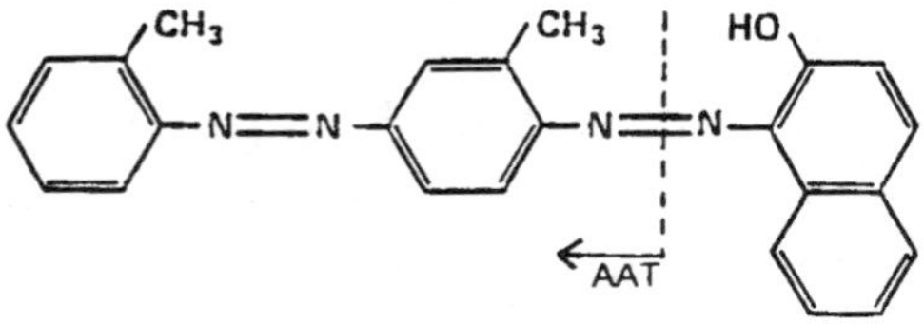

Fig. 27 AAT in Sudan IV

A Little DAB Can Do You In

p-dimethylaminoazobenzene (**DAB**) is even more carcinogenic than Sudan IV or AAT. One researcher stated "For efficient tumor induction DAB has generally been fed to rats in the diet at a level of about 0.06%..."[74] This led to as much as 100% tumor induction in as little as six months!

At one time it was allowed as a butter colorant, hence its popular name Butter Yellow. I find every patient blood test that shows an elevated alkaline phosphatase has an accumulation of DAB in the vital organs and in their fat reservoir.

---

72 Lawson, T.A., *The Effect of Prolonged Feeding of Ortho-Aminoazotoluene on Binding To Cellular Constituents in Mouse Liver*, Chem-biol. Interact., v. 2, 1970, pp. 9-16.

73 *Some aromatic azo compounds,* IARC Monographs, v. 8, 1974, p. 66.

74 Greenstein, J.P., Haddow, A., eds., *Advances In Cancer Research v I*, Academic Press Inc., 1953. Miller, J.A., Miller, E.C., *The Carcinogenic Aminoazo Dyes*, p. 342.

Sudan Black B

Sudan Black B accumulates in any organ, penetrating the nucleus of many cells, making it the most difficult of dyes to remove. It has three azo portions in the molecule, making it the most difficult of dyes to detoxify, too. While it is concentrated inside the tumor, it slowly leaks out, being taken up by the liver and other vital organs. It causes part of the LDH rise so commonly seen in advanced cancer patients. Did Sudan Black B cause a mutation that overproduces LDH or lactic acid? LDH and alkaline phosphatase are often seen to be linked on the blood test. The dyes, Sudan Black B and DAB, are both present when both enzymes are elevated. When only one test is elevated, only one dye is found present.

It requires large doses of coenzyme Q10, vitamin B_2 and glutathione (this is part of the 21 Day Program) to detoxify our azo dye collection. When we track carcinogenic dyes with the Syncrometer, we see them appear in the kidneys and bladder afterward. It still takes a special effort to dislodge them here.

Hair dye and food dye are considered to be far apart in terms of danger to the body by our government agencies. It is assumed that the hair, being external to the body, does not transmit its dye or other chemicals to the body. Nothing could be further from the truth. Hair dye is immediately absorbed by the scalp and remains there in a large reservoir to be slowly absorbed for six weeks! By then, a new batch of dye is applied. For this reason, hair dye should be non-carcinogenic and easily excreted by the body. If you have used hair dye you must begin to detoxify it and use only all-herbal dye in the future (see *Sources*).

Additional note: never, never get your skin tattooed. Long ago, when vegetable dyes were used, it may have been safe. But now, tattoos seep synthetic dye at a steady rate.

Fast Green FCF

Fast Green FCF is also known as Food Green 3. It is not an azo dye, it is a legal food color. I find fruits and vegetables that are dyed to give them extra appeal in the supermarket are saturated with Fast Green. Even eggplants and bananas are "colored", suggesting a combination of pesticide and dye was used. Fast Green brings with it the lanthanide metals (thulium, gadolinium, lanthanum, etc.). Both dye and lanthanides are very tightly stuck to the food. Two hot water washes are needed to clean the surface enough to risk cutting the fruit. Remember, wherever the lanthanides arrive in your body, immunity is immediately dropped. This allows parasite eggs to survive, as well as *Streptococcus* bacteria, the pain causers. If you can not get pain relief, it would be wise to avoid all fruits and vegetables for a few days, except watermelon, cantaloupe, honeydew melons, and the thick-skinned squashes or pumpkin.

The lanthanides polluting this dye could be the way children initiate cancers even when they do not have tooth fillings.

More Dastardly Dye Deeds

The Syncrometer detects a major disturbance in vitamin A metabolism in whatever organ Sudan IV and the other azo dyes are found. The bone marrow is particularly affected. We have genes for vitamin A receptors and binding proteins. A mutation at these genes could result from a translocation similar to "The Philadelphia Chromosome," characteristic of leukemia, a bone marrow cancer. At the bone marrow the Syncrometer detects abnormal vitamin A products like 13-cis-retinoic acid instead of the normal 9-cis. While at the bladder 9-cis is present but 13-cis is normal for this organ. Such exchanges could result from mutations induced by dyes. Meanwhile, the proper vitamin A members, like *all-t-retinoic acid* and the retinoic acid receptor *RARα*, are missing, as is *retinol binding protein*.

These vitamin A members are probably important in the growth regulation for which vitamin A is known. This could also explain why vitamin A, given to cancer patients, was found to inhibit tumor formation many times in the past. Here are just five examples from the research literature:

- Antitumor Action of Vitamin A in Mice Inoculated With Adenocarcinoma Cells[75]
- Concentration-dependent effects of 9-*cis* retinoic acid on neuroblastoma differentiation and proliferation in vitro[76]
- An Inhibitory Effect of Vitamin A on the Induction of Tumors of Forestomach and Cervix in the Syrian Hamster by Carcinogenic Polycyclic Hydrocarbons[77]
- Inhibition of the Growth and Development of a Transplantable Murine Melanoma by Vitamin A[78]
- Prevention of chemical carcinogenesis by vitamin A and its synthetic analogs (retinoids)[79]

Azo dyes are responsible for missing oxidizers![80] Remember that azo dyes are also responsible for an elevated alkaline phosphatase[81] and LDH on the blood tests. If yours are elevated, let this galvanize you into action. These dyes accidentally contaminate the safe dyes: annatto seed and riboflavin. Avoid <u>all</u> dyes. Children consume more dairy products, jello, and cool-aid than older persons. Is this why leukemia is commonly seen in children? (Seventy-five percent of all leukemia is in children.) Do children get more azo dyes, causing more vitamin A mutations, causing more leukemia?

Avoiding dyes will not pose a new restriction on your diet. It was already restricted to unprocessed (undyed) food. Now you must pay closer attention to natural food to be sure it has not been dyed. Which dye is used is irrelevant, since it is nearly all contaminated with Sudan IV, Sudan Black, DAB, and other azo dyes as detected by the Syncrometer. By avoiding all dairy products besides processed foods and washing natural foods

[75] Rettura, G., et. al., *Jour. Nat. Cancer Inst.*, v. 54, no. 6, June 1975, pp. 1489-91.

[76] Lovat, P.E., et. al., *Neuroscience Letters*, v. 182, 1994, pp. 29-32.

[77] Chu, E.W., Malmgren, R.A., *Cancer Res.*, v. 25 (6), pt. 1, pp. 884-95.

[78] Felix, E.L., et. al., *Science*, v. 189, Sep. 12, 1975, pp. 886-87.

[79] Sporn, M.B., et. al., *Federation Proceedings*, v. 35, no. 6, May 1976, pp. 1332-38.

[80] Greenstein, J.P., Haddow, A., eds., *Advances In Cancer Research v I*, Academic Press Inc., 1953. Miller, J.A., Miller, E.C., *The Carcinogenic Aminoazo Dyes*, p. 378.

[81] Woodward, H.Q., *The Glycerophosphatases of the Rat Liver Cancer Produced by Feeding* p-Dimethylaminoazobenzene, Cancer Research, v. 3, 1943, pp. 159-63.

twice in hot water, this risk from carcinogenic dyes will be gone. This is the main reason for removing dairy products from the diet during the 21 Day Program. After your tumors are gone and health has returned, you can begin to detoxify food dyes by adding vitamin B_2 to the food itself.

Don't Eat Carcinogenic Metals

Even though our bodies need copper, cobalt, germanium and perhaps even vanadium, it is needed in <u>organic</u> form. The inorganic form is toxic. The toxicity is subtle. It builds up slowly. Certainly, the body has detoxification mechanisms, but these use up your glutathione and precious metabolites. As you age, we have less ability to detoxify.

Although the body can often make the organic form out of inorganic metal that you eat, this does not justify eating it. Eat only the organic forms of germanium (aloe, garlic, hydrangea root), chromium (thyme, chromium-yeast). Ultratrace minerals can be found in fish, eggs and whole seeds.

- Cook in glass or ceramic pots, not stainless steel, which releases chromium and nickel, two of the most carcinogenic metals.
- Change copper or galvanized (source of cadmium) water pipes to PVC plastic. Perhaps the practice of grounding the house electricity is partly to blame for so much corrosion.
- Change glasses frames to plastic.
- Switch to non-metal jewelry. Wear no metal that touches the skin. (For solid jade rings, see *Sources*.)
- Use no metal tooth repairs

No Isopropyl Alcohol or Benzene

The FDA requires, and rightly so, that processed food, extracts, supplements, in fact everything that is put into a bottle or a package, must be essentially free of bacteria. This is very difficult to achieve, since even dust carries bacteria and fungal spores. Even plain water develops bacteria in a bottle. A manufacturer is very tempted to overdo the antiseptic, for your protection and their legal protection. The antiseptics used are not required to be disclosed. Nor is rinsing or drying required. In fact, what is required is a thorough drenching of bins without rinsing or drying.[82]

The cancer patient must have no isopropyl alcohol which is the most common antiseptic. For this supremely compelling reason the cancer patient must not eat bottled, canned, or packaged food (with a few exceptions as noted in this book).

Benzene comes into the food supply in huge amounts. It is part of petroleum residue. Wherever pesticide is used, the Syncrometer detects benzene. Although the pesticide has a specific chemical that is the active ingredient, this is usually just a few percent. The bulk of the pesticide is a petroleum-derived "vehicle" or base. This is the source of the benzene. Over half of all the greens (lettuce, spinach, parsley) on supermarket shelves that I tested were positive for benzene, implicating pesticide. Organic produce was only slightly better, testing negative only if in its original plastic package.

That is why I do not emphasize greens in the diet. It is sad for the vegetarian especially, and those health-minded individuals who promote juice-making, raw vegetables, and a natural diet. And for the cancer victim.

Although I have found an antidote to benzene, vitamin B_2, effective both in your body and outside it, this is far from satisfactory. The toxic compounds formed (phenol and others) have not been studied. How to detoxify all your foods is given in *Food Rules*.

---

[82] Block, S.S., *Disinfection Sterilization & Preservation*, 1983. p. 838. Discusses FDA regulations and their interpretation to the food handler.

Even after avoiding benzene to the best of your ability, detoxifying food with B_2 is essential for the cancer patient.

Don't Eat Asbestos

We are familiar with airborne asbestos, and the whole nation has made great efforts to remove it from our buildings. But this source of exposure is minor compared to the huge amounts we are eating daily! The Syncrometer detects it on apples, plums, pears, rolled oats, rice, and many other foods. It can be washed off some foods, but not off others. There are large amounts in sugar, which explains its presence in all sweetened foods. It can be filtered out of a light syrup made from sugar, using a coffee filter. Coffee, too, is contaminated with asbestos but can be cleared by filtering. What these foods have in common is rolling along conveyor belts. I suspect many conveyor belts, especially old ones, contain asbestos. Avoiding asbestos and learning to remove it are part of the instructions given in *Food Rules*.

Asbestos does special harm to us. Our white blood cells quickly eat it up themselves to protect our vital organs. But once the white blood cells are filled up, their lysosomes are speared and damaged, letting out their ferritin and the iron metal contained within. Ferritin reaches the surface somehow, where it coats the white blood cell all over the outside, covering up its precious receptor sites. Now it no longer recognizes bacteria, viruses, toxins or even its friendly neighbors. It can't even unload its toxic cargo to get it on its way for excretion. The immunity in this tissue (our white blood cells) is fatally reduced.

And even after the asbestos is removed from the tissues, by restoring immunity, the cells are left with the remains: a large pile of useless oxidized iron, the "ferric" form. It will take gigantic amounts of vitamin C to reduce it and remove it.

Unsaturated Fat Risks

Acrylic acid is a small bit of unsaturated fat. It is also a bit of polymer prepared by industry. Unsaturated fats have several double bonds in their molecular structure. We have been told they are good for us nutritionally. Consequently, we have been frying our foods in corn oil, canola oil, safflower and a host of new oils, instead of the old fashioned butter, lard, chicken fat and olive oil. We were not told that heat can disintegrate the unsaturated oils, leaving bits of acrylic acid that our bodies do not digest but instead escape from the intestine to enter our tissues and disturb DNA production.

In fact, the corn oil, canola oil, cottonseed oil on the grocery shelves, even <u>before</u> they are used to fry, contained acrylate molecules, according to the Syncrometer. This included the "cold pressed" varieties. Only olive oil and coconut oil, both fairly saturated, did not. Frying food to near-blackness with butter, lard, olive oil or coconut oil did <u>not</u> produce acrylates either. But microwaving coconut oil <u>did</u>, whereas microwaving did not make acrylate out of butter, lard or olive oil.

The more unsaturated the oil, the more easily it is broken up into acrylate bits, it seems.

Acrylic acid is detoxified in the body by adding methyl groups. The Syncrometer detects <u>methylmethacrylate</u> (the same as your denture plastic!) at the same locations as acrylic acid is found. Some acrylic acid is metabolized to malonic acid! Acrylates are dangerous molecules. Even the *IARC* concluded there is "<u>sufficient</u>" evidence for the carcinogenicity of ethylacrylate (similar to methacrylate) in animals.

Quick and easy Rules for baking and frying without making acrylic acid are given in *Food Rules*.

Don't Eat Moldy Food

Moldy food pervades the normal diet in "civilized" countries. As any food is stored, mold invades because mold spores are everywhere. After food is dried, pickled, spiced, smoked or treated with chemicals, any moldy flavor is covered.

We have seen how easily the advanced cancer patient is overwhelmed by a few bacteria in dairy foods or raw foods. We must prevent fungus invasion, too. Fungus growth is always seen at a tumor site. Fungus makes very toxic *mycotoxins* right there on site. The three I have studied are *aflatoxin, patulin*, and *zearalenone*.

Aflatoxin is a powerful mutagen, very much studied by scientists. It is present on nuts and grains. By baking your own bread and avoiding all nuts (except coconut), you can avoid it. Soaking nuts or grains in Dental Bleach or HCl detoxifies it and it may then be rinsed off.

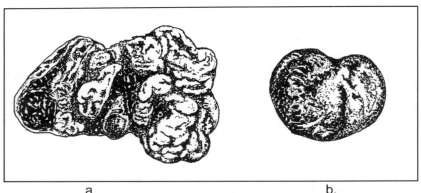

a.   b.
(a) Enlarged tumor-filled liver of rats fed aflatoxin. (Drawn from photo[83].) (b) The liver returns toward normal after giving glutathione (100mg/day). But this is equivalent to 25 gm/day for a human!
Fig. 28 Glutathione combats aflatoxin liver damage

If your blood test shows that the total bilirubin is at the top of its range, you are already suffering some aflatoxin damage to the liver. White bread fresh from a bakery never had aflatoxin in my tests. (But the bottom of loaves from a bakery must now be trimmed ¼ inch [½ cm] to get rid of synthetic, petroleum-based grease with silicone [!] used to coat the bread pan). Aflatoxin is

---

83 Novi, A.M., *Regression of Aflatoxin B1-Induced Hepatocellular Carcinomas by Reduced Glutathione*, Science, v. 212, May 1981, pp. 541-42.

not removed by boiling, or preserving. Peanuts are the most notorious aflatoxin carriers. Eat no nuts of any kind until you are well. There is one exception, the recipe for Almond Milk.

Patulin is present on any bruised fruit, and in fruit juice made from such fruit. Make your own juice; peel your fruit so all bruises are easily seen and removed. Patulin is also a carcinogen.[84] It is detoxified by cysteine.[85],[86] I also find that rinsing in hydrochloric acid water removes it.

Zearalenone is the mycotoxin that is associated with benzene in our bodies. In fact zearalenone is detoxified into benzene in our body fat.[87] Benzene is a pervasive immune lowering agent.

Zearalenone, itself, is estrogen-like. This means that our society has been exposed to two powerful new estrogens in the past half century: zearalenone from extra-moldy foods and bisphenol-A in plastic tooth replacements. Surely this could cause sexual dysfunction of various kinds for both men and women. And a furtherance of cancers of the breast, ovaries, uterus, and prostate. Zearalenone is plentiful in Russet potatoes, potato chips, brown rice and popcorn. Immersion in hydrochloric acid-water (not for potatoes or chips) detoxifies it.

Help From The Health Department

We should be able to trust the food we purchase to be free of truly harmful bacteria and parasite eggs. We should not expect it to be sterile—only reasonably free of filth.

---

84 Hatey, F., Moule, Y., *Protein Synthesis Inhibition in Rat Liver by the Mycotoxin Patulin*, Toxicology, v. 13, 1979, pp. 223-31.

85 Von Wright, A., Lindroth, S., *Lack of Mutagenic Properties of Patulin and Patulin Adducts Formed with Cysteine in Salmonella Test Systems*, Mutat. Res., v. 58, 1978, pp. 211-15.

86 Dickens, F., Cooke, J., *Rates of Hydrolysis and Interaction with Cysteine of some Carcinogenic Lactones and Related Substances*.

87 Clark, H.R., *Syncrometer Biochemistry Laboratory Manual*, New Century Press, 1999.

Until now our health department standards have served us well. But now that immunity is lowered for large fractions of the population: cancer patients, HIV/AID patients, environmentally ill persons, our standards of sanitation need to be raised. There should be fewer cockroach parts in cocoa and chocolate, less patulin in apple juice, less aflatoxin in peanut butter, and tougher requirements in restaurants.

Most of all, milk should be sterilized, not just pasteurized. A few salmonella and E. coli bacteria do not make a healthy person sick, not in glass after glass. And swallowing tapeworm eggs, which will never mature into a tapeworm (only into a very small "bladder cyst" larva) has never been seen to cause anything. Nobody drops dead or even gets sick. Yet here is the mysterious beginning of our tumors. Perhaps they will stay benign and never become aggressive. But without them, we would not even have to think about it.

Kosher is cleaner. Milk, cheese and butter purchased at Kosher grocery stores usually did not have tapeworm eggs, *Ascaris* eggs, Rabbit fluke, or filth-bacteria. Nor were they sterilized! Evidently, cleanliness is possible in the dairy industry. Amish-made products were similarly much safer. Yet, the cancer patient can not take chances. When dairy foods are finally allowed in your program, they must still be sterilized.

We can, of course, sterilize all our milk ourselves—and must do so. But if it were done as part of the regular sanitation procedure for milk, we would automatically have safe cheese, ice cream, yogurt, etc. Presently these are all slightly contaminated with parasites, bacteria, and carcinogenic dyes, and off limits to the cancer sufferer.

The Health Department should increase compliance in restaurants. We should feel secure that gloves were used to handle food. And hands washed after bathroom use. The security system should include an electronic message if the sink is not used between door openings. Better yet, the Health Department should develop and require testing sticks for *Salmonella* and *E. coli* for restaurant use.

Best is to choose homemade food. If you must eat in a restaurant you must take extra precautions. After your food arrives, pile it all on one plate and ask to have it heated in the microwave uncovered for three more minutes. Also dot it with 15 drops of hydrochloric acid, mixing as well as possible. Accompany with a beverage that has another three drops hydrochloric acid added. Do not eat raw salads unless you can dunk them in Lugol's while dining. Take Lugol's iodine drops with you when eating out. Put 1 drop in a glass of water to sterilize raw food during the meal. (This advice is only for cancer patients, and only in restaurants, until they are well. Others would risk oxidizing too many food elements.)

Whenever one of our patients became bloated or gassy, we routinely identified the bacteria that were eaten. Then we located the source. It wasn't the dust in their room, their water, their fingers, nor was it a "bug that was going around." It came from the food they had recently eaten! Most of our patients' "mysterious" setbacks, like headaches, fever, abdominal pain, nausea, diarrhea, and pain in general turned out to be caused by food bacteria. So don't be too discouraged if you suffer a setback. Before you blame it on the cancer, go through the bacteria-killing recipe (see page 141); stop eating suspect food and throw out those leftovers!

Can The Government Protect Us?

Certainly the United States Government tries. An independent group of chemists was formed about 1969: the International Agency for Research on Cancer (IARC) Working Group on the Evaluation of the Carcinogenic Risk of Chemicals to Man. They have met regularly. They have assessed chemical risks in great detail, establishing criteria in the best scientific manner. But are these criteria the best for you?

For instance, suppose you are the Food And Drug Administration (FDA) and "The Big Corporation" wants you to allow their new additive, <u>saccharin,</u> in food. It's a miracle substance, says The Big Corporation, a substance that sweetens without calories! Millions of people will benefit! So being a conscientious FDA policy maker, you diligently check the IARC Evaluations and find that saccharin is classified in "Group 2B." This means that it is "possibly carcinogenic to humans."[88] So impartial scientists have <u>no proof saccharin is carcinogenic,</u> points out The Big Corporation, so it wouldn't be legal for you to deny approval. As an FDA official, you decide the "fair" decision is to allow saccharin to be used (as actually occurred). But as the parent of a six month old baby, would you let her eat food sweetened with saccharin?

Agencies and committees like the FDA, IARC, and others, can be expected to be very, very conservative; certainly not biased against any particular chemical. But where safety is the issue, an evaluation committee <u>should</u> be biased (in favor of safety). This bias would change the language used by the committee. For instance, an unbiased committee would consider carbon tetrachloride as <u>possibly</u> carcinogenic (because <u>not enough</u> human experiments were done, although animal experiments definitely showed cancer induction[89]) whereas the safety-biased committee would consider it <u>probably</u> or <u>undoubtedly</u> carcinogenic (because <u>some</u> human experiments were done and these showed cancer induction besides the results from animals).

I think the IARC working group has failed. Despite their distinguished personnel, they have made a classification system that confuses and demoralizes the public that relies upon it. Their Group 1 category, which lists agents that "are carcinogenic to humans," has both benzene (indisputably carcinogenic) and nickel (used in our coinage and stainless steel cookware and

---

88 *IARC Monographs on the Evaluation of Carcinogenic Risks to Humans, volumes 1 to 42, Supplement 7*, World Health Organization, 1987, p. 43.

89 Ibid., pp. 32, 43.

tooth fillings).[90] It contains mineral oil, which is legally allowed in food! And estrogen replacement therapy, prescribed to millions of women! How can a lawmaker trust such a list? I am suggesting that **lay people** (excluding all professionals) staff committees and set their <u>own</u> standards. Devise categories that make sense. Advise lawmakers what they feel comfortable letting their children eat. We might never see saccharin, azo dyes, mineral oil and lots of other chemicals even near our food and body products again.

Although finding what is carcinogenic for people is important for all of society, finding what carcinogens are in <u>your</u> tumors is most important to <u>you</u>. If you have a tumor removed, ask the surgeon to give it to you, it's yours, after all. If this is not allowed, agree to fill out the necessary paperwork to make it legal. It should be given to you, not as a biopsy slide, but as a specimen, preserved and safe for anyone to handle. New labs are springing up with the capability of testing for toxins. Find laboratories willing to analyze it for copper, cobalt, vanadium, lanthanum, gadolinium, thulium, asbestos, benzene, silicone, zearalenone, patulin, aflatoxin and azo dyes. After finding some of these common denominators in your tumor, search for them in your foods, dental fillings (those you saved!) and environment, using the same lab. Laboratory costs are about $30.00 to $50.00 per test. Eliminate the culprits permanently from your life.

With your new expertise in toxins and where they come from, <u>you</u> will be more qualified to sit on a standards committee than most people, even scientists!

---

[90] Ibid., pp. 40-41.

Now you are eating <u>safe</u> food!

- There is no malonic acid in it because you shop from the "good" list.
- There are no azo dyes contaminating it because you check the label for <u>all</u> dyes, and are not eating dairy products, for now.
- There is no asbestos or mold or Fast Green dye because you wash and peel fruits and vegetables carefully. There are no parasite eggs because all food is sterilized.
- There are no solvents because you don't buy canned or processed food (except occasional Kosher varieties), or waxed produce.

You look forward to mealtime because it reminds you of how your grandmother cooked!

Safe Surroundings

Your own home brought you cancer! Any place else will be safer. The easiest and fastest way to make a complete environment change is to <u>leave home</u>.

The pets brought you *Ascaris* worms; *Ascaris* eggs are in the carpet. The carpet must be sterilized, or removed. The bedroom carpet is most important, because you breathe the polluted dust for one third of the time! Throw rugs and bed blankets can be dry cleaned. Laundering does not kill *Ascaris* eggs. If pets have been on the bed, throw away the mattress.

The water pipes brought you copper. The refrigerator brought you freon. Freon is known to enhance the mutagenic action of PAHs.[91] New furniture and bedding brought you formaldehyde. The laundry room, besides food, brought you asbestos. Gas fixtures, besides plastic teeth, brought you vanadium. Concern for ants and roaches brought you arsenic-containing pesticides.

If you are the caregiver, take your precious patient anywhere but home. Even a hospital is safer, if it weren't for the treatments given.

Find a motel with plastic water pipes, ask for a non-smoking room and move in for one month. If you are better after one month, stay another month. Stay until your toxic home has been cleaned up. Choose a ground floor room for convenience. Heaters must be electric. Do not use the air conditioner. Sit outside as much as weather allows. Remove the linens and bring your own borax-washed replacements or immediately take motel linens out to launder in borax and bleach. Rent a small, non-freon refrigerator for your room, available at office supply stores. Bring home-cooked food to the motel. Take copper-free water from the motel to do cooking. The motel is your temporary spa. If friends and family do the shopping, you can do the cooking.

---

[91]Mahurin, R.G., Bernstein, R.L., *Fluorocarbon-enhanced Mutagenesis of Polyaromatic Hydrocarbons*, Environ. Res., v. 45, no. 1, 1988, pp. 101-07.

Do not accept offers of cooked or prepared food. You must see the food being sterilized and know what is in it. Only a weight gain is a sure sign of success with cancer. Until you have gained ten pounds you cannot be sure that you are on the road to health. Weight gain is the mysterious indicator that all is well with the body. Use scales twice a week. (If you are overweight, consider yourself lucky—do not lose a single pound.)

When searching for the safest haven, also emphasize linoleum floors, no gas heaters, no wall paper or paneling, no refrigerator (except your new one), and no recent paint (fumes have vanadium). Do your own housekeeping with borax. Dusting with plain water. Bathroom fixtures are sterilized with ethyl alcohol (the 750 ml or 1 liter size bottle only). The toilet is sterilized with regular bleach by someone else while you are out of the room. No pesticide is used. Arrange this with the motel beforehand.

No visitors may smoke. And no pets may visit. Keep extra warm: wear socks, long pants, long sleeves, and turtleneck top until your body temperature is normal, above 98.5. Take your temperature in the morning, upon waking, several times a week. Take showers and shampoos at bedtime to conserve body heat.

Your home should be made ready while you are in the motel "spa." It should be completely overhauled.

- Bedroom carpet pulled up, floor cleaned, throw rugs purchased (washed first). Don't put down a fresh coat of paint or polyurethane.
- Pets given away.
- Plastic water pipe run to the kitchen, bathroom, laundry facility. (A temporary line can be hooked up at an exterior valve). You may check into plastic-coating of metal pipes (*Sources*).
- No hair dryers used.
- Clothes dryer covered with large plastic bag to put it out of use. Use a Laundromat.
- Refrigerator changed to non-freon variety.
- Gas appliances changed to electric.

- Dishwasher and laundry routines changed to borax and white vinegar.
- Chemicals removed from bedroom, basement and kitchen.
- All body care items replaced with homemade substitutes. (See *Recipes*.)
- Read *The Cure For All Cancers* for more suggestions.

If all this seems needless and excessive to your family, you must stay at the safe motel. But if your family did the job so you can return home, give them a big hug and thank you!

Personal Products

Although they are not part of your home, clothing and body products are part of your surroundings, too. They will be sources for cancer-specific toxins until you correct them.

All clothing, even whites, have dyes stuck to them that are eagerly absorbed by your body. Washing them in borax removes most dyes, but not DAB or Sudan Black B. These are the very toxins that spell ultimate doom for the cancer patient by raising alkaline phosphatase, and LDH. Clothing constantly rubs these two toxins into our skin, day and night. Our skin fat absorbs them. The liver, in its constant vigilance over toxins, pulls them inward for detoxification in its microsomes. When it can't keep up with the barrage from food, hair dye, and clothing, they begin to accumulate in other organs, causing more and more mutations.

Chlorine bleach, even though it is itself polluted with these dyes, can remove them from your clothing.

As soon as you read this, wash all your clothing, including wig, turbans, hats, shoes, jackets, bedding, and towels. Use ½ cup bleach per washer-load of whites, like sheets, jackets, underwear, socks, shoes, scarves, outerwear. Everything else, like colored clothing, silk, leather, rayon, can be given ¼ cup bleach per cold washer-load. Don't mix white and colored items.

Leather goods should be removed after five minutes bleaching, rinsed and dried by stuffing with paper to avoid shrinking.

Your own hair, if dyed, can be detoxified with dental bleach, applied to the dry hair for 5 minutes. Then rinse out. Wigs can be similarly treated.

Now that you have clean, safe food, air, water, bedding, clothes, and body products, you may rest briefly. Your achievement is great. If you are now in less pain or feel better, your reward is already there.

So far, all your efforts have gone into **removing** things, not **taking** things. Because **removing** things gives back your body its lost immunity and missing metabolism. **Taking** things only covers up the problem, like adding more and more fuel to a furnace that has no draft and is broken. Vitamins, herbs, medicines, and chemotherapy all belong to the category of **things to take**. They are not totally useless. But if your goal is regaining your full life-expectancy (not just 5 years) you must **remove** harmful things first and **take** things second.

We will next discuss supplements, but in my discussion notice the difference between those that are given to **remove** things and those that represent **taking** things.

Supplements

I hope you have already started the 21 Day Program. You may have noticed that the first thing we do is kill parasites so they can not take advantage of the nutritional supplements that follow. Parasites are dead in hours and it is now safe, and necessary, to feed the recovering body tissues. I have not done many experiments where we fed large amounts of supplements <u>before</u> killing parasites and bacteria. But feeding the "bad guys" may explain why the research literature has conflicting results on the benefits of giving vitamins to cancer patients. Our instructions are safe.

Here is the comprehensive list of supplements, most of which you will use. No others should be used since purity from pollutants and antiseptic is a life-and-death issue now. Corporations selling supplements cannot vouch for, nor even identify the antiseptics used in their own products. Nor colorants, fillers, pump sterilizers, valve lubricants, moisture absorbers, capsule sealers, release agents, etc. Each of these leaves a trace behind, in the finished product. We are accustomed to thinking that a trace is "negligible." But even ultra-traces are not negligible when they are uranium, Sudan Black B or thulium! The Syncrometer detects them in crucial organs of sick people, so they could <u>not</u> be negligible. For this reason, untested supplements are off-limits to cancer patients. You could, of course, have your supplements tested by a testing lab (see *Sources*).

Not all of these supplements are available in all countries. Where possible, I have given alternatives.

Supplement List

Sulfur-Supplying Compounds (remove heavy metals)

- glutathione
- methionine
- cysteine
- pantothenic acid (as calcium pantothenate)
- taurine
- vitamin B_1
- thioctic acid

Urea Synthesis Cycle Expanders (remove ammonia)

- ornithine
- arginine

Respiration Supporters

- thyroid
- niacin
- niacinamide
- thioctic acid
- biotin
- vitamin B_2
- coenzyme Q10
- potassium gluconate

Oxidizers (remove bacterial and industrial toxins)

- inositol
- Lugol's iodine solution
- rhodizonate, sodium or potassium (in Mexico)
- benzoquinone (clinical treatment only)
- ozonated oil
- ozonated water
- iron (ferrous gluconate)

Reducers (remove toxins)

- cysteine
- vitamin C (L-ascorbic acid, only)
- glutathione

Enzyme Cofactors (repair metabolism)

- vitamin A and beta carotene
- vitamin B_1
- vitamin B_2
- vitamin B_{12} and folic acid
- vitamin B_6

Methyl Group Donors (repair metabolism)

- methionine
- betaine hydrochloride (remove *Clostridium*)
- glycine

Major Minerals (repair metabolism)

- calcium (as powdered calcium carbonate)
- magnesium (as powdered magnesium oxide)
- potassium (as potassium gluconate)

Trace Minerals (repair metabolism)

- boron
- manganese (only as yeast complex)
- selenium (as sodium selenite and coconut)
- germanium (only herbal forms)

Detoxifiers (remove harmful chemicals)

- glutathione (reduced)
- glycine
- L-cysteine
- D-glucuronic acid
- L-ascorbic acid (vitamin C)
- taurine
- vitamin B_2
- coenzyme Q10
- magnesium
- dimethysulfoxide (DMSO)

RNAse Inhibitors (remove RNAse)

- coconut oil
- chicken broth
- shark cartilage
- raw red beets

Immune Stimulants (remove immune blocks)

- hydrangea root
- a very weak magnet
- methyl sulfonyl methane (MSM)
- papain
- bromelain

Tumor Digesters

- pancreatin
- prepared horseradish (peroxidase and catalase)
- lipase

Miscellaneous

- essential amino acids
- non-essential amino acids
- high strength magnet
- oregano oil
- wintergreen oil, crude (not distilled or synthetic)
- hydrochloric acid
- inositol phosphate
- EDTA
- vitamin D_3

The supplements are numerous and the tumor-ridden body has no appetite for even the best of <u>real</u> food, let alone supplements. But you must find a way to conquer your own resistance: it is essential for survival. Although many of the supplements are available as injectables, bypassing the need to eat them, this is not advised. Intravenous solutions and injectables are often contaminated with bacteria or polluted with solvents, heavy metals and dyes. They are not worth the risk unless there are only days remaining for you or the blood test shows clinical failure of some vital organ.

Additional Supplements Used For Special Purposes

Bloating and Gassiness

This is caused by food bacteria, *E. coli*, *Shigella*, and *Salmonella*. Take:

- turmeric, six capsules, (one teaspoon), three times a day.
- fennel, six capsules, (one teaspoon), three times a day.

These herbs can be purchased in bulk. Mix with water and a little vinegar or water and a little honey to make a cocktail.

- Lugol's iodine 6 drops in ½ glass water taken after meals and bedtime. **Not if allergic to iodine.**

If there is no relief in 24 hours, you are continuing to reinfect from food.

Intestinal Blockage or Bleeding

- Moose elm (also called slippery elm), one to two tablespoons a day, made into "cocoa" (see *Recipes*).
- Sodium alginate, two teaspoons powder a day added to one pint boiling water (see *Recipes*) or simply blended in cold water.

These two can heal the intestinal wall where tumorous growths have caused bleeding, ulceration and pain. They may be combined with any food or each other. Use both.

Bleeding

- Chinese Herb, Yunnan paiyao, (see *Sources*) ¼ teaspoon, three times a day, up to one teaspoon, three times a day, if bleeding is severe. This is outstanding in effectiveness for chronic bleeding, but not to be solely relied on for hemorrhage.

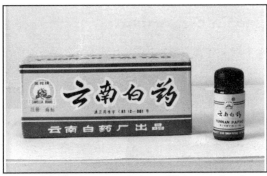

Fig. 29 Yunnan paiyao, Chinese herb to stop bleeding

- Ice cubes, emergency treatment for stomach hemorrhage. Swallow a dozen cubes quickly en route to the hospital's emergency room.
- Cayenne, swallow 20 capsules as quickly as stomach allows, in event of any hemorrhage. Follow with bread to reduce heat sensation en route to the hospital's emergency room.

Clinical help must be found in an emergency.

Poor Digestion

- Multiple digestive enzymes, two to three with each meal. Helps food leave the stomach to relieve "full" feeling. Relieves heartburn and hiatal hernia.
- Hydrochloric acid (5%), 15 drops distributed in food and beverages at mealtime. Stir while adding. Never put drops straight in mouth because it dissolves tooth enamel! Check blood chloride levels after six weeks. Do not exceed 45 drops a day (not including cooking routines).

Diarrhea and Constipation

Both are caused by the toxins produced by bacteria (the wrong bacteria) in the intestine. Killing them is the fastest way to relief.

Start with the antibacterial program: Lugol's (6 drops in ½ glass water). Ten minutes later turmeric (1 tsp. or 6 caps stirred into water), plus fennel (1 tsp. or 6 caps stirred into water). Later: 10 drops HCl (5%, USP) in a glass of water. Later: 20 drops oregano oil in an empty capsule, with food.

At the same time start taking sodium alginate (2 tsp. blended in 1 cup cold water). Sip it during the day. It helps both diarrhea and constipation.

Do not use anti-diarrhea drugs except as a last resort, since the bacterial problem will worsen while peristalsis is slowed.

If constipation continues, use Cascara sagrada capsules (as directed). Also try Epsom salts (as directed on package). Also try *lactulose* available at pharmacies. Since you will be giving yourself an enema at bedtime, the constipation will do little harm.

Anemia

"Building" blood can be the single most important task for you. If you have already begun getting transfusions, you know there is something terribly wrong with your blood-building organ—your bone marrow. It all hinges on <u>iron</u>.

Iron is more precious than gold to your body, as well as to bacteria, our iron "burglars." They try to get it for themselves. The body's strategy to keep it away from looting bacteria is to tie it tightly to two proteins: *transferrin* and *lactoferrin* ("fer" means iron.)

Transferrin is the protein molecule that transports iron in the blood like a custom-made raft. It must sail on this raft to the bone marrow where it is used to make hemoglobin. If other metals take over this raft, iron can't find its way to the bone marrow. Lactoferrin is another raft, but found in milk, tears, bone marrow, saliva, bronchial secretion, intestines, bile, urine, cervical mucous—obviously to keep iron away from the bacteria that enjoy living in these fluids. Both transferrin and lactoferrin are missing in cancer patients. This could be due to missing *xanthine oxidase*, a common oxidizer enzyme.

Making xanthine oxidase is somehow dependent on *xanthine*. (The Syncrometer detects their presence and absence together.) Xanthine is one of the purines (quite similar to nucleic acid bases) typically missing in cancer patients due to clostridium bacteria. To restore your purines you must kill the invading clostridium bacteria. As soon as this is done, within twenty-four hours, everything is back in place. And transferrin is busily transporting iron again from your body's storage piles.

Lactoferrin must be <u>eaten</u> before it gets reestablished. It is present in raw cows' or goats' milk and is not destroyed by sterilizing. Even one glass a week keeps lactoferrin reinstated. (Remember, though, that no dairy products are allowed in your 21 Day Program, so start this on day 22.) Goat milk does not have malonic acid and need not have vitamin C added.

To get your lactoferrin during the 21 Day Program, choose a small beef bone with marrow in it. Place in water or broth. Boil 5 minutes. Then add HCl drops to sterilize. Eat it at least once a week. <u>It is a delicacy</u>.

Iron is necessary for your body in many ways, besides making hemoglobin for your red blood cells. Muscle activity depends on *myoglobin*—much like hemoglobin; it contains iron. Detoxification of cholesterol, hormones, assorted amines, even industrial chemicals that have entered the body is done by enzymes called *cytochrome P-450s*. They require iron. Nearly half the enzymes in the Krebs cycle need iron. The enzymes catalase, peroxidase and various dehydrogenases also contain iron.

Iron must not be in competition with <u>copper</u>, either. Copper water pipes and copper seeping from metal or plastic dentalware keep blood iron levels too low. So <u>even when transferrin and lactoferrin are present</u>, your body may be starved for iron.

Yet cancer patients cannot simply be given iron supplements…even if blood levels are low. It could do more harm than good.

To be useful, iron must be in its special state, called <u>ferrous</u>. There is no benefit in having a large pile of iron in the <u>ferric</u> state. ("Ferrous" has an "o" like "good," to help you remember.) This is why the correct form of an iron supplement is ferrous, as in ferrous gluconate. Even this cannot be given safely.

While transferrin and lactoferrin move iron from place to place, *ferritin*, stores it.

Ferritin is a roundish ball of protein with tiny holes in the sides. Protein is sticky. Ferritin balls stick to old, worn out red blood cells, persuading them to give up their iron atoms which slip into the tiny holes to be trapped inside as <u>ferric</u> iron.

But here, ferric iron can do no harm, even though thousands of molecules pile up inside. Ferritin is equipped to handle it just like a hive is designed to hold bees. Ferritin then proceeds to store this rather dangerous iron until it can be recycled. This occurs mainly in the spleen and liver. But all cells have some ferritin; it is in their lysosomes.

Unfortunately, ferritin has an enemy, <u>asbestos</u>. Our bodies are riddled with tiny tufts of asbestos. We have inhaled some, no doubt, but we have <u>eaten</u> most of it in food. Our bodies are able to excrete a great deal of it in spite of its needle-like shapes. But the body uses ferritin, our sticky iron-storage protein, to coat and bundle-up these asbestos tufts (as discussed on page 30). That bursts open your ferritin molecules.

Ferritin is full of recycled iron waiting to be converted to the ferrous form. Both reducers, cysteine and vitamin C, can do this[92] but the Syncrometer detects <u>they don't work</u> in the presence of asbestos. Undoubtedly asbestos has oxidized cysteine and vitamin C, ruining their reducing power. But a supplement of methyl sulfonyl methane (popularly called *MSM*), a strong reducing agent, can substitute for them, and in just a few days

---

[92] Williams, W.J., Beutler, E., Erslev, A.J., Lichtman, M.A., *Hematology* 3rd Ed., McGraw-Hill, 1983, p. 308.

reduce enough ferric to ferrous iron to correct the anemia and save the day.

Lanthanide metals block the availability of iron even when large stock-piles of iron exist. I believe the lanthanides simply stick to them magnetically since the Syncrometer detects them in the same place and both are removed together by wearing a weak magnet.

A lot can go wrong with iron! And it's not over yet. Even if you fix all the problems mentioned so far, iron may still be secretly stolen by a silent chelator of iron: 1,10-phenanthroline. This is a very large molecule, similar to other PAHs that are made by *Ascaris*. Phenanthroline travels throughout the body attracting iron to itself, which turns it into *ferroin*. The Syncrometer detects ferroin and 1,10-phenanthroline whenever *Ascaris* is present—even as far away as the bone marrow!

And considering that 1,10-phenanthroline is powerful enough to suck the iron right out of the center of enzyme molecules, it can probably suck up our "good" copper the same way. Double harm is being done. Simply killing *Ascaris* gets rid of the ferroin and phenanthroline.

With parasites and other toxins gone, the iron level promptly rises and may reach forty from a value below 35 in the first five days, getting to a more normal level of 50 to 60 in three weeks.

The moral of the story is: chances are you have plenty of iron already so you should only take an iron supplement in a life threatening situation. Excess iron could be dangerous.

The low iron level in cancer has been known a very long time and is referred to as "anemia of chronic disease," which includes "anemia of malignancy." I find the same things that cause cancer cause anemia, namely parasites, dyes, and toxic metals. It is, more accurately, "anemia from *Ascaris, Clostridium*, copper, germanium, lanthanide and asbestos toxicity." It is the unavailability of iron in the midst of plenty (of iron) that strangles the cancer patient's metabolism and ultimately causes fatality in roughly half the failing cases I see, not the tumors themselves. Fortunately when you clean up the causes of cancer, you automatically clean up the causes of this anemia.

Cancer sufferers have to be especially careful about taking iron supplements because some research indicates inorganic iron (including ferrous gluconate) promotes tumor growth. Yet, as stated already, exceptions to this rule exist, and when the blood level falls below 20 while at the same time the RBC is below 3.5, we supply it as ferrous gluconate, 33 mg (one a day for only 5 days).

All anemic persons should:

- Kill clostridium bacteria to restore purines, including xanthine, so xanthine oxidase can be made again, restoring transferrin.
- Restore lactoferrin by drinking raw milk (which you sterilize) or eating bone marrow.
- Never drink water from copper plumbing; remove metal dental materials from your mouth.
- Use safe sweeteners. Sugar has asbestos which damages ferritin.
- Take MSM to reduce ferric iron into good ferrous iron.
- Kill *Ascaris* to eliminate 1,10-phenanthroline which robs iron.

As you can see, iron has a very complex story. It's like a million dollars. You need an armored truck (transferrin and lactoferrin) to get it to the bank safely. The truck must be running well (not malfunctioning due to clostridium using up all the xanthine). Once in the bank vault (ferritin), you must keep safecrackers (asbestos) away. If a customer withdraws some cash, your teller must not rip (oxidize) the bills, otherwise they are no good (ferric iron). When that happens, the teller should fix them with tape (reducers) so they are usable again (ferrous iron). Once out of the bank, the customer must protect his money from pickpockets (like 1,10-phenanthroline). Then the money can be spent wisely (on hemoglobin to carry oxygen in your bloodstream)! Cancer sufferers are especially prone to iron thefts because the same high "crime" neighborhood that makes tumors also causes anemia. Fortunately they both clean up together, too.

Insomnia

<u>All</u> insomnia I have seen is due to bacteria in the brain. The supplements given here do not correct the problem (only killing bacteria at their source does), they only give relief. Make sure you are correcting the problem at the same time as getting relief. Do not take vitamins or supplements at bedtime (except Lugol's, calcium, magnesium) because they tend to energize you. A hot shower is helpful, too, as is chamomile tea.

- Ornithine 500 mg, take six or eight for a strong effect.
- Melatonin 2 mg, take two for a strong effect.

They may be taken together.

Lymphoma

In the lymphomas, butyrates are absent in the lymph nodes. They represent the oil of butter. They are present in healthy people. It is known that the enzyme, tributyrinase, is very low (10%) after feeding the azo dye DAB.[93] This could account for low levels of butyrate. The Syncrometer detects the absence of butyrates in the lymph nodes if toxic germanium is present or isopropyl compounds (isopropylidene nucleic acids) are present. This suggests that the absence of good germanium allows isopropyl-caused mutations to occur preferentially at a butyrate-related gene such as the tributyrinase enzyme. Giving a supple-

---

[93] Langemann, H., Kensler, C.J., *Cholinesterase and Tributyrinase Activity of Rat Liver and Rat Liver Tumors*, Canc. Res., v. 11, 1951, p. 265.

ment of butyrate to lymphoma patients was already advanced in 1982.[94] The dose is 3 gm daily (see *Sources*).

Liver Cancer

These are commonly used by alternative cancer doctors. Try some or all.

- Silymarin (milk thistle concentrate, see *Sources*), take 2 three times a day.
- Cesium chloride, 3 to 6 gm a day after meals (provided clinically only). May give side effects like nausea. Intended to push excess sodium out of cells to rehabilitate them.
- Urea powder (provided clinically only), 3 to 6 tsp. a day, dissolved in beverages.
- Raw beef liver juice, sterilized with hydrochloric acid, 1 oz. daily. (See *Recipes*.)
- Raw bitters (foraged greens), sterilized with hydrochloric acid. (See *Recipes*.) Use raw peeled aloe vera if other herbs not available.
- Glycyrrhizin (licorice extract), 2 capsules three times a day.

Bone Cancer

To heal bone, you need calcium, magnesium, and bone hardeners: manganese and boron.

- Calcium carbonate, 500 mg, take one a day. Do not take calcium if blood test shows calcium level is over 9.6. Take with meals. Capsules are preferred, so you can dissolve more of it. Be sure your brand is lead-free. (Ask for a lead analysis.)

---

[94] Bradford, R., Culbert, M.L., Allen, H.W., *International Protocols For Individualized, Integrated Metabolic Programs In Cancer Management*, 2nd ed., The Robert W. Bradford Foundation, 1983, p. 109.

- Magnesium oxide, 300 mg, take one 3 times a day at beginning of meals. Capsules are preferred.
- Boron, 1 mg, take one with each meal, twice as much if in pain.
- Manganese, 10 mg, take one a day for one month. Then stop.
- By prescription *Clodronate* (or equivalent), two tablets, three times a day. This is sodium diphosphonate; it stops further dissolving of bones.
- Vitamin D, 25,000 IU per day for 10 days, then 25,000 IU twice a week only. Do not use vitamin D if blood test shows calcium level is over 9.6. Vitamin D is a <u>differentiator</u>, meaning it causes cells to return to their normal work. It causes inositol phosphate to appear in tumor cells and remove calcium deposits so the digestion-flag can be raised. Excess is toxic!

A Reason For Everything

This book is empirical in approach, not medical or clinical, which is based on protocol. Empirical means, whatever <u>works</u> will be accepted. <u>How</u> it works, <u>why</u> it works, and <u>when</u> it works are interesting aspects, that can ultimately lead to a real understanding, but not necessary at first. Like the person with a sore toe, I tried many solutions, keeping those that worked for our cancer patients. Consequently, <u>nothing</u> is used in our 21-Day Program without a basis, <u>not</u> merely because it has a history of use, <u>not</u> because it is touted as having value, <u>not</u> simply as a generalized application of "good nutrition". The actual experiments supporting the use of each supplement are too voluminous to be included here. But some are described in my *Syncrometer Biochemistry Laboratory Manual*.

When a lot of variables, such as these supplements, are in use, the scientific aspect of the design is very complex. The human brain cannot cope with many variables and see results that can be attributed <u>to one combination</u> and not another. For this reason, science, including medical science, phrases its questions <u>one variable</u> at a time. For example, a lab rat may be given asbestos <u>or</u> carcinogenic dye <u>or</u> methyl cholanthrene <u>or</u> urethane <u>or</u> copper and so forth, but never more than one of these. The results may be minimally tumor inducing. Anti-tumor treatments are given one by one, too. But the human counterpart gets hundreds of tumor-inducing substances at the same time—quite a different situation. Experimental animals are not eating asbestos-laden dyed food, nor getting metal and plastic tooth restorations nor thulium-polluted vitamin C. This is how medical science <u>missed</u> finding the causes and cures of our tumor growths. <u>Any single</u> entity <u>does not work alone,</u> not in causation, nor in cure. Only a specific <u>set</u> is the correct set.

In the 21 Day Program a selection is made to provide the most effective <u>set</u> of these supplements. Their effectiveness was monitored by the Syncrometer, blood tests, scans and assessing the general well-being of patients. As our research advances this set will change, becoming more effective and more manageable.

Here are the explanations.

Make Mitochondria

Thyroid. Since <u>all</u> cancer sufferers need thyroid hormone supplementation for a number of purposes, it is advisable to start this immediately, as soon as it can be obtained. Remember, the Syncrometer detects <u>no</u> thyroxine in tumors, thereby crippling recovery until it is obtained.

Thyroid hormones come in natural form as desiccated (dried) thyroid gland, or as synthetic L-thyroxine (T_4) or other synthetic varieties. The natural form is easy to regulate without a doctor's assistance. For this reason I recommend obtaining desiccated thyroid (see *Sources*). But it should be treated by dusting with vitamin B_2 to detoxify any dyes or solvents present. Dip in water that has two drops of HCl per cup added to provide sterilization. Pills come in various sizes from one grain to three grains. Begin with a dose of one grain the first morning upon rising. This lets you know if it will agree with you—that you are not allergic to it. On the next day take two grains upon rising. It is not too much, so that it disables your own gland, but enough to reach the tumor cells with a significant impact.

The main purpose of taking thyroid is to stimulate the mitochondria of the tumor cells to divide and grow larger. These will be more capable of taking up oxygen so respiration can intensify to produce ATP energy. ATP energy will help make the enzymes and other cell chemicals needed to differentiate (do their kind of work). You can expect to feel an energy increase and a need to breathe faster. But this may take several weeks.

Another purpose for taking a thyroid supplement is to raise your body temperature. You may begin to feel warmer, even hot and sweating. The heart will beat faster to carry the extra oxygen all over your body. All these signs are good—unless overdone. If the pulse goes higher than one hundred, cut back on the thyroid to half the dose. This protects you from overdosing, although the results are not life-threatening. It takes about three weeks for the mitochondria to respond to the thyroid stimulation, so the sooner you can begin, the better your chance of early success. The use of thyroid was advised by early cancer researchers[95] and is still in use by some alternative therapists. Much higher doses were documented by Loeser, up to 25 grains daily for four to six weeks. They are no doubt beneficial when tolerated but should only be taken under the watchful eye of a physician.

A thyroid test of the <u>blood</u> can not show a deficit that is specifically present in the <u>tumorous</u> organ. It is, therefore, wasteful and even misleading to do the test. That is why it is not included in our blood tests. How long should you stay on thyroid supplementation? Until your tumors are gone. This may be three weeks or three months. Be patient with your body. It is working miracles for you.

Lugol's iodine solution is more than an antiseptic that kills *Salmonella*. It stimulates the thyroid to make more thyroxine, a

---

[95] Loeser, A.A., *A New Therapy For Prevention of Post-Operative Recurrences in Genital and Breast Cancer, A Six-Years Study of Prophylactic Thyroid Treatment*, Brit. Med. Jour., v. 6, 1954, pp. 1380-83.

vital part of every patient's recovery. The dose is six drops in ½ glass of water (not beverages) after each meal. Taken this way it serves both purposes at once. <u>Do not take Lugol's solution if you are allergic to iodine.</u>

Bust Malonic Acid

Vitamin B_{12} and Folic Acid. After seeing the sudden appearance of malonic acid in a tumor within minutes after eating some, I first tried doses of vitamin C to detoxify it. Nothing happened. I gave individual amino acids and a long list of other supplements. There were no changes. I gave vitamin B_{12} alone or folic acid alone. Nothing happened. But when I gave B_{12} and folic acid together in large amounts the malonate disappeared and methyl malonate was in its place within ten minutes. We could begin to mend the metabolism of the tumorous organ by giving 6 mg vitamin B_{12} and 25 mg folic acid. Anything less would allow malonic acid to persist.

Vitamin B_{12} is needed in amounts much larger than was thought necessary in the past. In fact, cancer patients have a serious deficit. Some of the body's deficit is due to constant malonate detoxification. But some may be due to *Ascaris* parasites. They eat it—even turning pink from it! After eating it, the organic cobalt in the B_{12} molecule is turned into toxic inorganic cobalt. A flood of cobalt in the liver causes globulin levels to rise (leading to multiple myeloma). For this reason B_{12} is not given until your *Ascaris* parasites have been killed—on Day 1. The Syncrometer detects no B_{12} in the tumorous organ until 6 to 12 mg have been given for several days. A new sense of well being is often noticed by the patient after taking B_{12}. It has been believed that B_{12} will not be absorbed if given by mouth. This may be true for certain "pernicious anemia" cases, but cancer patients make good use of it. The injectable variety is too often polluted with antiseptic to risk.

Vitamin B_{12} and folic acid have been extensively researched in connection with cancer. Deficiencies are conducive to tumor

151

formation[96] according to most researchers. Since both vitamins are essential for cell health and cell division, a popular <u>clinical</u> approach to cancer treatment is to withhold them until tumor cells die. This works as long as the body is strong enough to recover from the systemic effects. But at the "terminal" or "hopeless" stages this no longer makes sense. It is wiser now to turn around at lightning speed and supply all the nutrients in massive amounts. Survival should come first.

Rapid Rescue

Glutathione (GSH), single-handedly can improve a semi-comatose condition. The powerful chemistry in this molecule can be seen when the terminal event has already begun. It can be compared to water. The power in the simple water molecule can <u>only</u> be seen in a severely dehydrated person, someone who has collapsed on the desert without water to drink. Only <u>water</u> cures and the amount must be large. The amount of glutathione must also be large.

When a dying patient cannot be fed by intubation or IV and only one supplement can realistically be given, glutathione is the choice. Thirty capsules, 500 mg each, can be quickly snipped with scissors and dumped into straight honey to make a goop or honey-water to be drunk. This is 15 gm. Given daily, it can salvage a loved one more quickly than any other non-clinical treatment.

The molecule is just a simple tripeptide, meaning only three amino acids are linked together to form it (glutamic acid, cysteine, glycine). It is known that the body makes it readily; therefore, there should be no need to supplement. Yet, for the extremely ill cancer patient, glutathione is a necessary supplement, and in very large amounts.

Glutathione detoxifies metal, somehow raises immunity, and supplies sulfur.

---

[96] Eto, I., Krumdieck, C.L., *Role of Vitamin B₁₂ and Folate Deficiencies in Carcinogenesis*, Adv. Exp. Med. Biol., v. 206, 1986, pp. 313-30.

Supply More Sulfur

Cysteine and Methionine. Text books teach that methionine can be converted to cysteine and only methionine would really be needed. Yet, in a very ill cancer patient, I find giving methionine <u>does not</u> produce cysteine. Both must be given. It takes rather large amounts, not skimpy amounts as in regular supplementation. The criterion of effectiveness used is when the Syncrometer detects its presence—and its staying power—in the sick organ. Cysteine gives a quick diuretic effect, too, very good for any sick person. Cysteine can trigger the liver to quickly regenerate, so new normal liver is made to tide over the liver cancer patient while tumors are being shrunk. We typically see a lot of regenerated liver on a scan after three weeks of this supplement. A liver full of tumors is not lethal as long as some good liver is present to do the body's manufacturing. Cysteine was researched by scientists decades ago and found beneficial in certain cancers.[97] We use it to supply reducing power, detoxifying power, a sulfur source, an iron mobilizer, and as a parasite killer! It kills parasites and bacteria whether inside the body or outside, provided a correct dose is taken. Methionine supplies methyl groups. A shortage of these was found to be particularly severe when weight loss had set in, a fact also noted in recent research.[98]

Taurine is thought to be made from cysteine. But in the cancer patient, taurine is deficient even <u>after</u> giving cysteine. The body needs taurine—at least to detoxify cholesterol and steroids. It is even possible that a deficiency of taurine <u>allows</u> the mis-biochemistry of *Ascaris* parasites to occur, so mutagens are formed. Perhaps if there were plentiful taurine, cholesterol would be detoxified properly. Taurine is especially helpful in

---

[97] Connor, C.L., Carr J.L. and Ginzton, L., *Cysteine in Jensen's Sarcoma*, Proc. Soc. Exp. Biol. And Med., v. 34, 1936, pp. 374-76.

[98] Sengeløv, H., Hansen, O.P., et. al., *Inter-relationships Between Single Carbon Units' Metabolism and Resting Energy Expenditure in Weight-losing Patients with Small Cell Lung Cancer. Effects of Methionine Supply and Chemotherapy*, Eur. J. Cancer, v. 30A, no. 11, 1994, pp. 1616-20.

lung cancer when formaldehyde has been one of the toxins in the home.

Crank The Krebs Cycle

Pantothenic acid, or pantothenate, is another sulfur compound. It is used by the body to make coenzyme A. Without coenzyme A many links to the Krebs cycle are missing. Coenzyme A is regularly missing in tumors, according to the Syncrometer. It is probably being siphoned off as malonyl CoA, oxidized by phenol to a useless oxidation product, or disabled by cobalt toxicity. To make more coenzyme A–much more–pantothenate is given in teaspoon doses.

Coenzyme Q10 and thioctic acid are part of the oxidation chain (respiration) in our cells. This means they can accept an electron that has been pulled away from a food molecule, hold it for a moment and pass it to another molecule willing to accept it. The electron is being passed along like a hot potato and with each change of hands, more energy is released to our advantage. A large dose of Q10 (three to four grams) can also kill tapeworm stages and detoxify dyes! When dyes have accumulated in our fatty tissues such as the skin, it must be taken in a large dose daily.

Biotin is a factor needed to make certain enzymes work. It is necessary to make fat and to use stored fat. It is missing in tumorous organs. It must be taken in large amounts before it becomes detectable here by the Syncrometer, though it is present in all other organs. By large amounts I mean several milligrams (mg), whereas most biotin supplements are in micrograms (mcg, which is one thousandth of a mg).

Niacin and Niacinamide. Both forms can be used by the body to make the NADs. NADs work with enzymes that do oxidizing and reducing, and are essential. The NADs actually handle the electrons, pulling them away from some compounds and giving them to the next oxidizer in the chain. We have two major NAD systems: NAD and NADP (NAD-phosphate). The N stands for niacin. The A stands for adenine, a purine base.

After an electron (plus its partner, hydrogen, H) has been picked up, it is written NADH or NADPH (which are reduced NADs).

The Syncrometer never detects NADH or NADPH in a healthy organ in the morning. Evidently, the electron (and hydrogen) are passed on to the next recipient so fast that it is never in the reduced state long enough to be detected. But in a tumor, the reduced forms are always present. Obviously, there is a serious slowdown of oxidation. Late in the day, after 5 PM, even healthy organs in elderly people can build up some NADH and NADPH showing, perhaps, the effect of age on our metabolism.

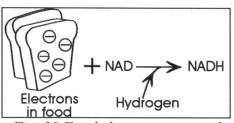

Fig. 30 Food electrons captured by oxidized NAD

Often a tumorous tissue shows <u>neither</u> the oxidized NADs <u>nor</u> the reduced NADHs. This suggests an absolute shortage. Low NAD levels were the result of feeding the dye, DAB, to animals in 1940.[99] Although our 21 Day Program removes all synthetic dyes, perhaps the damage is done and the parts are now missing that are needed to make the NADs. Fortunately the N-portion is easy to provide.

The N-portion can be provided by a supplement of either niacin or niacinamide. The problem with taking niacin is the "niacin flush." Some people flush with a dose as small as 25 mg. The face feels hot and turns red. Neck and arms may turn red and itch also. All this lasts five to ten minutes, sometimes followed by chills. It is harmless and perhaps even beneficial. But for this reason, only a small dose is given, a pinch, three times a day, with food. Niacinamide does not cause flushing and can also increase NAD levels. So a larger dose of niacinamide is given, 500 mg, twice a day. The problem with niacinamide is that it is a methyl acceptor. It seems wise to minimize supple-

[99] Kensler, C.J., Sugiura, K., Rhoads, C.P., *Coenzyme 1 and Riboflavin Content of Livers of Rats Fed Butter Yellow*, Science, v. 91, 1940, p. 623.

ments that use up methyl groups since there is a general short-age of these.

These doses of niacin and niacinamide lead to prompt re-plenishment of both NAD and NADP levels. Of course, this does not correct the oxidation flaw.

Raise Reducing Power

Vitamin C detoxifies methyl malonate, restores ferrous iron, and adds reducing power to your body's chemistry. But it should be balanced with the use of oxidizers (which we do).

Vitamin C is known to prevent scurvy in humans by making strong connective tissues like bone and skin. About a dozen more functions have been studied by scientists.

Vitamin C is probably the most popular and frequent sup-plement used. So I want to discuss safety for a moment. Any supplement used daily should be as safe as food and water. Even the smallest amount of pollutant becomes more important due to daily accumulation of whatever toxins are present. Food and water have a safety feature built into them—they are both changed in source and variety during the day. A vitamin or min-eral tablet, on the other hand, stays the same, bringing with it the same processing pollutants day after day after day.

Processing <u>must</u> introduce pollutants. It is in the very nature of processing, even when so simple a process as just mixing is done. The bins and vats must all be cleaned and sterilized. The sterilizing solutions themselves are not safe and pollute the product in trace amounts. No one should be given supplements that have not had a <u>final</u> analysis for heavy metals (particularly lanthanides), solvents, and synthetic dyes. (See list of laborato-ries who do such testing given on page 593) Cancer patients, especially, suffer from the least amount of toxicity; it's a matter of life and death for them.

There are a lot of vitamin C varieties on the market, but I can only recommend L-ascorbic acid (straight vitamin C) be-cause it has the least amount of processing. I don't even rec-ommend the tablet form of plain vitamin C because the extra ingredients that must be added to make tablets may inadvertently pollute the product.

Vitamin C is often marketed for children. Be particularly cautious of those. Is that flavored, chewable, or "better than regular vitamin C" really worth taking a risk?

Thulium pollution, especially, concerns me. Both the Syncrometer and independent laboratories have detected it in some vitamin C varieties. Thulium is a rare earth (lanthanide) metal. Lanthanides have recently been shown to cause extensive mutations, with thulium in the lead.[100]

There is yet another reason for sticking to plain vitamin C. As soon as you do any kind of chemistry with it, like "buffer" it with calcium, you create oxidation products. These are sometimes called ascorbic acid "metabolites," and have not been well researched. But excessive oxidation products of vitamin C have been found in the blood of diabetics, in the lens during cataract formation, and in aging in general.[101] Adrenal and kidney tumors have been implicated, too. You take vitamin C for its reducing power. Why ingest a form that is partly oxidized?

Oxidize the Bad Guys!

Although the current emphasis is on reducing chemistry, (antioxidants), at least one early researcher thought the problem in cancer was a missing Mystery-oxidizer. Dr. William E. Koch thought that older persons lacked certain oxidizers that children had in abundance. This allowed toxic amines to interfere with regulation of cell division. So he designed three "super oxidizers" that could be taken safely in microgram (homeopathically small) amounts: benzoquinone (BQ), rhodizonic acid, and glyoxilide. I have seen that a single dose of BQ can kill fluke, *Ascaris* and tapeworm stages, all bacteria, and can destroy my-

---

100 Jha A.M., Singh A.C., *Clastogenicity of Lanthanides: Induction of Chromosomal Aberration in Bone Marrow Cells of Mice in Vivo*, Mut. Res., v. 341, 1995, pp. 193-97.

101 Nagaraj R.H., Monnier, V.M., *Protein Modification by the Degradation Products of Ascorbate: Formation of a Novel Pyrrole from the Maillard Reaction of L-threose With Proteins*, Biochimica et Biophysica Acta 1253, 1995, pp. 75-84.

cotoxins, as well as oxidize metals, truly a magic bullet. Unfortunately, the cancer patient is not strong enough to survive such a "blitz"—a serious crisis might follow. I prefer rhodizonic acid which is less powerful and without after-effects. A 10 mg dose in $^1/_8$ cup water is held in the mouth for 5 minutes before swallowing. Six doses a day is typical.

The Syncrometer does indeed detect BQ and rhodizonic acid in children and healthy tissues of adults, but never in the presence of *Ascaris*.

Busy B's

Vitamin B$_1$ is thiamin. Since slow oxidation of food limits the availability of ATP energy, helping food oxidize in any way is important. Cancer patients become emaciated as the disease becomes terminal. Part of this is due to not eating. There is no appetite. In fact, there may be revulsion toward food. The patient shoves everything away except water. The liver dictates this behavior. Perhaps it knows it can't digest. It takes a large amount of thiamin and other digestive "help" to persuade the liver it can digest food. It takes 500 mg taken with each meal to increase appetite.

Vitamin B$_2$ is riboflavin. Besides being part of the oxidation chain that metabolizes food, B$_2$ has a number of other activities. It is a detoxifier of azo dyes[102] and benzene. The Syncrometer detects the disappearance of benzene within minutes after taking a large enough dose of B$_2$. But it is only changed to phenol, halfway to complete detoxification. So vitamin B$_2$ is taken with magnesium to detoxify phenol as well. Phenol is extremely destructive, oxidizing our vitamin C, our sulfur-based enzymes, and even vitamins.

Vitamin B$_6$ helps enzymes that transform amino acids, called transaminases. It is a vital function of the liver. In fact, if transaminase levels in the blood are high, it shows these enzymes were dumped by the liver—due to dying liver cells. Un-

---

102 Miller, J.A., Miller, E.C., *The Carcinogenic Aminoazo Dyes*, Advances In Cancer Research, Greenstein, J.P., editor, Academic Press Inc., v. 1, 1953, pp. 346-47.

fortunately, bacteria also make much use of B$_6$, so we have kept this supplement low, only 250 mg, twice a day.

Assist P450s

Glucuronic acid: This is used by the body as a detoxifier, especially for the hemoglobin salvaged from old worn out red blood cells called bilirubin. It helps the liver detoxify bilirubin and avoid jaundice. It is said to be present in the popular Kambucha tea. Such tea if used should be prepared very carefully, to prevent bad molds from growing. Glucuronic acid also assists the P450 system of detoxification inside cells.

Kill Bacteria

With the immune system down, a cancer patient is as helpless as an infant in a burning building. So food and fingers must be sterilized before eating. Use these five systems to kill the truly harmful parasites and bacteria.

Lugol's iodine. This is curative for *Salmonella* infection, the most common cause of stomach discomfort or bloating. <u>Do not take if allergic to iodine</u>. Also use Lugol's as mouthwash, hand wash and general disinfectant, diluting 1 drop in a cup of water.

Colloidal silver, home made (see *Sources*). Six drops on tooth brush after meals. One tablespoon as mouthwash, gargle. Swallow. Is particularly effective against *Clostridium*. Use one to four tbs. for pain, up to ½ cup in acute situations.

Oregano oil, of the variety *Oreganum vulgare* specifically kills *Clostridium*. To penetrate a tumor, though, you must use 20 drops three times a day for several days. To avoid burning your tongue, put them in an empty capsule and swallow. Any drops on the outside should be washed off. You may have bread and a beverage with it.

Cysteine. $^1/_8$ teaspoon per quart clear liquid kills parasites and bacteria. Use twice as much if liquid has particulate matter.

This will not kill *Toxoplasma* or *Leishmania*, though, which are also found in plain dirt. To kill these an equal amount of salt must be added. Cysteine and salt is particularly compatible with buttermilk, yogurt, blended cottage cheese, and eggs. One tsp. cysteine (4000 mg) by mouth kills many parasites and bacteria internally; consume within ½ hour, may cause temporary side effects at this dosage. Eat solid food afterward to reduce side effects.

Hydrochloric acid (HCl 5%), 3 drops in a glass of water three times a day kills bacteria in the stomach, but also reaches the gall bladder to help the liver kill its bacteria. Do not take straight in mouth—it dissolves teeth.

Kill Leftover Pathogens

Betaine hydrochloride. This is the only supplement we know that can clear the intestinal tract of clostridium bacteria; therefore it is essential to your recovery. Betaine will not clear clostridium from your teeth. It is also a methyl group supplier.

Ozonated oil can distribute itself to locations where ozone as a gas or ozonated water cannot reach. It can detoxify benzene in the body (changing it to phenol) similar to the action of vitamin B_2. We have seen it kill various bacteria and viruses when monitoring with the Syncrometer. Even *Leishmania* and malaria parasites have disappeared after several weeks' use but more research is needed to confirm this, and also to establish a mechanism of its action, as well as a level of safety.

I have found that it does not oxidize vitamin C into breakdown products in the body. But it does oxidize some vitamin E. For this reason a supplement of vitamin E should be taken 5 hours after taking ozonated oil. If it is taken sooner than this, the ozonated oil is neutralized before it has completed its action. Until more is known, caution is advised; use only with the mop-up program and liver cleanse (not as an ongoing supplement).

It must be sterilized, preferably before ozonating (2 drops HCl per cup, shaken), since most oils on the market are contaminated with *Ascaris* eggs and larvae.

Inositol is a sugar-like compound with unique features. It is ultra-oxidized in having six molecules of oxygen attached to itself. It is missing in organs that are infected with bacteria. But when inositol is eaten, it is immediately transformed into two new molecules. The Syncrometer now detects rhodizonic acid and L-ascorbic acid!

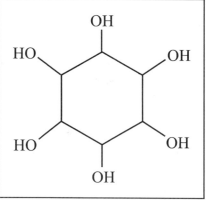

Fig. 31 An inositol molecule, pretty as a snowflake!

Could eating inositol regularly provide this "mystery oxidizer" that seems to be lacking in adults, just as Dr. Koch imagined? And would it keep us deparasitized and detoxified automatically?

It is also baffling in a second, more obvious way. We have been taught that humans cannot make their own ascorbic acid. Yet here we see it appear from a precursor compound. It is as if internal oxidation-reduction occurred in the inositol molecule, producing rhodizonic acid, an oxidizer and ascorbic acid, a reducer. More research is needed to confirm this.

Inositol Phosphate is formed after six phosphate molecules have combined with inositol, one at each OH. This makes the new molecule (popularly called IP6) quite acid and able to combine with the calcium deposits created by lanthanides. Remember, calcium deposits prevent the digestion flag to appear. Tumor cells do not have IP6, although others do. Although removing lanthanides is most important, we can speed up removal of calcium deposits by giving IP6, also called phytic acid. Take 10 drops of a 50% solution, three times a day, in ½ cup plain water before meals or water with inositol added.

Wintergreen oil (natural only, not distilled or synthetic) is another mysterious helper that needs more research. I believe it seeks out tumors, turning them into cysts with liquid centers, as

161

seen on a scan. Take three drops, three times a day (excess is toxic). It is also a traditional tumor shrinker.[103]

Restore Major Minerals

Calcium. There is a serious deficit of calcium in all cancer patients even when tumors themselves have too much and blood levels are much too high! But we cannot give more while blood levels are too high, called hypercalcemia. The problem in this case is in the thyroid gland. As soon as the thyroid problem, itself due to toxins and bacteria from teeth, is corrected, the calcium level may plummet, revealing the true shortage. Only repeated blood tests would show you this sudden change, in time to treat the hypocalcemia (low levels) that suddenly develops. The amounts we recommend are in the 21 Day Program. Don't exceed the Program because taking too much calcium could precipitate it in the wrong places. Excess calcium could even trigger cell division in some settings. Be sure yours is lead-free (ask for an analysis).

Magnesium (oxide) should be taken as a powder, like calcium, to help it dissolve in the stomach. Taken as a powder, it does not cause diarrhea. It is a major enzyme activator. There is a severe deficit in cancer patients. Magnesium helps to detoxify phenol. Phenol is produced by *Streptococcus* bacteria, and also comes from benzene. Phenol is even produced during digestion by the liver. High doses of magnesium are needed during the time when benzene, dyes, and plasticizers are being mobilized from the body tissues and newly opened tumors. After this, a lower dose may be taken. Take at the beginning of meals. Magnesium also reduces anxiety, relieves pain, protects the heart, and stops spasms of many kinds.

Potassium gluconate. There is a severe deficiency of potassium in the tissues of a cancer patient. Even ½ teaspoon of potassium gluconate powder, which contains 240 mg potassium,

---

[103] Strong, L.C., *Possible Effect of Oil of Gaultheria in Diet of Mice Susceptible to Spontaneous Carcinoma of the Mammary Gland*, Am. J. Cancer, v. 28, 1936, pp. 550-58.

taken three times a day does not bring up the level to its correct value for several weeks. The level should be 4.6 or 4.7. <u>But no higher</u>. For this reason, you should not exceed ½ teaspoon three times a day, and <u>must</u> monitor your blood at least every three weeks.

All cancer patients need supplementation with potassium <u>even when</u> the blood level is not seriously low, for example, 4.1. The blood level does not tell the whole story—that cellular levels are really much too low. But when the blood level is above 4, a lower dose of ¼ teaspoon, taken three times a day with food (it has a slightly salty taste) is more suitable.

Potassium is a respiration stimulant, causing increased uptake of oxygen, exactly what is wanted to restore health to the tumorous organ. After a blood level of 4.7 is reached, <u>stop</u>. Never take potassium gluconate for more than 3 weeks without getting a new blood test.

To find the equivalent dose in capsules, empty capsules into a measuring spoon and record the number used.

Always use a <u>measuring</u> spoon to portion out powdered supplements.

Get the Ammonia Out

Ornithine and Arginine. When an organ is besieged by bacteria it is overwhelmed by the ammonia they make. Ammonia is the same fume that comes from a diaper pail. Our livers can detoxify it very quickly, but not other organs because they can't do the chemistry called the *urea synthesis cycle*. Other organs must ship any ammonia made in them to the liver.

In the urea synthesis cycle two molecules of ammonia are pinned together with a carbon dioxide molecule to make a single *urea* molecule. Urea is odorless, tasteless, and harmless. Urea can be excreted easily into the bladder, but it is useful in several ways before it is excreted. It helps to keep the osmotic strength of the blood up so liquid cannot seep out and cause edema. Urea in pure crystalline form (28 grams in a liter of water in one day) is often given by mouth to cancer patients in alternative treatment centers, especially for liver cancer (provided the blood level of BUN is not already too high). It is well tolerated and does not raise the BUN for several weeks, after which it can be stopped.

Ornithine and arginine both play a role in the urea synthesis cycle probably expanding it and speeding it up and thereby helping the liver detoxify the whole body from ammonia. It is like supplying more trucks and wagons to do a hauling job. Removing ammonia returns each cell to a less alkaline state, giving strength to the cells' own ability to kill bacteria (lysosomes must keep themselves acidic). Arginine is particularly beneficial in combating clostridium bacteria. But it takes a lot of arginine to keep up with the ammonia production of a moderate clostridium infection. Three tablespoons was needed at first to control *Clostridium* in tumors. After finding the real source of *Clostridium* (Rabbit fluke and tooth microleakage) and getting rid of them, we could reduce the dose to one sixth of that!

There may be an actual shortage of ornithine and arginine in the tumorous tissue because these amino acids are consumed in the manufacture of *polyamines*. During cell division large quantities of *diamines* and polyamines are made to somehow satisfy the needs of chromosomes. The enzymes, arginase and ornithine decarboxylase, makers of these polyamines, are always working overtime (remember that cobalt stimulates arginase) in cancer patients and using up arginine and ornithine. This way a shortage of arginine and ornithine could easily develop and stall the urea synthesis cycle. This would worsen the ammonia buildup, ruin cells' immunity, and allow a runaway *Clostridium* infection.

When you begin to feel sleepy by daytime, the ornithine dose can be reduced but not the arginine dose.

Supply Amino Acids

Essential and Nonessential Amino Acids. Amino acids are the building blocks for protein. <u>Essential</u> amino acids are the ones that the body can't make. <u>Non-essential</u> are the ones that it can (when the person is healthy). But cancer patients have a considerable handicap in interconverting (making) amino acids. Often none or just a few are detected in the tumorous organ. This could also be due to lack of ATP energy to operate the transport mechanisms that pull them into the cells. To heal, cells <u>must</u> have amino acids, they cannot wait for health to improve first. So don't be deceived, even the "non-essential" ones are essential to you right now.

The recipe for a "mix" is on page 569. There are 19 ingredients altogether. It takes large doses before they are detectable by Syncrometer. And they will not <u>stay</u> present unless taken daily for a few weeks.

Both shark cartilage and chicken broth help cells replenish their amino acids in days, not weeks; perhaps this is due to the RNAse inhibitor they contain.

Shark Cartilage helps replenish RNAse inhibitor and amino acids as well as providing other factors. But it must be sterilized with cysteine-salt water ($^1/_{16}$ teaspoon each per cup liquid) or by adding HCl drops (see *Recipes*). Not many brands have RNAse inhibitor present. It must be a casualty of processing. For this reason we always add chicken broth to the cancer program besides shark cartilage.

Glutamic acid is a very versatile amino acid and can be transformed into other amino acids. By picking up ammonia it changes to glutamine which has further uses. One use is making purines, which in turn makes uric acid. So when your blood uric acid level is low it indicates a need for glutamic acid. I recommend taking glutamic acid separately from the "mix" because so much more is needed. A large dose, 1 tbs. three times a day, often brings a sense of well being immediately.

Glycine is the simplest of all amino acids and for this reason can be made from others, and it should therefore never be low

165

according to classical textbooks. But I find cancer patients don't have it! Glycine is used to make creatine, which in turn makes creatinine. So when your blood creatinine is low, I believe there is a shortage of glycine. In addition to the "mix," take ½ tsp. three times a day if creatinine levels are below 0.8.

Stop p53 Mutations

Organic germanium (not inorganic) can stop p53 mutations. **Hydrangea root** is one, but not the only, source of organic germanium. Garlic and ginseng are said to have a lot. Most plants have a tiny bit. And we should not need a lot. The Syncrometer finds it also prevents hCG from appearing even in the presence of isopropyl alcohol, suggesting that this, too, is the result of a mutation. So it is wise to supplement. Remember, good germanium can be turned to bad just by getting a dose of benzene or asbestos. And the bad germanium may be cooperating with dyes to cause enzyme mutations—raising LDH and alkaline phosphatase while lowering tributyrinase and blood iron. So it is wise not to supplement too much. Commercial varieties of organic germanium were found to be impure and are not recommended.

Organic germanium is known to reduce T-suppresser cells and elevate T-helper cells. It also produces interferon. The Syncrometer detects that it controls viral integrase, the enzyme that can lock out viruses from your DNA.

You may make the hydrangea root into a tea, as in the kidney herb recipe, doubling the amount of hydrangea. Or use as powder for three weeks.

Return Immunity

Papain and bromelain are plant enzymes often used to help digestion. I use them because they can digest the ferritin off white blood cells (at least papain has been studied in this regard,[104] bromelain was discovered by Syncrometer). Previously when we discussed ferritin, it was the hero that sacrificed itself to surround the villain asbestos. Why are we now trying to digest it? Because there is a drawback to using ferritin. Ferritin as it coats and smears the outside surface of white blood cells inadvertently "blinds" them.[105] Their surface has the receptors which sense enemy molecules, acting as their "eyes and ears." Digesting ferritin lets the white blood cells regain their "sight." They can now find other white blood cells to pass their toxic cargo to,[106] which is the normal method.

Now tissues can be cleared of asbestos much more quickly. And excess damaged ferritin is no longer present, exposing its ferric iron, which was oxidizing good germanium. Immunity has returned.

We give 1 tsp. papain twice a day in a beverage before meals. (Be careful not to inhale it, you could start an allergic reaction.) Bromelain is much more palatable, though less effective. You can use 1 tsp. (4000 mg) two times a day instead of papain. But in serious illness use both.

Selenium can be detected by the Syncrometer as sodium selenite in healthy organs, never as selenate (so I assume that is the beneficial form). But in the presence of ferritin coated white blood cells or phenol or *Ascaris* produced chemicals, only the selenate form is detected. It switches back to selenite as soon as the above abnormal oxidizers are gone. Lack of selenite stalls the unloading from White Blood Cells. They seem to be bursting with high bacteria and toxin levels soon after ferritin and lanthanides are gone, yet unable to dispatch and unload these until large amounts of selenite are consumed. It typically requires 3,000 to 4,000 mcg daily for 3 weeks. Fresh coconut is a

---

[104] Papenhausen, P.R., Emeson, E.E., Croft, C.B., Borowiecki, B., *Ferritin-Bearing Lymphocytes in Patients With Cancer*, Cancer, Jan. 15, 1984, v. 53, pp. 267-71.

[105] Pattanapanyasat, K., Hoy, T.G., Jacobs, A., Courtney, S., Webster, D.J.T., *Ferritin-bearing T-lymphocytes And Serum Ferritin in Patients With Breast Cancer*, Br. J. Cancer, 1988, v. 57, pp. 193-97.

[106] Fubini, B., Barceló, F., Areán, C.O., *Ferritin Adsorption on Amosite Fibers: Possible Implications in the Formation and Toxicity of Asbestos Bodies*, Jour. Tox. Env. Health, v. 52, 1997, pp. 343-52.

good source after that, when much smaller amounts are needed. Selenite can be detected now when one half coconut is eaten for three days straight. If raw coconut is not available, continue taking sodium selenite, but at a reduced level, 1000 mcg a day, for several months after all tumors are gone.

Bring Back Iron

Methyl sulfonyl methane (MSM) is a powerful substance that can return your ferric iron and bad germanium to ferrous iron and good germanium! Even while asbestos is still present and ferritin has coated the white blood cells! Use ½ tsp. twice a day for 3 weeks. Double this dose if severely ill. This will not remove asbestos or dyes.

Supply Missing Growth Regulator

Vitamin A is a growth regulator. The gene that allows it to be transported and absorbed is always mutated when azo dyes are present, according to the Syncrometer. Vitamin A, *retinol binding protein* and *retinoic acid receptor* α are all absent in the tumor.

The truly effective dose is 100,000 I.U. a day. It forces open the cells' lysosomes so powerful enzymes are released, your oxidizers. Palmitate and acetate forms are usable. You <u>will</u> certainly get hypervitaminosis A (scalded looking skin or peeling) from this dose taken daily; it is the result of so many opened lysosomes, not truly serious. But you can also get good results from taking this dose intermittently, such as 3 days ON, 3 days OFF. Do not exceed this dosage without a doctor's assistance.

Beta carotene is the precursor to vitamin A. Phenol produced by streptococcus bacteria oxidizes it so no vitamin A can be made. Correcting the phenol problem allows instant return of both beta carotene and vitamin A. This conversion <u>does</u> require zinc. But experiments with zinc supplementation are not complete. So it is wiser to eat zinc-rich food (sunflower seeds, oysters, and fish). Since vitamin A is so easily destroyed even after supplying it as a supplement, it seems wise to give beta carotene as well.

Lick the Lanthanides

Although heavy metals will leave by themselves after using ozonated water and many sulfur-containing supplements, lanthanides will not. The lanthanides are a group of 15 elements listed in the periodic table beginning with lanthanum: lanthanum, neodymium, praseodymium, samarium, gadolinium, cerium, terbium, europium, dysprosium, holmium, erbium, thulium, ytterbium, lutetium, promethium. They have special properties: their magnetic nature[107], their high molecular weight, their similar chemistry (so similar they can hardly be separated from each other), and their affinity for tumors.[108] Their magnetic properties is why lanthanides are used to make "ceramic" magnets, much more powerful than iron and steel magnets of the same size. That is also why they are used as "contrast" materials for MRI and CT scans, especially gadolinium. Surprisingly, the Syncrometer detects not only gadolinium, but all the lanthanides together in contrast materials. Were they never truly separated in the production process? Each cancer patient is getting dose after dose of all the lanthanides by injection!

Lanthanides do special damage.[109] They cause calcium to deposit in cells. This triggers the enzyme, protein kinase. And this signals cells to divide! At the same time, white blood cells that begin to eat up the lanthanides are disabled by the very same calcium buildup and must stop eating them. So lanthanides accumulate. Cells that are filled with calcium deposits get stiff—too stiff to move about. And too stiff to put up the acute distress signal. The signal, a molecule of *phosphatidyl serine*,

---

[107] Lee, E.W., *Magnetism*, Dover Publications, Inc., New York, 1970, p. 103.

[108] Yokoyama, A. and Saji, H., *Tumor Diagnosis Using Radioactive Metal Ions and Their Complexes in Metal Ions in Biological Systems*, Carcinogenicity and Metal Ions, H. Sigel (ed.), v. 10, ch. 10, p. 321.

[109] Das, T., Sharma, A., and G. Talukder, *Effects of Lanthanum in Cellular Systems A Review*, Biological Trace Element Research, v. 18, 1988, pp. 201-28.

should be sticking out of the cell surface to attract pancreatin. Normally, pancreatin would digest such a cell and no tumor could form. We never detect pancreatin in lanthanide-loaded cells, although it is present in all other tissues, especially high after eating. So neither white blood cells nor pancreatin is capable of removing a tumor! Not without special help. Yet the Syncrometer has found what helps.

- A very tiny patch of low strength magnetic material (see *Sources*), and
- a high strength magnet.

The small patch should not be too strong (not over 100 gauss, which is the unit of measurement for magnetic field strength). It should be ½ inch wide and about 1 inch long. It should be placed lengthwise over the center-line that you can draw along your spine. The back of your neck is convenient. The North side of your patch is placed against your skin. Tape it down securely with cellophane tape. Patches as small as a few gauss need recharging by a high strength magnet after several days. Patches as high as 100 gauss might last a year before needing a charge.

The high strength magnet should be a ceramic block with a strength between 1000 and 4000 gauss. Keep it away from delicate instruments since they could be instantly ruined.

Determine which is the North side of your magnets even if they come already labeled. This means the side that attracts the end of a compass needle pointing North. You must be certain of this; place the compass on a table; it will soon settle down and point northward. Identify the tip that points North. Now bring your magnet, slowly, toward the compass, with one side of your magnet facing the compass. Find which side of your magnet pulls the compass needle tip pointing northward. Label this side of your magnet North. The opposite side is South. (These instructions are using the "biological convention" in labeling.)

The main purpose of the small magnet is to pull iron and lanthanides out of your tissues; this includes excess ferritin that coats your white blood cells. These two effects raise your immune power. Soon bacteria can be devoured again and the white blood cells fill up with asbestos, lanthanides and bacteria, evidence for their ability to devour them again.

The high strength magnet has more purposes. It will stop DNA production by *Clostridium* without disturbing your own. To achieve this you must <u>sit</u> on the N pole for ½ hour daily (not more).

<u>Do not position the magnet over the heart. Do not use the high strength magnet if you have a pacemaker.</u>

Remove Calcium Deposits

Vitamin D can induce inositol phosphates IP6, IP2 and IP3 to appear in the correct ratios even when none were there before. This results in disappearance of calcium deposits much faster than if using only the magnet. A hard bony tumor may begin to soften in a few days. Use 25,000 units of cholecalciferol daily for 21 days. No more. It can be toxic. Use only if calcium levels are below 9.7.

Digest the Tumor

Enzymes, including pancreatin, lipase, DNAse, peroxidase, and catalase are produced by the body in large amounts. The Syncrometer detects all these in <u>every</u> organ. But not in the tumor or <u>its</u> white blood cells.

We have been taught that digestive enzymes stay in the digestive tract. And that eating them would do no good since they would be themselves digested. This may be partly true, but only partly. The tumor can be deluged with pancreatin and lipase by taking 1 tsp. of each between meals 3 times a day. "Enzyme therapy" was discovered long ago by cancer therapists and was built into several alternative programs. But will the flood of enzymes digest the tumor? Only if lanthanides and the calcium deposits they cause are gone, so the cell "flag" may be raised, saying "I am ready for digestion…come and get me." The flag, phosphatidyl serine appears on the cell surface when calcium deposits, particularly calcium triphosphate, are gone. At this point the enzymes are exceedingly swift. In one week a large bite can be missing from the tumor.

We use horseradish sauce (Heinz brand) to supply peroxidase and catalase since the dried herb is missing catalase. Use three tsp. daily on food.

Intravenous (IV) Supplements

If you are a caregiver, you might notice that in spite of all the good intentions your patient has to eat and take supplements, day after day passes and it simply does not happen. There are reasons beyond anyone's control for not eating. If your patient continues to lose weight, they are <u>not eating enough</u>. Provide the richest, highest calorie food you can. Prepare it in the most appealing way you can. But if they have not eaten food for two days, you must give IV feedings. The IV feedings should include fat and protein, not merely sugar. It is common practice to give terminal cancer patients dextrose-water (glucose/sugar) alone as nourishment. Perhaps it seems justified to clinical personnel since better nutrition would only delay the final event. I recommend an intensive feeding program including a liquid amino acid mixture and a fat emulsion (see *Sources*). If blood albumin levels are low (below three), a bottle of albumin should be given daily as well (alternate days as condition improves). Along with these nutritional IVs, hefty doses of vitamins and minerals should be given (see IV *Recipes*).

Unfortunately, I find that the IV bags and bottles of injectable supplements are often polluted with antiseptics, heavy metals, bacteria and even *Ascaris* eggs and larvae! The bags themselves seep plastic because the Syncrometer finds polyvinyl chloride inside (a carcinogen!). For this reason we use only <u>glass</u> IV bottles. Since you cannot test easily for bacteria, you should give each 500 ml IV bottle one ml of ethyl alcohol (either 76% or 95%) to kill Coxsackie viruses that are often present. To eliminate bacteria and parasites, run the IV tube through a five micron (5μ) syringe filter placed "in line." As for isopropyl alcohol or benzene, you are taking a chance—it is simply a gamble. But it is better than doing nothing.

This is our "minimum nutrition" list for IVs.

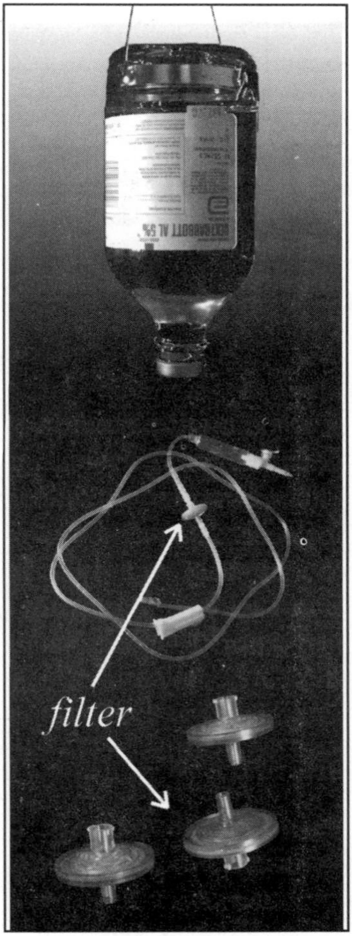

Fig. 32 Good IV bottle and filter

- Fat emulsion (1,000 ml, Intralipid™ 10% see *Sources*) Use ½ or whole bottle a day.
- Magnesium (10 gm/20ml) use 2 gm in a day. Gives pain relief. Stops spasms.
- Potassium chloride (149 mg/ml) use 2 to 4 ml a day.
- Vitamin B-100 complex, use 5 ml a day.
- Amino acid solution (1,000 ml, with electrolytes). Give ½ or whole bottle in a day.
- Vitamin C (L-ascorbic acid, 500 mg/ml), 25 gm up to 100 gm in critical cases. Use calcium and magnesium injectables to neutralize acidity.
- Calcium gluconate 10% (50 ml) use 25 ml when blood level is below the normal range. Use together with vitamin C to help neutralize the acidity.

173

Note: if you do not sterilize the vitamin C, amino acids, B-complex, and fat emulsion, and filter them, you will be <u>intro-ducing</u> the very pathogens you are trying to clear!

These supplements are added to IV bottles of saline (salt) or

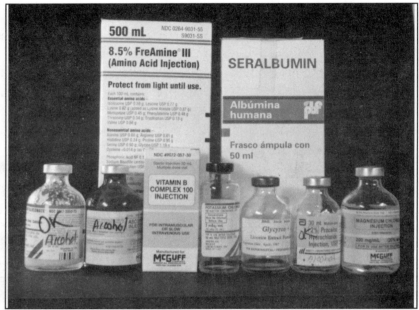

Each bottle must be tested separately for heavy metals, dyes and solvents.

Fig. 33 Assorted supplements given by IV

dextrose (sugar) depending on which is lowest on the blood test. If both are low, glucose (50%) is added to a saline IV bottle to give both at once.

Note that no oxidizers are included in this regimen, nor sulfur compounds. It is quite inadequate, but may tide your patient over the first few days, when a small improvement makes the critical difference. As soon as your patient is willing to drink chicken broth instead of water, you have gained ground.

Additional IV treatments may be used in other situations.

- Procaine, use 5 to 10 cc of 2% solution (the preferred pain killer).

174

- EDTA, single dose, (3 gm) to remove heavy metals.
- Laetrile (also called amygdalin, 3 gm/ampoule) use 2 to 3 ampoules a day. Available in Mexico.
- Vitamin K, 5-10 mg a day to reduce bleeding.
- Vitamin A (25,000 to 100,000 IU/day).
- Albumin (use a one dose bottle, 12.5 gm in a day).
- Rhodakem, 2 to 6 vials a day (can also be taken by mouth) (product includes rhodizonate). Available in Mexico.
- Glycyrrhizin, 30 ml, especially good for liver cancer.
- DMSO, 5 ml (100%) increases penetration of other supplements. Differentiates (normalizes) tumor tissue.[110]
- Cesium chloride, 3 gm a day at first. Then 6 gm daily unless nausea occurs.
- Insulin, rapid acting, 15 to 30 U along with 100 ml of 50% glucose. (Must watch patient for signs of hypoglycemia.)

IV treatments speed up tumor shrinkage. They are life-saving when the liver can no longer detoxify what is coming out of the tumors as evidenced by rising LDH, alk phos, GGT, etc. If you are very ill, choose IV therapy to help your body survive each opened tumor; it could take 5 weeks!

Many details of good IV therapy are given in the book *Intravenous Nutrient Protocols in Molecular Medicine* by Majid Ali, MD, Denville, NJ, USA, 1994.

How To Take Your Supplements

Taking some supplements out of the capsule reduces the queasiness and discomfort from dozens of capsules bouncing around in your stomach. Capsules can be cut in half with scissors and dumped into foods or mixed with straight honey or maple syrup to make "candy". Always add spices (natural herbs

---

[110] Collins, S., Ruscetti, F., Gallagher, R., and Gallo, R.C. *Terminal Differentiation of Human Promyelocytic Leukemia Cells Induced by Dimethyl Sulfoxide and Other Polar Compounds*, Proc. Natl. Acad. Sci. USA, v. 75, no. 5, May 1978, pp. 2458-62.

only, commercial varieties may have added dyes!) to such a concoction. But you need to be warned which supplements taste like burning rubber tires or worse so you can leave these in their capsules. Here is my assessment of taste.

Supplements that taste terrible: glutathione, methionine, thioctic, amino acids, niacinamide, papain.

Supplements that taste quite bad: taurine, B vitamins, ozonated oil, vitamin C, shark cartilage, MSM.

Supplements that taste okay: cysteine if dissolved in broth or grapefruit juice, pantothenate, ornithine, arginine, coenzyme Q10, potassium gluconate (salty), beta carotene, vitamin A, wintergreen, folic acid, Chinese herb (Yunnan paiyao), biotin, niacin, betaine, calcium, magnesium.

Supplements that taste good: inositol (sweetish), fennel, turmeric, moose elm.

More do's and don'ts about supplements:

- Always wash a color-coated tablet under the kitchen faucet to remove the dye. (Close sink first). Dunk in vitamin B_2 powder and set to dry on paper towel.
- Take coenzyme Q10 in the morning upon rising, before or after thyroid.
- Lugol's must be taken by itself with water at end of meals to avoid oxidizing your vitamins and food.

Supplements can be mixed together, stirred into cereal, mashed potatoes, pudding, or rice and gulped down at beginning of meal.

Always keep bread nearby when taking supplements. If one should stick in your throat eat a bit of bread.

If nausea threatens, eat bits of bread, not liquid. Take two drops of mint oil (see *Sources*).

If a stomachache threatens, sip hot water.

For spasms of intestine, sip hot water or take one niacinamide.

Don't take supplements at bedtime, especially B vitamins, because they are too energizing. But calcium and magnesium with hot moose elm are soporific.

The actual amounts of supplements to take are given in the next chapter.

Choose IV therapy if supplements "won't go down." But remember, IV therapy does not take the place of green black walnut hull, cysteine, ozonated oil, and all the rest.

21 Day Cancer Curing Program

Your supplements have been divided into manageable "packages"; every day some new ones are added to those you are already taking. You will be on the full program in about a week. By then your body will be sufficiently cleared of toxins to begin "tumor drainage." This takes up the second week. In the third week, the body is cleaned up again to start the actual shrinkage. Tumors that can be seen or felt are given a topical treatment, too (see *Recipes*, page 572).

You may want to quickly check the section on special problems (page 139) to see if there are any extra supplements you wish to add.

Check the *Recipes* or *Sources* chapters for many of the items used below.

Many persons can consume these dosages easily. But if your frame is small, your appetite poor and there is no room for supplements, **just do the best you can**.

Caution: The dosages recommended here are for cancer patients only, and then only for 3 weeks. DO NOT use this cancer curing program to PREVENT cancer or for other diseases. I have not evaluated these dosages when taken for a prolonged period of time.

Day 1

1. Kill all your parasites in a single day. This includes mopping-up after tapeworm stages, flukes, and *Ascaris* worms. Take:

- 2 tsp. green black walnut hull tincture extra strength
- 9 capsules cloves (500 mg each)
- 9 capsules wormwood (200 to 300 mg each)

Mix the tincture with fruit juice (hand squeezed) or tap water and spoon it down carefully or sip slowly. You may add sweetening and cinnamon. Don't let it stand after mixing, it begins to lose its potency after twenty minutes. Keep the stock bottle refrigerated. Take the capsules afterward, one at a time. You may take these later in the day if you wish. Keep a bit of bread nearby, to swallow if a capsule sticks. If you have stomach cancer or liver cancer, the alcohol could be harmful. There are some powdered black walnut hull capsules on the market, but beware! Some have no potency, while others are extremely potent. Ones I have tested are listed in *Sources* along with the number of capsules to be taken.

Later in the day, when you are comfortable, mop up after shielded parasites and viruses that still survive. Use cysteine and ozonated olive oil (more information on page 52).

- L-cysteine 500 mg, take two capsules, twice within ½ hour. You may snip open and empty capsules into broth or other tart beverage (like lemonade). This avoids tummy twinges from the undissolved crystals. Stay seated until side effects wear off (a half hour). Do not drive a car.
- Add 4 drops HCl (5%) to a cup of olive oil. Ozonate for 25 minutes, using a ceramic or wooden aerator. Then cap tightly and store in freezer until used. If it will be used the same day, store in refrigerator. Take 1 tbs. at least 5 hours after the cysteine. If you take it sooner, it will undo some of the benefit of cysteine. It is quite palatable mixed with mashed potatoes or pasta. Do not gulp it straight since this could give you nausea.

If you do not have cysteine yet, take the ozonated oil anyway. If you do not have an ozonator to make ozonated oil, take the cysteine anyway. Catch up as missing ingredients arrive.

Repeat the whole parasite program daily.

The amount of black walnut tincture extra strength may be increased to 10 tsp. if there are only days remaining, especially for brain and bone marrow cancers which are hard to reach. You may take it in 2 tsp. doses five times in a half hour or all at once. Another effective schedule is 8 tsp. followed by a one hour rest, then another 8 tsp. Choose what is easiest for you. Only 9 capsules of cloves and wormwood are needed, though. Try to avoid nausea by eating bits of bread afterward, with a drop or two of sterilized mint oil. You might wonder why there is a need for repeat treatments at all if these doses are truly effective. The explanation is that parasites tightly encased inside a tumor with little circulation are very hard to reach. They continually emerge to reinfect the body and must be promptly killed.

2. Zap every day (page 51). This will gradually remove ferritin from your white blood cells. It also brings North pole magnetic fields into your body which remove lanthanide metals, besides outright killing of parasites and bacteria. Zap more often if extremely ill.

3. Start your dental work. If you have only weeks left, but can sit in a dentist's chair, take the first appointment available and have all your teeth with metal or plastic fillings extracted. You do not have time to wait for the tedious task of cleaning up teeth that have small fillings. Do not waste a day deliberating over any teeth! You may request general anesthesia if the dental surgeon agrees.

Be sure to clean out cavitations that can be seen on X-rays. Hidden cavitations can be cleaned up later.

[Note: If your red blood cell count is 3.2 or less, you should request a transfusion first, to make up for the minor blood loss during extraction. You should also be off any blood thinner and not use aspirin for pain the day before and during dental work. If your platelet count is below 10,000, you should request a dose of platelets first to protect you.]

If you have more than three weeks remaining, take the first appointment available to extract all teeth with large metal or plastic fillings, and teeth that are capped, or have root canals. After healing for five days to let the gums close, get a digital X-ray exam of the front teeth. Plastic fillings can be identified and drilled out. Your recovery now depends on <u>perfection</u> practiced by your dentist; the tiniest speck of plastic remaining will still show its poisonous effect on your next blood test and will prevent recovery (high LDH, alkaline phosphatase, globulin, low iron). Leave the fresh cavities open until the blood test results have become normal. Keep them sanitary by brushing after eating with colloidal silver and oregano oil (see *Sources*).

Rinse your mouth at bedtime with dental bleach, for one month. Start the Dental Aftercare program (page 83) carefully and meticulously, on the same day as the dental work.

4. Treat all your essential medications as if they were contaminated by dyes, benzene, and isopropyl alcohol. Treat them as described in the Safer Painkillers section (page 65).

5. Start your tumor shrinking diet (page 97). Choose malonate-free foods. Remove asbestos, dyes, lanthanides all together with 2 hot water soaks separated by a 10 minute cooling.. Sterilize everything afterward except water (see page 517). Every food is given a few drops of hydrochloric acid (5%, USP) after serving on your plate; stir in well. Total drops of hydrochloric acid added not to exceed 45 drops daily, not counting those used in kitchen preparation.

6. Throw away all your cosmetics, lotions, salves, deodorant, shaving supplies, shampoos, hair dyes, eye liner, soap, mouthwash, toothpaste, nail polish, absolutely everything that goes on or in your body. Switch to our recipes (page 544). More are given in *The Cure For All Cancers*. Take a shower and shampoo the chemicals out of your hair with borax and citric acid. Do not use a hair blower and keep very warm by dressing in extra clothes.

You may use a henna variety of hair dye purchased in bulk (see *Sources*). If your hair is already dyed, wash in dental bleach for 5 minutes. This will not affect color. Rinse with citric acid. Launder clothing in straight borax. Bleach all clothing once to get out azo dyes and the metal germanium. Toxins, except for hair dye, will leave your body in the first week. But toxins <u>inside</u> your tumors are marooned and require a special seven day program which begins in the second week.

7. Start glutathione, 500 mg; take two, three times a day, to be completed before supper time to avoid having too much energy at bed time. Take them before meals so it can act on the tumorous organ as a reducer. If you are bedridden, double this dose. If only days remain, take thirty capsules daily. Take all at once stirred into honey or maple syrup (each treated with HCl first to sterilize). If this causes diarrhea, take with food in several doses.

8. Start Lugol's iodine. Take six drops in ½ glass of water at the end of each meal (three times a day). Take it at bedtime, too, if bloating is present. No HCl needed.

9. Start thyroid: one grain in the morning upon rising. Increase to two grains in the morning after that. If you were on a thyroid medication previously, be sure to come up to at least that dosage. (A pharmacist can help you convert your brand to grains). Remember to treat tablets with vitamin B_2.

10. Schedule blood test (SMAC 24: must include serum iron) and scan (see the Reading Your X-rays chapter for advice on scans, page 243).

11. Set kidney herbs to soak overnight per recipe (page 560).

12. Do the same for liver herbs (recipe page 562).

End of Day 1

You have accomplished a lot. You will probably feel better tomorrow. If you had to omit some instructions, catch up on them as soon as the supplies arrive. Day one instructions have the highest priority.

On each day more supplements will be added. <u>Do not stop taking those</u> that were scheduled on previous days.

Day 1 At A Glance

Before breakfast	2 tsp. black walnut tincture extra strength, 9 wormwood capsules, 9 clove capsules, 2 glutathione (500 mg each), thyroid (one grain).
Breakfast	follow guidelines so it is malonate-free, sterilized, dye-free, asbestos-free, etc. Finish with Lugol's (six drops) in ½ cup water. (No HCl.)
Midmorning	make dental appointment. Schedule blood tests. Zap when convenient. "Clean" up all essential medications. Throw out all commercial body products.
Before lunch	2 glutathione (500 mg each)
After lunch	Finish with Lugol's (six drops) in ½ cup water.
Afternoon	4 cysteine (500 mg each). Ozonate some sterilized olive oil 25 minutes to take later. Launder with borax and bleach all your clothes and bedclothes.
Before supper	2 glutathione (500 mg each)
After supper	Finish with Lugol's (six drops) in ½ cup water. Set to soak kidney herbs and liver herbs.
Bedtime	1 tbs. ozonated olive oil with food

Day 2

Capsules of supplements may be emptied, mixing all together in a closeable container; then taking one third with each meal. We will call such a mixture "vitamix." Supplements that are particularly bad tasting should be flavored. It is important not to feel revulsion toward your supplements. You may use the spice-like supplements (fennel, turmeric, beet cocktail, oregano oil, wintergreen oil) to mask the bad tasting ones (shark cartilage, MSM, papain, DMSO and others).

1. Start kidney herb recipe (1¼ cups a day) and liver herbs (2 cups a day). This will improve kidney and liver function so toxins can be detoxified and flushed out rapidly. Leave out the magnesium because there are separate in-

structions below. Stir two drops hydrochloric acid into each cup at time of drinking.

2. Coenzyme Q10, 400 mg, take ten in the morning, upon rising, before or after the thyroid pill. Repeat this high dose on Day 7 through Day 14, and on Day 19. On other days take one capsule daily. This will begin to destroy the azo dyes accumulated in the spleen and body fat, particularly Sudan IV, DAB, and Sudan Black B. You may snip open the capsules and mix powder with straight honey or put powder directly in mouth. Take it 5 hours away from the reducers cysteine, glutathione, and vitamin C; that is why early morning is best.

3. Start vitamin B_2 and magnesium. Take two B_2 (300 mg each) capsules and one magnesium oxide capsule (300 mg) three times a day. This will destroy the benzene and phenol that has accumulated in your spleen and body fat as well as helping to detoxify azo dyes there.

4. Betaine hydrochloride (about 300 mg), take three, three times a day with meals. This kills *Clostridium* in the colon.

5. Start vitamin B_{12}, 1000 mcg, take two, three times a day, at mealtime. This vitamin hatches *Ascaris* eggs; make sure you have already taken cysteine and ozonated oil previously, have zapped and are adding HCl to each food. If not, postpone this.

6. Vitamin C, 2000 mg (same as 2 gm, or ½ teaspoon), three times a day. No "mineral ascorbates" or other vitamin C like products due to toxic oxidation by-products. You may take more.

7. Chicken broth, one pint a day (see *Recipes*) alternating with shark cartilage , two tablespoons or more a day. Each beverage will receive two drops of hydrochloric acid before consuming.

8. Start bromelain or papain, four 1000 mg capsules, twice a day. If extremely ill use both. This will digest and clear the ferritin coating on your white blood cells to recover immunity. Take well before meals (at least 15 minutes).

9. Turmeric and fennel. Take six capsules (or one teaspoon) of each, three times a day. Don't mix with food like I recommend for other supplements because these are so flavorful they will overpower your food. You may mix them with sweetened water if you wish. Sterilize with 2 drops HCl for each.

10. If you have tumors you can see or feel, use the Topical Tumor Shrinker on page 572.

Day 2 At A Glance

Before breakfast	Ten coenzyme Q10 (400 mg). Repeat parasite program, 2 tsp. black walnut tincture extra strength, 9 wormwood capsules, 9 clove capsules. Thyroid (two grains). Open six glutathione capsules, six 300 mg B_2 capsules, three 300 mg magnesium oxide capsules, nine 300 mg (approximately) betaine hydrochloride capsules, and six 1000 mcg vitamin B_{12} capsules to make today's vitamix. (You could leave this all in capsules or tablets and take separately, but we find this is a lot easier, even though a few bites of your meal won't taste as good.) Take 1 tsp. bromelain or 1 tsp. papain stirred into a beverage to make a "cocktail" (they may also be encapsulated). Use both if very ill. Sterilize all concoctions as well as food.
Breakfast	Take 2 gm vitamin C. Mix a third of your vitamix with part of your breakfast and gulp down. Distribute 15 drops of hydrochloric acid in your foods and beverages. Take six fennel capsules and six turmeric capsules. Finish meal with Lugol's (six drops).
Midmorning	Make kidney herb recipe (sip 1¼ cups throughout day). Make liver herbs (sip 2 cups throughout day). Add 2 drops hydrochloric acid to each cup. Zap when convenient.
Lunch	Take 2 gm vitamin C, another third of your vitamix, 15 drops of hydrochloric acid in your food. Take 6 fennel and 6 turmeric capsules. Take six drops Lugol's after meal.
Afternoon	Repeat mop-up, 4 cysteine (500 mg each). Make a big pot of chicken broth and freeze all except today's portion. 1 tsp. bromelain or papain or both if very ill.
Supper	Supper should include chicken soup, at least one pint. Take 2 gm vitamin C and the final third of your vitamix, 15 drops of hydrochloric acid in your food. Take six fennel capsules and six turmeric capsules. Take six drops Lugol's after meal.
Bedtime	Finish mop-up, 1 tbs. ozonated sterilized olive oil. Apply topical tumor shrinker if you have tumors you can see or feel.

Critical Blood Tests

If you got your blood tested on the first day, you can expect your results on day two or three, because laboratories only take 24 hours. If you haven't been notified of your results by now, call your doctor and ask that they be read or faxed to you. You may be feeling quite well but any result outside the normal range should get immediate attention.

As soon as they arrive, review them yourself. It is the custom in the American medical community <u>not</u> to share these results, <u>not</u> to explain them, and in fact, to minimize testing. I believe all this is intended to avoid embarrassing questions by the patient such as, "Why didn't I improve?" or "Why is my LDH so high?" With this attitude, liver enzymes, serum iron and even the LDH are often omitted completely by physicians (make sure to request them).

As soon as you have results, find the ones that are too high or too low, and take appropriate action as described in the chapter *Reading Your Blood Test Results*.

Day 3

1. Start folic acid, 25 mg per day (that is 25 one milligram or 0.9 mg capsules). You may have been on chemotherapy that used anti-folate compounds. Their purpose was to kill your cancer cells. If you are now considered a terminally ill cancer patient, you may agree that such clinical treatments failed for you and are not worth pursuing at this point. My approach is the opposite—we will shrink the tumors and rehabilitate the nearby tumor-like tissue, letting the body select those cells it will digest. You should decide to cease anti-folate chemotherapy if you plan to use folic acid.

2. Raw beet juice, 2 Tbs. before each meal. Add 1 teaspoon to 1 tablespoon vinegar as desired. This reduces phenol

formation during digestion. Sweeten and dilute to taste. You may add other supplements.

3. Niacin, a pinch, three times a day, with meals. (If you take too much, you may experience the "niacin flush", a sensation of heat and red itchy skin followed by chills. It lasts about 20 minutes and is harmless.)

4. Vitamin A (retinyl palmitate or retinyl acetate) comes as tablets and liquids, in various strengths. You need 100,000 units daily. This <u>will cause</u> a mild hypervitaminosis A (too much vitamin A) in three weeks even if accompanied by vitamin E. Expect a rash, headache, itchy skin, peeling or flaking, loss of numerous skin blemishes and warts. If symptoms appear, go off for 3 days, resume again and repeat. Put drops directly in mouth, tablets may be crushed for the vitamix if that is more convenient. **Do not exceed this dose or length of time without a doctor's supervision.**

5. Vitamin E. Take about 100 IU if not already included with vitamin A.

6. Start powdered hydrangea root, 1 tsp. two times a day to supply good germanium.

7. Measure your daily urine output. Get a gallon jug, fill with 2½ quarts or liters of water, mark the outside, and empty it again. You may also need a plastic funnel, and a pint container for collection. Catch all urine for 24 hours. If it doesn't reach the 2½ quart/liter mark, start over and drink more liquids. High volumes are needed to expel asbestos and freon. Check urinary pH upon rising in the morning. Keep notes.

8. Begin daily enemas (alternate Lugol's and black walnut tincture extra strength). If you have pain, you may use a coffee enema (filtered coffee only). These reduce bacteria levels in the bowel. Take one a day (two if very ill) using 1 pint liquid each time. See instructions, page 558.

Day 3 At A Glance

Before breakfast	One coenzyme Q10 (400 mg). Repeat parasite program, 2 tsp. black walnut tincture extra strength, 9 wormwood capsules, 9 clove capsules. Take thyroid (two grains), vitamin A (100,000 units), and vitamin E (100 IU). Open six glutathione capsules, six B_2 capsules, three magnesium oxide capsules, nine betaine hydrochloride capsules, six vitamin B_{12} capsules, 25 1 mg folic acid capsules, and $^3/_{16}$ tsp. of niacin to make today's vitamix. Mix 1 tsp. bromelain or papain and 1 tsp. powdered hydrangea root and 1 Tbs. shark cartilage and 1 fennel capsule with ½ cup water, pinch of B_2, 4 drops HCl and sweetening. Drink promptly.
Breakfast	Take 2 gm vitamin C. Mix a third of your vitamix with part of your breakfast and gulp down. Add 15 drops of hydrochloric acid to your food, putting 3 drops in each food and beverage, except water and Lugol's. Take 5 fennel capsules and 6 turmeric capsules. Finish with Lugol's (six drops).
Midmorning	Prepare the kidney herb concoction (1¼ cups) to sip throughout the day. Pour 2 cups of liver herbs to sip, too (can be combined with kidney herbs for convenience). Make a pint or more of beet juice from the recipe. Zap when convenient. Start collecting urine.
Lunch	Take 2 gm vitamin C. Mix a third of your vitamix, 15 drops of hydrochloric acid in your food, 2 Tbs. beet juice, six fennel capsules, six turmeric capsules, six drops Lugol's afterward.
Afternoon	Repeat mop-up, 4 cysteine (500 mg each). Mix 1 tsp. bromelain or papain and 1 tsp. powdered hydrangea root and 1 Tbs. shark cartilage and 1 fennel capsule with ½ cup water, pinch of B_2, 4 drops HCl and sweetening. Drink promptly.
Supper	Take 2 gm vitamin C. Add the final third of your vitamix, 15 drops of hydrochloric acid to your food, 2 Tbs. beet juice, six fennel capsules, six turmeric capsules, six drops Lugol's after meal.
Bedtime	Finish mop-up, 1 tbs. ozonated olive oil. Do an enema.

Day 4

1. Calcium, 500 mg per day. It should be taken with an acid beverage. (Your beverages are already acidified with either vitamin C, vinegar, or hydrochloric acid.) Do not take calcium supplements if your blood value is over 9.6.
2. Methionine, 500 mg, take two, three times a day.

3. Methylsulfonylmethane (MSM), 4 capsules (800 mg each) twice daily to reduce bad germanium and ferric iron to good germanium and ferrous iron.
4. Ozonated water, 2 glasses a day. This detoxifies heavy metals as they are mobilized from body fat and tissues, and kills streptococcus bacteria. It also removes acrylic acid and acrolein.
5. Vitamin B_1, 500 mg, take one, three times a day (if appetite is good, take one a day).
6. Vitamin B_6, 250 mg, take two a day.
7. Potassium gluconate, ½ teaspoon (this is 240 mg potassium), three times a day until blood potassium reaches 4.7. Then stop. Use as salt on food. Blood potassium must be monitored at least every 3 weeks.

Day 4 At A Glance

Before breakfast	One coenzyme Q10 (400 mg). Repeat parasite program, 2 tsp. black walnut tincture extra strength, 9 wormwood capsules, 9 clove capsules. Take thyroid (two grains), and vitamin A (100,000 units) plus vitamin E, 100 units. Open six glutathione capsules, six B_2 capsules, three magnesium oxide capsules, nine betaine hydrochloride capsules, six vitamin B_{12} capsules, 25 folic acid capsules, $^3/_{16}$ tsp. niacin, one 500 mg calcium capsule, six 500 mg methionine capsules, three (or one) 500 mg vitamin B_1 capsules, and two 250 mg vitamin B_6 capsules to make today's vitamix. Combine bromelain or papain and powdered hydrangea and four 800 mg MSM capsules and fennel or spice and sweetening in ½ cup water. Drink.
Breakfast	Take 2 gm vitamin C. Mix a third of your vitamix with part of your breakfast and gulp down. Add 15 drops of hydrochloric acid to your food, 2 Tbs. beet juice, six fennel capsules, six turmeric capsules, six drops Lugol's afterward. Potassium gluconate has a slightly salty taste, so "salt" your breakfast with ½ tsp. if your blood test potassium is below 4.7.
Midmorning	Prepare the kidney (1¼ cups) and liver (2 cups) herb concoctions to sip throughout the day. Zap when convenient. Empty the urine jug. If you had less than the mark, drink more liquids today and continue collecting. If you had more than the mark, continue to drink as much liquids and you can stop collecting urine. Ozonate a glass quart jar of water for about ten minutes. Drink a glassful now (no need to add hydrochloric acid).
Lunch	A pint of chicken soup, 2 gm vitamin C, another third of your vitamix, 15 drops hydrochloric acid on your food, 2

	Tbs. beet juice, six fennel capsules, six turmeric capsules, six drops Lugol's afterward. "Salt" with ½ tsp. potassium gluconate if your blood test is below 4.7.
Afternoon	Repeat mop-up, 4 cysteine (500 mg each). Combine papain, etc.
Supper	Take 2 gm vitamin C. Add the final third of your vitamix, 15 drops hydrochloric acid to your food, 2 Tbs. beet juice, six fennel capsules, six turmeric capsules, six drops Lugol's afterward. "Salt" with ½ tsp. potassium gluconate if your blood test is below 4.7.
Bedtime	Finish mop-up, 1 tbs. ozonated olive oil. Do an enema.

Day 5

1. Arginine, 500 mg, take two, three times a day.
2. Inositol, 500 mg, take two, three times a day.
3. Ornithine, 500 mg, take two, three times a day.
4. Glutamic acid, one teaspoon, three times a day (increase to heaping tsp. for liver cancer).
5. Schedule blood test five days after first one if a previous result was critical, ten days if poor, three weeks later if initial results were good.
6. Pantothenate, one teaspoon, three times a day.
7. Taurine, 500 mg, take one, three times a day.
8. Set small magnet, about 100 gauss on a ½ x 1 inch (1 x 2 cm) square of magnet cloth (see *Sources*); apply North side over the center of your spine, at base of neck. Tape on. Apply another one over the center of your spine just above the waist. Sit on N pole of strong magnet (1000 to 5000 gauss) for 30 minutes daily (see page 170).

Day 5 At A Glance

| Before breakfast | One coenzyme Q10 (400 mg). Repeat parasite program, 2 tsp. black walnut tincture extra strength, 9 wormwood capsules, 9 clove capsules. Take thyroid (two grains), and vitamin A (100,000 units) plus vitamin E, 100 units. Open six glutathione capsules, six B_2 capsules, three magnesium oxide capsules, nine betaine hydrochloride capsules, six vitamin B_{12} capsules, 25 folic acid capsules, $3/_{16}$ tsp. niacin, one calcium capsule, six methionine capsules, three (or one) vitamin B_1 capsules, two vitamin B_6 |

	capsules, six 500 mg arginine capsules, six 500 mg inositol capsules, six 500 mg ornithine capsules, 3 tsp. glutamic acid, three tsp. pantothenate, three 500 mg taurine capsules to make today's vitamix. Combine papain or bromelain, MSM, and hydrangea powder and shark cartilage. Drink at once. Assemble magnets and apply with tape. Sit on N side of big magnet for ½ hour; may zap at same time.
Breakfast	Take 2 gm vitamin C. Mix a third of your vitamix with part of your breakfast and gulp down. Distribute 15 drops hydrochloric acid on your food, 2 Tbs. beet juice, six fennel capsules, six turmeric capsules, six drops Lugol's after meal. Use ½ tsp. potassium gluconate as salt.
Midmorning	Prepare the kidney (1¼ cups) and liver (2 cups) herb concoctions to sip throughout the day. Zap when convenient. Ozonate a glass quart jar of water for about ten minutes. Drink a glassful now (no need to add hydrochloric acid).
Lunch	Take 2 gm vitamin C. Take another third of your vitamix, 15 drops hydrochloric acid on your food, 2 Tbs. beet juice, six fennel capsules, six turmeric capsules, six drops Lugol's afterward. "Salt" with ½ tsp. potassium gluconate.
Afternoon	Repeat mop-up, 4 cysteine (500 mg each). Drink another glass of ozonated water. Combine papain or bromelain, powdered hydrangea, MSM, and shark cartilage. Drink at once.
Supper	Take 2 gm vitamin C. Add the final third of your vitamix, 15 drops hydrochloric acid on your food, 2 Tbs. beet juice, six fennel capsules, six turmeric capsules, six drops Lugol's afterward. "Salt" with ½ tsp. potassium gluconate.
Bedtime	Finish mop-up, 1 tbs. ozonated olive oil. Do an enema.

Day 6

1. Amino acids, both essential and nonessential (see *Sources*), two teaspoons total (6 size 00 capsules), three times a day.
2. Glucuronic acid, 250 mg, take one, two times a day.
3. Wintergreen oil (natural only), three drops, three times a day. (Placed in empty capsule or on bread is the easiest way we have found to take it.) Do not exceed dosage; it can be toxic.
4. Biotin, 1 mg, take one a day.
5. Selenium, as raw coconut, ¼ of a coconut daily (see *Recipes*) or as sodium selenite, 500 mcg (micrograms), take six a day.
6. Niacinamide, 500 mg, take one, two times a day.

7. Oregano oil, 20 drops placed in an empty capsule, three times a day. Eat bread with it. Brush teeth with one half drop.

Day 6 At A Glance

Before breakfast	One coenzyme Q10 (400 mg each). Repeat parasite program, 2 tsp. black walnut tincture extra strength, 9 wormwood capsules, 9 clove capsules. Take thyroid (two grains), and vitamin A (100,000 units) plus vitamin E, 100 units. Open six glutathione capsules, six B_2 capsules, three magnesium oxide capsules, nine betaine hydrochloride capsules, six vitamin B_{12} capsules, 25 folic acid capsules, $^3/_{16}$ tsp. niacin, one calcium capsule, six methionine capsules, three (or one) vitamin B_1 capsules, two vitamin B_6 capsules, six arginine capsules, six inositol capsules, six ornithine capsules, 3 tsp. of glutamic acid, three tsp. pantothenate, three taurine capsules, two 500 mg niacinamide capsules, six tsp. amino acids, two 250 mg glucuronic acid capsules, and one 1 mg biotin capsule to make today's vitamix. Combine papain or bromelain, powdered hydrangea, MSM, and drink. Drink coconut beverage or add 6 500 mcg sodium selenite capsules to vitamix. Take 20 drops oregano oil.
Breakfast	Take 2 gm vitamin C. Mix a third of your vitamix with part of your breakfast and gulp down. Sprinkle 15 drops hydrochloric acid on your food, 2 Tbs. beet juice, six fennel capsules, six turmeric capsules, six drops Lugol's afterward. Use ½ tsp. potassium gluconate as salt. Have a piece of bread or empty capsule with three drops wintergreen oil. Sit on magnet.
Midmorning	Prepare the kidney (1¼ cups) and liver (2 cups) herb concoctions to sip throughout the day. Zap when convenient. Ozonate a glass quart jar of water for about ten minutes. Drink a glassful now.
Lunch	Take 20 drops oregano oil. A pint of chicken soup with 2 gm vitamin C, another third of your vitamix, 15 drops hydrochloric acid on your food, 2 Tbs. beet juice, six fennel capsules, six turmeric capsules, six drops Lugol's afterward. "Salt" with ½ tsp. potassium gluconate. Have a piece of bread or empty capsule with three drops wintergreen oil.
Afternoon	Repeat mop-up, 4 cysteine (500 mg each). Drink another glass of ozonated water. Combine papain, etc.
Supper	Take 20 drops oregano oil. Take 2 gm vitamin C. Add the final third of your vitamix, 15 drops hydrochloric acid on your food, 2 Tbs. beet juice, six fennel capsules, six turmeric capsules, six drops Lugol's afterward. "Salt" with ½ tsp. potassium gluconate. Have a piece of bread or empty capsule with three drops wintergreen oil.
Bedtime	Finish mop-up, 1 tbs. ozonated olive oil. Do an enema.

Day 7

1. Beta carotene, 15 mg (2400 units), once a day.
2. Thioctic acid, 500 mg, one a day. I think this tastes too bad too put in the vitamix. I suggest taking it separately.
3. Phytic acid (inositol phosphate, "IP6"), 50% solution, take 10 drops in a cup of water, three times a day before meals.

For prostate cancer add linseed (flax seed), 1 tablespoon daily. Rinse in bleach water (dental bleach is fine) to destroy aflatoxin and zearalenone. Then add a pinch of vitamin B_2 to remove benzene. Soak them in a beverage for 10 minutes; then stir into cereal or casserole dish. Or you may blend them in a blender. Do not use purchased linseed oil. Sterilize final serving. Also take zinc gluconate 10 to 30 mg daily.

For bone cancer add boron, 3 to 6 mg daily.

For liver cancer add silymarin, a milk thistle product. Take two, three times a day. Also drink green bitters and raw liver cocktail (see *Recipes*) once a day.

For lung cancer add "lung tea", a mixture of comfrey and mullein. Also eat one small clove of raw garlic with each meal.

Day 7 At A Glance

Before breakfast	Ten coenzyme Q10 (400 mg). Repeat parasite program, 2 tsp. black walnut tincture extra strength, 9 wormwood capsules, 9 clove capsules. Take thyroid (two grains), and vitamin A (100,000 units), plus vitamin E, 100 units. Open six glutathione capsules, six B_2 capsules, three magnesium oxide capsules, nine betaine hydrochloride capsules, six vitamin B_{12} capsules, 25 folic acid capsules, $3/16$ tsp. niacin, one calcium capsule, six methionine capsules, three (or one) vitamin B_1 capsules, two vitamin B_6 capsules, six arginine capsules, six inositol capsules, six ornithine capsules, 3 tsp. glutamic acid, three tsp. pantothenate, three taurine capsules, two niacinamide capsules, six tsp. amino acids, two glucuronic acid capsules, one biotin capsule, one 15 mg beta carotene to make today's vitamix (bone cancer add 3-6 mg boron), (liver cancer add silymarin). Combine papain or bromelain, powdered hydrangea, MSM, shark cartilage, and drink. Make coconut beverage or add

	six sodium selenite (500 mcg) to vitamix. Check magnets for snug fit against skin. Sit on big magnet.
Breakfast	Take 10 drops phytic acid in cup of water. Then take 20 drops oregano oil in capsule with bread; then take 2 gm vitamin C. Mix a third of your vitamix with part of your breakfast and gulp down. Sprinkle 15 drops hydrochloric acid on your food, 2 Tbs. beet juice, six fennel capsules, six turmeric capsules, six drops Lugol's afterward. "Salt" your breakfast with ½ tsp. potassium gluconate. Have a piece of bread or empty capsule with three drops wintergreen oil. Take one 500 mg capsule of thioctic acid.
Midmorning	Prepare the kidney (1¼ cups) and liver (2 cups) herb concoctions to sip throughout the day. Zap when convenient. Ozonate a glass quart jar of water for about ten minutes. Drink a glassful now. (Liver cancer make some green bitters and raw liver cocktail and drink as soon as made.)
Lunch	Take 10 drops phytic acid in cup water, then take 20 drops oregano oil; then take 2 gm vitamin C. Take a third of your vitamix, 15 drops hydrochloric acid on your food, 2 Tbs. beet juice, six fennel capsules, six turmeric capsules, six drops Lugol's afterward. "Salt" with ½ tsp. potassium gluconate. Have a piece of bread or empty capsule with three drops wintergreen oil.
Afternoon	Repeat mop-up, 4 cysteine (500 mg each). Drink another glass of ozonated water. For prostate cancer soak one tbs. linseed to eat with supper and take zinc gluconate. Combine papain or bromelain, powdered hydrangea, MSM, shark cartilage, and drink.
Supper	Take 10 drops phytic acid in cup water, then take 20 drops oregano oil; then take 2 gm vitamin C. Add the final third of your vitamix, 15 drops hydrochloric acid on your food, 2 Tbs. beet juice, six fennel capsules, six turmeric capsules, six drops Lugol's afterward. "Salt" with ½ tsp. potassium gluconate. Have a piece of bread or empty capsule with three drops wintergreen oil.
Bedtime	Finish mop-up, 1 tbs. ozonated olive oil. Do an enema.

Done With The First Week

You have now cleared your body tissues and body fat of parasites, bacteria, metals and carcinogens. Many tumors—those with thin walls around them—have been cleaned up, too. If you have been using the Topical Tumor Shrinker (for tumors close to the surface) you may have seen these shrink already. (If you are experiencing hypervitaminosis A symptoms, like rash, headache, redness, itchiness, flaky skin, you may wish to take a break from the topical treatments, <u>and also oral vitamin A</u>, for at least three days.)

But tumors that are hard to reach, in brain or bone marrow, or with tough coats around them have <u>not even begun</u> to spill their contents. This is fortunate since the vital organs need special protection from the tumor contents. It will be like opening the cages of lions and tigers at a zoo. Your special protectors will be glutathione, ozonated water, oregano oil, ozonated oil, and the parasite program. Because within the tumors, and <u>only within them</u>, *Fasciolopsis*, *Ascaris*, Rabbit fluke, and *Clostridium* are still alive!

We will next begin to drain the tumors, killing and detoxifying everything that emerges.

We will start with a high dose, 12 gm, of riboflavin (vitamin B_2) which will saturate the tissue around the tumor. Lower doses cannot do this. (A dose of DMSO will help the B_2 penetrate and toxins get out but is not essential.) Suddenly all the toxins break free and flow out of the tumor—into your body! Aflatoxin, zearalenone and benzene are set free; asbestos and heavy metals are set free; carcinogenic plasticizers and dyes are now free; silicone from old toothpaste and duster spray is set free; acrylic acid and acrolein are set free; the malonates are now free; flukes and *Ascaris* are set free. We will also use a magnet to set the lanthanide metals and iron free.

The flood gates have been opened. There must be enough B_2 now to combine with <u>all</u> the dyes, benzene, and acrylic acid, enough glutathione to protect the liver from <u>all</u> the aflatoxin, enough magnesium to detoxify <u>all</u> the phenol. There must be enough ozonated water to combine with <u>all</u> the metals and enough ozonated oil to kill whatever viruses escape. And, of course, all escaping parasites and bacteria must be promptly killed. Finally, there must be enough magnetic power to attract the lanthanides and the iron. After this the calcium deposits can be dissolved again with the help of phytic acid and vitamin D, letting the "digest me" flag, phosphatidyl serine, go up. Pancreatin and lipase arrive to digest both the protein portion and the acrolein fat residue remaining. Peroxidase and catalase appear, too. This tumor has now been drained and is busy being digested. Soon it cannot be distinguished from normal tissue.

Meanwhile, the more urine is produced, the faster asbestos, silicone and urethane leave the body.

If no more asbestos or dyes are eaten, you can unload one tumor-full in two to three days. During the toxic flood, vanadium will cause a globulin elevation, dyes will cause vitamin A mutations and dyes will also cause enzyme mutations that raise LDH and alk phos. Released copper, phenanthroline, and toxic germanium will lower blood iron so not enough can reach the bone marrow. So the benefit of shrinking a tumor turns into a disadvantage to your white blood cells, liver, and other vital organs who must carry the burden. We must proceed slowly. And if the LDH or alk phos rise too high, you should use IVs to help with detoxifying. Fortunately the white blood cells are regaining their power to help by "eating" everything again. This way, much less needs to be detoxified.

The liver herbs will help to send the entire toxic team on to the kidneys. And the kidney herbs will send them to the bladder. That is why you stay on these herbs as well as all the supplements.

Yet the bladder will keep them tightly stuck, allowing them to circulate back into the body unless a large amount of urine is produced. The next week you must drink enough beverages to produce <u>one gallon</u> of urine in 24 hours.

Day 8

To make it easier to take these special high doses this week you may reduce your Day 7 vitamix to $^1/_3$ (or one meal only). Each vitamix now lasts three days.

1. Glutathione, 40 capsules (20 gm) in a single dose, stirred into honey. This protects the liver from the coming aflatoxin flood which then avoids a bilirubin rise.
2. DMSO, 25% in water (optional). Take one tsp. as a mouthwash, twice daily. Swish slowly over gums. Hold several minutes. Swallow for maximum effectiveness. This "pushes" your supplements into your tissues. It also helps to draw toxins out of cavitations. You may add your wintergreen drops to this mouthwash. (50% DMSO is preferred, if available.) Must be edible quality.
3. EDTA, $^1/_8$ tsp. (750 mg) three times a day in 1 cup hot water. This chelates the heavy metals for excretion, before they can get stuck in another tissue.
4. Vitamin C, 12 gm. Take 2 gm with each meal and also between meals.
5. Vitamin B_2, 40 capsules (12 gm) stirred into honey or maple syrup (sterilized) and taken in a single dose. Take these about one hour after the glutathione. **This opens the tumors, even without DMSO or EDTA.**
6. Ozonated oil, 1 tbs. (sterilized), taken 5 hours or more after B_2. This kills viruses.
7. Black walnut tincture extra strength, 10 tsp. (or 2 freeze dried capsules four times daily, see *Sources*). 9 capsules cloves and 9 capsules wormwood once a day. Also take mop up cysteine and ozonated oil. This kills shielded parasites and emerging viruses.
8. Magnesium, 1 three times a day with meals. This detoxifies phenol produced from liberated benzene.
9. Exchange bromelain or papain for pancreatin (1 tsp.) plus lipase (1 tsp.). This will begin to digest (shrink) the tumors. Take twice a day.
10. Levamisole, 50 mg, take one three times a day. Kills *Ascaris* and keeps ferritin off white blood cells.
11. Vitamin D_3 (cholecalciferol) 25,000 units daily, to soften tumors by removing their calcium deposits.

Each high-dose day will be followed by a lower-dose day.

Day 8 At A Glance

Before breakfast	Ten coenzyme Q10 (400 mg each). (One Q10 capsule on Days 16, 18 and 20.) Take thyroid (two grains), and vitamin A (100,000 units) plus vitamin E, 100 units. Kill parasites with 10 tsp. black walnut tincture extra strength (or 2 capsules freeze dried), 9 wormwood and 9 cloves today. Take 2 gm vitamin C. Do DMSO mouthwash. Take $\frac{1}{8}$ tsp. EDTA in water. Take one Levamisole, 50 mg. Open three magnesium oxide capsules, nine betaine hydrochloride capsules, six vitamin B_{12} capsules, 25 folic acid capsules, $\frac{3}{16}$ tsp. niacin, one calcium capsule, six methionine capsules, three (or one) vitamin B_1 capsules, two vitamin B_6 capsules, six arginine capsules, six inositol capsules, six ornithine capsules, 3 tsp. of glutamic acid, three tsp. pantothenate, three taurine capsules, two niacinamide capsules, six tsp. amino acids, two glucuronic acid capsules, one biotin capsule, one beta carotene to make today's vitamix (bone cancer add 3-6 mg boron), (liver cancer add silymarin). Combine six 500 mg pancreatin, six 500 mg lipase, powdered hydrangea, MSM, and drink. Make coconut beverage and drink or take sodium selenite, 500 mcg. Take one drop vitamin D (25,000 units). Take 40 500 mg capsules of glutathione (only 20 capsules on days 15-21) stirred into a beverage.
Breakfast	Take 10 drops phytic acid in cup water, then take 20 drops oregano oil, then take 2 gm vitamin C. Mix a third of your vitamix with part of your breakfast and gulp down. Sprinkle 15 drops hydrochloric acid on your food, 2 Tbs. beet juice, six fennel capsules, six turmeric capsules, six drops Lugol's afterward. "Salt" your breakfast with ½ tsp. potassium gluconate. Have three drops wintergreen oil. Take one 500 mg capsule of thioctic acid.
Midmorning	Take 40 300 mg capsules of vitamin B_2, stirred into honey or sterilized maple syrup (only 20 capsules on days 15-21). Prepare the kidney (1¼ cups) and liver (2 cups) herb concoctions to sip throughout the day. Take another 2 gm vitamin C. Zap when convenient. Empty the urine jug and start collecting again. Drink more liquids today because your goal is one gallon! Ozonate a glass quart jar of water for about ten minutes. Drink a glassful now. (Liver cancer make some green bitters and raw liver cocktail and drink promptly.) Take $\frac{1}{8}$ tsp. EDTA in a cup of hot water. Take one Levamisole, 50 mg.
Lunch	Take 10 drops phytic acid in cup water, then take 20 drops oregano oil, then a pint of chicken soup with 2 gm vitamin C, 15 drops hydrochloric acid on your food, 2 Tbs. beet juice, six fennel capsules, six turmeric capsules, six drops Lugol's afterward. "Salt" with ½ tsp. potassium gluconate. Have three drops wintergreen oil.
Afternoon	Take 4 cysteine (500 mg each). Drink another glass of ozonated water. For prostate cancer treat and soak one tbs. linseed to eat with supper, also take zinc gluconate. If you are getting low on chicken soup, make some more.

	Combine pancreatin, lipase, powdered hydrangea root and MSM and drink with another 2 gm vitamin C. Take $\frac{1}{8}$ tsp. EDTA. Take one Levamisole, 50 mg.
Supper	Take 10 drops phytic acid in cup water, then take 20 drops oregano oil, then take 2 gm vitamin C, 15 drops hydrochloric acid on your food, 2 Tbs. beet juice, six fennel capsules, six turmeric capsules, six drops Lugol's afterward. "Salt" with ½ tsp. potassium gluconate. Have three drops wintergreen oil. Do DMSO mouthwash.
Bedtime	Take 1 tbs. ozonated olive oil. Do enema. Sit on magnet.

Day 9

Clear the toxins that emerged from your tumors yesterday using a "low dose" of glutathione and vitamin B_2. Coenzyme Q10 remains at a high dose to continue catching dyes and other toxins being released from tumors.

1. Coenzyme Q10, 10 capsules (4 gm).
2. Glutathione, 10 capsules (5 gm).
3. Vitamin C, 12 gm a day.
4. Vitamin B_2, 10 capsules (3 gm).
5. Magnesium, 1 three times a day.
6. Ozonated water, 2 glasses a day.
7. Ozonated oil, 1 tbs. a day.
8. Parasite program.

Day 9 At A Glance

Before breakfast	Ten coenzyme Q10 (400 mg each). (Only one Q10 capsule on Days 15, 17 and 21.) Take thyroid (two grains), and vitamin A (100,000 units) plus vitamin E, 100 units. Kill parasites with 10 tsp. black walnut tincture extra strength (or 2 capsules freeze dried), 9 wormwood and 9 cloves. Take 2 gm vitamin C. DO DMSO mouthwash. Take $\frac{1}{8}$ tsp. EDTA. You have 2 days of vitamix leftover from Day 8, so no need to make any. Take one 50 mg Levamisole and 1 drop vitamin D. Combine pancreatin, lipase, powdered hydrangea, MSM, shark cartilage, and drink. Make coconut beverage and drink or take six 500 mcg sodium selenite. Take <u>10</u> 500 mg capsules of glutathione stirred into honey (20 capsules on days 15-21).
Breakfast	Take 10 drops phytic acid in cup water, then take 20 drops

	oregano oil, then 2 gm vitamin C. Mix a third of your vitamix with part of your breakfast and gulp down. Sprinkle 15 drops hydrochloric acid on your food, 2 Tbs. beet juice, six fennel capsules, six turmeric capsules, six drops Lugol's after meal. "Salt" your breakfast with ½ tsp. potassium gluconate. Have a piece of banana or bread with three drops wintergreen oil. Take one 500 mg capsule of thioctic acid. (Liver cancer add silymarin.)
Midmorning	Take <u>10</u> 300 mg capsules of vitamin B_2, stirred into honey or sterilized maple syrup (20 capsules on days 15-21). Prepare the kidney (1¼ cups) and liver (2 cups) herb concoctions to sip throughout the day. Take another 2 gm vitamin C. Zap when convenient. Empty the urine jug. If you had less than <u>one gallon</u>, drink more liquids today and continue collecting. If you had more than one gallon, continue to drink as much liquids and you can stop collecting urine. Ozonate a glass quart jar of water for about ten minutes. Drink a glassful now. (Liver cancer make some green bitters and raw liver cocktail and drink promptly.) Take $^1/_8$ tsp. EDTA. Take one 50 mg Levamisole.
Lunch	Take 10 drops phytic acid in cup water, then take 20 drops oregano oil, then 2 gm vitamin C, 15 drops hydrochloric acid on your food, 2 Tbs. beet juice, six fennel capsules, six turmeric capsules, six drops Lugol's afterward. "Salt" with ½ tsp. potassium gluconate. Have three drops wintergreen oil.
Afternoon	Take 4 cysteine (500 mg each). Drink another glass of ozonated water. For prostate cancer, soak one tbs. treated linseed to eat with supper. Combine pancreatin, lipase, powdered hydrangea, MSM, shark cartilage, and drink with another 2 gm vitamin C. Do DMSO mouthwash. Take $^1/_8$ tsp. EDTA. Take one 50 mg Levamisole.
Supper	Take 10 drops phytic acid in cup water, then take 20 drops oregano oil, then 2 gm vitamin C, 15 drops hydrochloric acid on your food, 2 Tbs. beet juice, six fennel capsules, six turmeric capsules, six drops Lugol's afterward. "Salt" with ½ tsp. potassium gluconate. Have three drops wintergreen oil.
Bedtime	Take 1 tbs. ozonated olive oil. Do an enema. Sit on magnet.

Day 10, 12, 14

Repeat day 8.

Continue to alternate high dose and low dose vitamin B_2 and glutathione treatments.

Make a quadruple batch of vitamix (12 days' worth) for convenience.

Don't forget to go for your blood tests. Continue wearing the magnets and sitting on the big magnet.

Day 11, 13

Repeat day 9.

Day 15 To 21

Continue repeating Day 8 on even days (16, 18, 20) and Day 9 on odd days (15, 17, 19, 21), except change glutathione to 10 gm (twenty 500 mg capsules), and vitamin B_2 to 6 gm (twenty 300 mg capsules) every day. This is a compromise between high and low doses in order to accomplish some of each. Also reduce coenzyme Q10 to one capsule (400 mg) except Day 19.

If you were using the Topical Tumor Shrinkers, and you took last week off (because of hypervitaminosis A) you may be ready to resume (including oral vitamin A).

How Well Did You Do?

How do you know you have opened and detoxified all your tumors? Each high dose day drains one tumor, so five tumors require about 10 days. Numerous small ones occasionally open together. If you have 4 or 5 large tumors, chances are they will open one at a time; this is an advantage. You should wait till the liver and kidney have recovered somewhat as seen on a blood test (steady transaminases, GGT, and bilirubin) before opening the next one. The proof that tumors are gone is only seen on a scan. The proof that toxicity is gone is only seen on the blood test (LDH, alkaline phosphatase, globulin and iron are completely normal). This will not happen unless even small leftover bits of dyes, asbestos, inorganic germanium and lanthanides have left the body. They may be stuck in the lysosomes or nucleus of the liver cells or tumor cells, still causing mutations and still keeping the blood levels abnormal. Continue the program until these tests are normal. The chance is quite good that it will happen by the 21st day!

It is time to assess the results.

---

1. Review your latest blood test.
2. Review a new scan.
3. Compare pain level.
4. Compare functional level, appetite, and energy.

All these results should show beginning improvement. If they did not, you reinfected too frequently with parasites or bacteria. If dental work is not complete, this could explain the bacterial reinfection. You should also assume you are reinfecting with parasites from raw unsterilized food. If you are not in absolute control of this, stop eating raw food. Start over again. Repeat the parasite killing program, plus mop-up on the same schedule as before. Assume you still have a tooth infection even if the pain is somewhere else. Find a dentist using digital X-rays to be sure there is no leftover plastic or a tattoo. If you see a suspicious site, use DMSO again as mouthwash, plus EDTA and vitamin C as before to draw out the toxins. Be sure to include the magnet therapy. If your mouth has the odor of decay, water pick for a whole day, one half hour on and one half hour off. Stop taking any supplement that is not listed. Stop using any herb or spice or supplement from a can or bottle unless it is treated with vitamin B$_2$ and hydrochloric acid. Stop using a cosmetic or hair dye for which you did not find a substitute. Wear no unwashed, unbleached clothing. Of course, you have been reinfecting from your own draining tumors, too, which is unavoidable. Continue the high-dose, low-dose alternating regimen for vitamin B$_2$ and glutathione during the third week if the scan still shows the original tumors. If diarrhea occurs, reduce glutathione to half and take with meals (also see page 141 for diarrhea).

Continued Care

If symptoms have subsided and the scan and blood test show improvement, continue the supplements at a reduced level of your own choosing. Half doses are suitable for a second three week period. But vitamin B$_2$, glutathione, vitamin C, and coenzyme Q10 should be continued as in the third week, until the blood test is perfect.

Occasionally, the blood test does not become normal due to an unforeseen toxin. Lead from polluted supplements are responsible for high transaminases. Vanadium, lanthanides and dyes from dental plastic will keep globulin, LDH and alkaline phosphatase high. Reinfection with *Ascaris* will keep iron low. Search teeth for remaining plastic using digital X-rays. Then use DMSO and EDTA again along with magnet therapy. It is now time to focus on gaining weight. Weigh yourself twice a week.

Gaining weight is the single mysterious event your body can accomplish if it is well. Only the body knows what this means. We must try to listen and hear our bodies' requests.

Your body may crave sugar now. Your liver is not yet able to make and store sugar or change stored sugar to blood sugar. You must eat often, plenty of simple starches and fats. This means potatoes, sweet potatoes, home made bread, pasta, fruits, and vegetables, and their juices. 4000 calories per day is a proper goal! Adding dairy foods (Kosher only, properly sterilized), will help you reach this.

Getting your appetite back is a very good sign. Hopefully, this happened in the first week. If not, be sure to stay on the B vitamins.

Eat to gain weight. Even one pound of weight gain indicates a return of health. Digestive enzymes (see *Sources*) can help greatly in relieving an over-full feeling, especially when supplements take up so much "room". Take 3 or 4 with each meal.

Take them between meals, too. But hydrochloric acid helps digestion most. Do not stop using this to sterilize your food (even Kosher food). Often you must force yourself to eat, if you plan to become healthy. Use whatever tricks and entreaties work for you. Aim to gain two pounds a week after the first three week program is completed.

Congratulations!

You have accomplished what few others have. Throw yourself a party when the last tumor is gone! And buy a truly exceptional gift for your caregiver.

What if it fails? What if LDH and alkaline phosphatase keep rising? What if liver enzymes keep rising? Or any other blood value keeps worsening? This can happen if detoxification can't keep up with tumor drainage. In spite of taking "bushels" of supplements to detoxify, it may not succeed. In this case, seek out IV therapy. Use the entire set of IVs (filtered) listed every day. Keep urine flow high. Do more enemas. It may take three weeks of daily IVs to catch up on opening tumors, but it <u>will</u> happen.

Reading Your Blood Test Results

You can help your doctor or health professional immensely by learning to understand your own blood test results. You might also wish to remain discreetly silent about it in order not to offend him/her. There is an element of mystique created around test results in order to keep them off-limits to patients and hold them hostage. I believe this practice is archaic. Not only can you learn to interpret blood test results, you can learn not to panic or take up doctors' time needlessly. Sharpen this new talent on all the blood test results given for the case histories, and then apply it to yourself. Remember, though, not to add your state of psychological distress over reading your own blood test to your doctor's burden. Find solace in the fact that you are going to learn to solve most problems yourself, right now!

Your blood test results are easy to understand, although the form looks complicated. In one column, your results are given. In another column the expected "normal" results are given. The normal results will be given as a <u>range</u> because healthy people can be expected to vary to some extent. Your first step is to fit your result into the normal range given on your printout to see whether it is above, below, or in the middle of it.

The Perfect Blood Test

<u>Photocopy the next page</u> and use it as a bookmark and reference while reading this chapter and the case histories (*True Stories*) that follow.

Fold in half twice lengthwise then across middle.

Test	Healthy range by our clinic standard	Units	Our lab range (for comparison)
WBC	5.5 - 7.5	thous/uL	4.0 - 10.0
RBC	4.4 - 4.7	MIL/mm^3	4.5-6.5
platelet count	200- 300	thous/uL	150-450
eosinophils	<3	%	
blasts	0	%	0
glucose (fasting)	85-95	mg/dL	65-115
BUN	15 - 16	mg/dL	5.0-26.0
creatinine	0.9 - 1.0	mg/dL	0.6-1.4
AST or SGOT	12	U/L	0-55
ALT or SGPT	12	U/L	0-55
GGT	12	U/L	0-57
Total bilirubin	≤ 1.0	mg/dL	0.1-1.8
uric acid	3.0 - 4.0	mg/dL	2.2-7.7
cholesterol	200 plus your age	mg/dL	130-200*
triglycerides	100 - 200	mg/dL	30-180
sodium	138 -142	m Eq/L	133-145
potassium	4.5 - 4.7	m Eq/L	3.3-5.6
chloride	98 - 104	m Eq/L	95-111
calcium	9.1 - 9.6	mg/dL	8.5-10.4
phosphorus	3.0 - 4.0	mg/dL	2.2-5.6
Total protein (T.p.)	7.0 - 7.4	gm/dL	6.3-8.3
albumin	4 - 4.6	gm/dL	3.9-5.1
globulin	2.5 - 2.8	gm/dL	2.0-5.0
LDH	125 - 160	U/L	91-250
alkaline phosphatase (alk phos)	75 - 85	U/L	39-117
total iron (serum)	75 - 105	ug/dL	30-170
HGB		gm/dL	13.5-18.0
carbon dioxide		m Eq/L	12.0-33.0

*Cholesterol range not statistically set, see text.

Common abbreviations

alk phos	alkaline phosphatase	HGB	hemoglobin
ALT	alanine amino transferase	K	potassium
AST	aspartate aminotransferase	LD or LDH	lactic dehydrogenase
BUN	blood urea nitrogen	Na	sodium
Ca	calcium	P	phosphorus
chol	cholesterol	plt	platelet
Cl	chloride	RBC	red blood corpuscles
CO$_2$	carbon dioxide	T.b.	total bilirubin
creat	creatinine	T.p.	total protein
FBS	fasting blood sugar or glucose	trig	triglycerides
GGT	gamma glutamyl transpeptidase	WBC	white blood cells

Blood Sugar

Take *glucose* (blood sugar), for example. The range given by our lab was usually 65 to 115 mg/dL. If your value was 95, using this range, it is exceptionally good. To understand the meaning of a result using a different range, you should know how the range was decided.

One of the very large testing labs analyses the blood sugar results for, say, the last 10,000 patients it has tested. It is assumed that they represent the healthy population (which is, of course, not true, since illness brought them to the lab for testing to begin with). The <u>average</u> blood sugar level is found. Then ninety-five percent of all these patients' results are clustered around this average to make a "normal curve". Five percent are thrown away as representing abnormal levels. The lowest and highest levels for these 95% are used to give the range.[111]

This is far from a true standard of good health. It assumes that 95% of the population is healthy. If, in reality, only 80% are healthy, very many people are not being attended and consequently not being alerted to the need for improvement because they are assigned to the "normal" group. Preventive health care is not being served.

A concept of "sick" or "not sick" depending on whether you fit into the values seen for 95% of the patient population is misleading. It is like defining overweight as over 500 pounds (200 kg)! A wrong concept such as this does a disservice to society. Don't let a physician's reassurance that "everything is normal" fool you into thinking you are normal (meaning healthy). Your standard should be higher than "statistically normal," your standard should be "healthy."

In this book, the true, healthy values will be given **as I perceive them**, together with their correct meaning, so you can take steps to help any organ that is weak. I determined them by observing at least two thousand patients closely, most with a series of tests that spanned a period from the time they arrived with

---

[111] Berkow, R., Ed., *The Merck Manual* 16th ed., Merck Research Lab., 1992, p. 2573.

illness to a later time when they were well again. It is based on judgment, not statistics, and it wouldn't surprise me if others disagree with me. However the body stays surprisingly constant when it is healthy, making the task of identifying healthy values fairly easy.

Sometimes your laboratory will have a wildly different range for a particular test than the ranges I have listed, even though the units are identical! That is because there are different types of tests for the same substance. You should scale your result, then, before comparing it to the ranges in my chart. For example if your lab's range goes from 240 to 380 but our lab's range goes from 120 to 200, you can assume that your lab's procedures roughly double the results. Therefore you must divide your result in half before comparing it to our lab's range.

Let us return to the blood sugar, glucose. It should never be lower than 80 mg/DL whether you have fasted before the test or not. The liver should always be able to make blood sugar for you, even if you have not eaten recently. The liver stores a reserve of blood sugar for this purpose. If yours is below eighty, the liver is not able to keep your level up, either because its stores are empty, or for other reasons.

Cancer patients have a special disability in that part of their liver metabolism that makes and stores blood sugar. At the same time, cancer patients use up more blood sugar than normal, healthy persons, so the blood sugar drops as cancer advances. As you recover, the liver will regain this function. If your blood sugar is already below seventy, you must eat throughout the day to re-nourish your body. Your body must be nourished to heal. You should eat the richest, most nourishing (but safe) foods you can find. If your blood sugar is over 90, you are still in good condition. You must work hard to eat enough high calorie, nutritious food to keep this figure from dropping.

There are only three categories of foods: carbohydrate, fat, and protein. All your carbohydrate foods, potatoes, rice, grains, pasta, vegetables, and fruit, are turned into blood sugar by the body's chief factory, the liver.

Why couldn't we simply eat glucose (also called dextrose, or confectioner's sugar) to supply it all? Because there are many food-factors packed into ordinary foods that you would miss by eating plain sugar. Nevertheless, if no food can be digested, a beverage of honey water or maple syrup in water will sustain you for several days, until you are able to eat. If vitamins, minerals, amino acids, fats, and a few extra nutrient factors are added, you can be sustained for six weeks, plenty of time for tumors pressing on the liver or intestine to shrink enough to let regular food pass again. If you are a caregiver and your patient refuses all food, make a "complete food" in beverage form (see *Recipes*).

If your blood sugar is much too high, due to diabetes, in addition to cancer, consider yourself lucky, especially if somewhat obese. This means you have not gone through your reserves yet. Do not try to lose weight even if you are overweight. Your diabetes will improve while on this program; it may even be cured. It is most important not to eat artificial sugar or calorie-reduced food. You must nourish your body better than ever before to heal from your cancer. You must eat three regular meals and three snacks a day to help your body heal itself. As your diabetes improves, your weight might drop drastically, effortlessly.

CBC

CBC stands for **complete blood count**. A small amount of blood is dispensed into the automatic counter to determine how many of each kind of blood cell you have.

There are three kinds, **white blood cells**, **red blood corpuscles**, and **platelets**, but they are all made from the same original "baby cells" in the bone marrow, called *stem cells*. Stem cells are constantly multiplying to provide us with these three kinds of blood cells.

White Blood Cells (WBC)

These cells are our defense team. One type has the ability to crawl (by means of pseudopodia!), squeeze through tiny spaces, respond to something dead or toxic far away by moving toward it, and simply eat it to destroy it. These are called **granulocytes** (and also called "segs" or "polymorphs" or "neutrophils") and should constitute about seventy percent of your total WBC. About twenty percent are smaller, rounder, and capable of destroying viruses; those are the **lymphocytes**. The lymphocytes are further divided into T and B lymphocytes, named after the thymus or the bone marrow. Lymphocytes get their "final training" at one of these two organs. The last 10% of your WBCs are other varieties.

Your total WBC count should not be below 5,000/mm^3 (same as 5,000/uL). Any amount below this implies a <u>toxin in the bone marrow</u>. Toxins abound. Heavy metals and azo dyes are especially attracted to your bone marrow probably because of its high fat content. (Metals and dyes are fat soluble.) Lead, mercury, thallium, nickel, germanium, copper, cobalt and vanadium are commonplace. These consume your sulfur supply, especially glutathione. Then bacteria and even parasites are allowed in. Many of these metals and dyes were found to be carcinogens decades ago.

Carcinogens have a special affinity for the stem cell line in the bone marrow that makes white blood cells, probably because they are constantly in mitosis. Scarlet Red dye (Sudan IV), Sudan Black B, DAB, and other dyes are commonly found here by the Syncrometer. Hydroxyurea is found here too if *Ascaris* is present. Hydroxyurea specifically <u>kills</u> stem cells. Copper[112] and lanthanide metals[113,114] cause very large mutations,

---

[112] Yamamoto, K., Kawanishi, S., *Hydroxyl Free Radical Is Not the Main Active Species in Site-specific DNA Damage Induced by Copper(II) Ion and Hydrogen Peroxide*, Journal of Biological Chemistry, v. 264, no. 26, 1989, pp. 15435-40.

[113] Eichhorn, G.L., Butzow, J.J., *Degradation of Polyribonucleotides by Lanthanum Ions*, Biopolymers, v. 3, 1965, pp. 79-94.

[114] Das, T., Sharma, A., Talukder, G., *Effects of Lanthanum in Cellular Systems, A Review*, Biological Trace Element Res., v.18, 1988, pp. 201-28.

breaking the chromosomes at characteristic places. This is, no doubt, how the "Philadelphia chromosome" and other translocations are induced. We have found that this mutation disappears when synthetic dyes are removed from food, teeth, hair and clothing, vanadium is removed from teeth, and copper water pipes are changed.

When the WBC count is much too high, over 15,000, it may represent leukemia. The simple step of changing copper water pipes often corrects the problem in its early stages. But when the WBC is over 30,000, much more must be done quickly. Removing all plastic and metal from teeth, killing parasites and bacteria can reduce the count to 20,000 in ten days. Removing all dyes brings it down further. At this point it is important to provide selenium and vitamin A. Your WBCs need these to battle pathogens.

Special caution to avoid benzene is essential to get back your normal WBC count, whether too high or too low. Benzene goes preferentially to the bone marrow and thymus where WBCs are "nesting". A list of benzene polluted foods and products is given in *The Cure For All Cancers*, however an easy rule of thumb is not to eat or use processed products, or ones that involve petroleum (as in pesticide residue and waxed fruit), nor to drink bottled water.

There should never be any **blasts** in your CBC. These are baby white cells, allowed out into the circulation before they are mature enough. It always signals overproduction (namely leukemia) in the bone marrow.

The healthy level of WBCs is 5.5 to 7.5 thousand per mm^3. (A mm^3, also written as uL, is about the size of a poppy seed.) While levels below five reflect a toxin in the bone marrow, levels above this range reflect overproduction. This could be due to stimulation by bacteria. This alerts you to an infection somewhere.

The **eosinophil** count should be ≤ (less than) 3%; higher values imply the presence of parasites, particularly *Ascaris* and your body's "allergic" response to them.

When the WBC is extremely low (below four) immunity is much too low. You are susceptible to any invader. Levels below three are life-threatening. But even levels as low as 1.5 have been quickly doubled (in six weeks) by avoiding benzene, doing dental work and killing parasites.

Red Blood Corpuscles (RBC)

The healthy level of red blood cells is 4.4 to 4.6 million per mm^3 for both men and women. We have been taught that 5 million is the perfect result, especially for men. This is not correct. All levels higher than 4.6 are the result of cobalt and/or vanadium toxicity! These toxicities are very common. The Syncrometer detects the element vanadium in the bone marrow, liver and other vital organs when fossil fuel is breathed chronically, as with gas or oil heat. Of course, the cleaner the furnace burns, the cleaner the air remains. A dust sample taken off the kitchen table in the morning can be tested for vanadium with the Syncrometer. Vanadium could come from the gas stove or leaking refrigerant. Humans should not be inhaling vanadium mist constantly. Although there is plenty of vanadium in the dust and dirt outdoors, it does not accumulate in us to a detectable level from this exposure. Even worse than fossil fuel pollution, is sucking on objects day and night that release vanadium, namely tooth prostheses (fillings, caps, root canals, crowns).

Cobalt causes the same deceptive elevation in the RBC level.

The RBC count is a <u>masked</u> value. Certain toxins elevate it, while other toxins lower it. If they occur together, a middle value is reached which appears to be in mid-range, and is, therefore, considered normal and "healthy." Carcinogenic food dyes target the bone marrow. *Anemia* (low RBC) results. The anemia is not noticed when the RBC count is artificially elevated by cobalt and vanadium. Are we a nation of anemic people, lulled into complacency by falsely high RBC levels?

The RBC level can rise to normal or drop to normal in five days, after removing cobalt and vanadium! We have been trained to believe that it moves very slowly, taking months to achieve a significant change. This is true when iron is being supplemented to <u>force</u> a rise in RBC level. When so many toxic forces are acting, the RBC level can only move very slowly. But when toxins and parasites are removed the RBC moves toward normal very swiftly.

When hydroxyurea and carcinogenic azo dyes are no longer bathing the bone marrow (after the parasite treatment and dental cleanup) an "anemia of long-standing" or "anemia of chronic disease" or "anemia of unknown origin", (such as an RBC of 3.4) frequently rises 0.5 units in five days! These "anemia" labels are given to indicate "mysterious" diseases but are simply caused by toxicities.

If the RBC falls below 3.0 a transfusion must be obtained promptly (the same day). Some hematologists focus on the <u>hemoglobin</u> level rather than the RBC to assess the need for transfusion. This might result in waiting too long. I recommend giving transfusions a bit too early rather than a bit too late.

When the RBC or hemoglobin drops too low, not enough oxygen is delivered to your tissues. If not enough oxygen reaches the heart, it can be permanently damaged. Heart failure is not far away. It is best to get two units of blood together and raise the RBC to a comfortable level for your body, rather than to skimp along on one unit received more often. To heal, your body needs <u>lots</u> of oxygen, not a survival amount. Use your transfusion time wisely; it is "borrowed". Hurry to clear parasites, bacteria, artificial teeth, and environmental toxins out of your body. You may request *erythropoietin* from your clinical physician to help build blood temporarily.

If your religion does not allow you to accept a blood transfusion, find a hospital that has experience with your circumstances—the Chamber of Commerce is always willing to help. If your bone marrow has been killed by radiation, a transplant may be necessary. Often your own marrow can still grow back if you make every effort.

Take vitamin E (400 units, see *Sources*) and calcium (1000 mg) daily if you are getting blood transfusions. It seems a wise policy to toughen the RBC walls and to support clotting. Be patient with your bone marrow. We have seen a patient recover after getting fifty transfusions.

Although we use "blood builders," they are not effective if the toxins still remain so all effort should be focused on removing toxins.

Platelet Count

You should have 200,000 to 300,000 platelets in a mm^3 (uL) of blood. A count below this implies a toxin in the bone marrow where they are made, or a destruction process going on after they arrive in your blood. An allergic response may cause platelets to burst and be suddenly gone, too. When platelets are sparse, not enough clotting action is present in blood. Surprisingly, our blood vessels spring leaks all the time, and must be patched by platelets. Numerous small bleeds do not get patched, and are allowed to develop, when the platelet count drops below 100,000. If dental work is necessary and platelets are below 100,000, a dose of platelets should be given just a few hours before the appointment (not sooner).

Platelets should be given before the mouth and gums are bleeding. Removing copper, cobalt, vanadium and azo dyes restores the bone marrow's ability to make platelets again.

As the platelet count drops below 10,000, emergency care is needed. Extra precaution against copper toxicity is now most important. Every food, every supplement, all water, every drug must be tested for copper before it is given to the patient as a double precaution against pollution. Large doses of magnesium (magnesium oxide, 300 mg, three a day) will slow platelet destruction.

Of course, dental extractions to remove the copper, cobalt, vanadium, and germanium will trigger the very bleeding that is necessitating platelet transfusions. But time is of the essence— every minute counts now. Without the dental clean-up, death is certain. With the dental work, survival is at least possible. Dental surgery should be done in a hospital where blood and platelets can be immediately given, bleeding stopped by clinical means and other emergencies attended to.

High platelet levels such as over 400,000 results in too much clotting activity; the blood will run sluggishly because it is too viscous and therefore does not deliver enough oxygen and food to the cells. A small amount of niacin ($^1/_{16}$ teaspoon or a pinch) and an equally small dose of aspirin (½ baby aspirin) are given three times a day to thin the blood in this case. Platelet counts of 500,000 to 800,000 tell us there is a small amount of bleeding going on chronically somewhere in your body (the body is trying to stop it by clotting it!) The bleeding should be searched for. However, often the platelet count does not go up, as expected, so bleeding must be guessed at by watching the RBC to see if it is steadily dropping.

BUN and Creatinine

BUN stands for **blood urea nitrogen**—namely, how much urea is in the blood. Since the kidneys excrete urea, we have mistakenly thought that high levels in the blood imply kidney disease and low levels imply extra-good kidney function. Neither concept is correct.

I have found that high urea levels imply a bacterial infection somewhere and low levels mean there is a block in its formation. When your body cannot form urea, there is serious trouble ahead; yet it has routinely been interpreted as "extra-good" kidney function.

The bacteria that raise the BUN most are the exceptionally bad ones, *Clostridium* varieties. Others add their part, too. Bacteria make copious amounts of ammonia which is extremely toxic to us. (It has the odor of a diaper pail.) So our bodies catch the ammonia and make urea out of it, so it can leave our bodies quickly. Urea is removed from the blood by the kidneys and bladder.

When your BUN is quite near or actually <u>over</u> the top of the range, you must quickly kill bacteria. The main sources, of course, are decaying teeth and your bowel contents. Use the techniques discussed; tooth extraction, betaine supplement, hydrochloric acid, enemas, Lugol's, turmeric, and fennel to quickly reduce your bacterial burden. Double or quadruple the kidney herb recipe until you can produce 1 to 1½ gallons of urine in 24 hours. The BUN should drop in a week.

A BUN that continues to rise becomes life threatening. At higher levels such as over 50, urea begins to damage the tissues, including the kidney itself. If the kidney becomes damaged, BUN will rise still further and dialysis must be used as a stop gap measure until kidney health recovers.

A BUN level over 55 often brings dizziness and delirium, yet some persons can endure a level of 80! There are many ways of clearing up this condition, even at this late stage. Take numerous (four) enemas in a day. Help the kidneys by stopping all malonate consumption—methyl malonate is <u>the</u> kidney toxin. Detoxify it with as much vitamin C as you can tolerate. Cysteine is a specific kidney helper (take two 500 mg capsules three times a day for several weeks). But first of all, kill parasites and start taking the increased amounts of Kidney Cleanse recipe. All the <u>clinical</u> techniques for lowering BUN (hydration, etc.) should be used, too.

BUN levels can be too low for many years without you being aware of it. A test result that is near the bottom of the range or below is too low. There is a block in the urea synthesis cycle somewhere, probably in the liver. Malonic acid can do some blocking; toxins produced by bacteria themselves may contribute; dyes also block urea formation.

In my observation, the ammonia that is blocked from making urea is forced to make pyrimidines—the very nucleic acids that unbalance the ratio of purine to pyrimidine bases.

If the BUN corrects itself, but then goes to an extreme again, search for the same causes as before—they have probably returned!

Creatinine is more truly a test of kidney function than BUN. Yet, creatinine formation can be blocked too, and be extra low. Again, this does not imply extra good kidneys!

Since creatinine is made from creatine, an extra low value could mean too little creatine is being made, or at least left in the body. Too little would be made if the necessary ingredients are in short supply. The ingredients are glycine, arginine and methyl groups donated by SAM. Malonic acid toxicity shortens the supply of these. Without enough creatine turning into creatinine, blood levels must be low.

Creatine is muscle food. Some cancer patients waste a lot of their creatine because the muscles are unable to use it. So it is excreted. Again, there is very little left to turn into creatinine, giving the appearance of "extra-good kidneys." The amount in your blood should not be less than 0.9. Even this value is "too good," since it is the level of young healthy persons. If you have cancer and yet have a creatinine level that is very low, you can guess that you are unable to make enough creatine or are wasting it in the urine. Stop eating malonic acid foods immediately and get the malonate (plastic) out of your dentalware. In the meantime, supplement yourself with shark cartilage and amino acids, both essential and non-essential.

Creatinine levels rise when the kidneys fail to clear it from the blood. A level of 1.4 should not be exceeded. If it goes above this, vigorous help for the kidneys should be obtained at once. The Kidney Cleanse, starting with the usual dose but doubling it (or quadrupling it) after a few days helps most. Lots of water (at least two quarts/liters a day) helps. Cysteine (three grams a day) and lysine (five grams a day) are especially useful supplements. Alkalinizing your body with ½ teaspoon baking soda or sodium/potassium bicarbonate mix (two parts baking soda, to one part potassium bicarbonate) at bedtime helps the kidneys, too. Sometimes a drug is responsible for kidney failure. To test this all drugs should be eliminated or substituted with an equivalent variety for at least a few days to see if the creatinine will fall. If the kidneys respond and creatinine levels drop, do not go back to earlier drugs. Even a creatinine level over 5.0 can be reduced to safe levels again in these simple ways.

But clinical help should be requested before it rises above 3.0. This will buy you a small window of time; use it wisely—to extract rotten teeth or get plastic out of teeth, kill bacteria and parasites, change diet, and find drug replacements.

Liver Enzymes

The liver is the body's main manufacturing plant so its health is reflected in our health. When the liver gets sick, we get sick. That is why nearly half of the blood tests done are actually liver tests, in some form. The liver can regenerate new cells and keep itself repaired! Old worn out cells must die to facilitate this rejuvenation. If the liver is injured chemically, many more cells will die. If they die, they release their enzymes into the blood stream. Three common enzymes are:

1. **AST** (aspartate amino transferase), also known as SGOT.
2. **ALT** (alanine amino transferase), also known as SGPT.
3. **GGT** (gamma glutamyl transpeptidase).

The two transferases go up quite readily when there is any kind of liver disease or when drugs are used, since drugs are toxins to the liver—meaning that liver cells are killed. If your transferases, also called transaminases, are going up, a liver toxin is present and you must search, even amongst your "natural" supplements for a toxin. The Syncrometer usually detects lead polluting vitamins or herbal concoctions in such cases. For this reason, only tested supplements are recommended for your use. If your transaminases are over 70, and rising, don't wait; try going off all supplements for five days to see if the transaminases will fall. If not, replace all your drugs, too, with substitutes for five days.

Sometimes an essential drug such as a heart drug or anti-seizure drug is responsible for the elevated transaminases. Even if the transaminases merely climb over 70 U/L, replacement prescriptions should be requested from your doctor.

Transaminases over 350 can still be brought down to safety, if you act quickly. But if they soar higher, liver failure is in progress. You must make every effort to help the liver. (Seek out IV therapy.)

The GGT reflects a different liver function. I have not yet found the cause of its elevation in cancer patients.

All three enzymes should be below 25 U/L. (It is unrealistic to expect to see the truly healthy level of 12 in a cancer patient. Some damage may be permanent.) If yours are elevated, try to find the cause. You can be pleasantly surprised just by stopping painkillers and substituting other anti-pain measures. Changing pain killers sometimes works. Using two or three different pain killers, each in a small amount, also may work to lower your liver enzymes. Don't give up, even if your GGT is over 1000; it can still be corrected.

Total bilirubin (T.b.)

It is the liver's job to detoxify the hemoglobin that is salvaged from old worn out red blood cells.

Since red blood cells have a life span of only 120 days, about one percent of them die each day, and must be trapped by the spleen in order to salvage certain parts. Their iron must be salvaged. Their hemoglobin must be conjugated (detoxified), and excreted as bilirubin in the bile. If the liver is not capable of conjugation or the bile ducts are blocked, raw (undetoxified) bilirubin builds up in the circulation. You can detect a yellowish tint first in the whites of the eyes. It is called *jaundice*.

There is no time to lose. If your T.b. is over 1.0, there is a serious problem. The problem can be corrected if the T.b. has not gone too high. Most of the time, the problem is aflatoxin toxicity. Stop at once eating all grains, including rice, bread, pasta, cereals, and popcorn. Only oatmeal and corn on the cob present no danger from aflatoxins. Also eat no food that could be moldy: all nuts and many fruits and anything fermented. Five days of complete relief will get the T.b. moving downwards.

You must stay on this restrictive diet until the T.b. is back to 1.0; then return to normal food slowly—watching the T.b.

If your T.b. hovers around 0.9 to 1.0, you are too close to the brink of jaundice. Reduce grains; go off nuts, whole wheat, and brown rice.

The most insidious source of aflatoxins is the inside of your own tumors. From here they leak out slowly to reach your liver where the harm is done. But this ends when the tumor contents are detoxified. Sometimes a high T.b. is due to obstruction of bile ducts by tumors pressing against them. This is a clinical emergency. A bypass (stent) can be put in place to help them drain again. While waiting for this surgery, do the entire tumor-shrinking program. Shrinkage can begin in twenty-four hours. When the bowel movement regains its dark color, you know the bile is draining again. HCl drops may be maximized to stimulate bile secretion. Coffee enemas also stimulate bile formation. Taking glucuronic acid as a supplement may help the liver do its conjugation.

When the T.b. reaches thirty, it can still be filtered out of your blood in a clinical procedure. It is important not to let it get higher, since it may damage your other organs. It also helps to give albumin by IV, one bottle (12.5 gm) daily to absorb some of it. Exposure to direct sunlight for one hour seems to help our patients. Raised levels of glutathione (20 gm per day) and vitamin C (3 tsp. or 15 gm per day) help the liver the most with this severe jaundice (if these levels give you diarrhea, spread them out over the day). Do not give up even if T.b. reaches fifty! You may be improving your situation, namely curing your cancer, and yet not losing your jaundice. The pigment seems tightly stuck in your tissues for some time. Be patient. Do the program meticulously.

Uric Acid

When a cell dies the body wisely recycles it by breaking it down, keeping what can be reused, and getting rid of the rest.

When the body breaks down nucleic acids, specifically, their purine bases are turned into uric acid, which must be excreted through your kidneys. Traditionally, a high uric acid level in the blood is thought to be bad (and even causes gout), while a low uric acid level is thought to be good, reflecting efficient kidneys.

But in cancer, the uric acid level is often <u>much</u> too low, and again, this is not due to having superior kidneys. I think it is because there is a lack of purine bases that uric acid comes from. Certainly the Syncrometer detects no purine bases in tumorous organs.

Why is your body short on purines? The correct answer must wait for more research, but five possible explanations come to mind:

1. Bacteria are eating the purines.
2. Excess ammonia is making too many pyrimidine bases. This in turn is using up an equal number of purines (all of them, in fact) when double strands of nucleic acid are being made.
3. Purines can't be made because they require glutamine, and glutamine is being destroyed by glutaminase, and glutaminase production is being stimulated by malonic acid.
4. A blocked <u>urea</u> synthesis cycle may be related to low uric acid levels. Cancer patients typically reveal low urea levels (BUN), implying cycle blockage, and when urea is fed, the uric acid level rises, too.
5. Maybe <u>some</u> purines exist, but the enzyme, xanthine oxidase, which transforms purine bases into uric acid, is missing.

It's even possible that <u>all</u> of the above are responsible in varying degrees! But if I had to pick a single culprit, it would be *Clostridium*. Every time the uric acid level is too low, the Syncrometer finds *Clostridium* bacteria present in some tissue. As soon as they are killed, purines and xanthine oxidase are again present, and the uric acid level rises to a more normal value!

Even if you are perfectly healthy, would having low uric acid levels be good? Maybe not. Uric acid is not a useless waste item, merely to be eliminated. In other animals it goes on to make allantoin, a healing agent. We are taught that this does not occur in humans. Yet, the Syncrometer routinely detects allantoin; it must surely occur at a low level. With very low levels of uric acid, perhaps we fail to make any of this beneficial and mysterious substance.

Another possible benefit of uric acid is that it is itself a purine, and as such would have solvent action on PAHs. Therefore uric acid may draw PAHs along with it into the intestines or kidneys and out of your body. The ultra low levels of uric acid in cancer patients may have allowed dispersal of PAH-like mutagens throughout the body.

Uric acid levels can be manipulated. Supplementing glutamine raises it by increasing purine synthesis. We prefer to give glutamic acid, though, since this turns into glutamine by picking up a molecule of ammonia, thereby helping to dispose of ammonia at the same time. It takes three to ten grams a day of glutamic acid to raise the uric acid level significantly in five days. Unless bacteria are removed, though, it will fall back down.

Folic acid lowers uric acid levels. If killing bacteria raises uric acid levels from too low to too high (above six), this is evidence for a folic acid deficiency. A daily intake of twenty-five to thirty-five milligrams will reduce uric acid levels to three or four, a value I consider correct. This is the same dose that the 21 Day Program uses to detoxify malonic acid on a daily basis. You are getting a double benefit.

Uric acid levels are another example of a "masked" result, where a folic acid deficiency can mask a glutamine deficiency, leaving uric acid levels looking normal. But it doesn't mean you are healthy. By the time a huge bacterial infection arrives, forcing low uric acid levels as we see in cancer victims, a lot of help is needed.

Without the disturbances of disease and deficiencies, we might not need a daily intake of twenty-five milligrams of folic acid. Stopping malonate consumption would reduce the need further. The maximum allowable supplement in the United States is one milligram. This is not nearly enough to correct our common health problems. The regulation is important, though, because taking a lot of folic acid can mask a B_{12} deficiency. A better solution would be to make it mandatory to provide B_{12} along with the larger amount of folic acid, all in the same dose.

Triglycerides and Cholesterol

Triglycerides are your blood fats. They are usually much too low in cancer patients. The reason is not yet understood by scientists. But it is easy to see that cancer patients are very malnourished, using up both blood sugar and fat to sustain the body. At the same time the patient feels neither hunger nor appetite, and loses weight steadily.

If your triglycerides are below one hundred, you must eat, eat, eat to catch up on lost calories and nutrition. Even if your triglycerides are above one hundred, you must struggle hard to keep this level up. Your food must be as rich in fat as your digestion allows. Five or six meals a day is the norm. You must force yourself to eat, even without appetite.

Triglycerides that are "too high," such as over 300, are a welcome sight in cancer patients. It shows there is plenty of energy reserve to support the sick body. Do not try to lower your triglyceride level by dieting. Your diet must be extra nutritious now, without regard for calories. As your health improves, especially kidney health, high triglycerides may suddenly drop by one hundred points, putting you on the brink of too low triglycerides!

Cholesterol levels tend to go with triglyceride levels, and are often much too low, as well. Since cholesterol is largely made in the liver, low cholesterol reflects a sick liver. Cholesterol is needed for every cell—it forms the outer coat or membrane. Old cholesterol must constantly be disposed of, and new cholesterol made. A healthy cholesterol level of "two hundred-plus-your-age" was established decades ago for Americans. It is not less true now, despite the current emphasis on cholesterol lowering. Cholesterol levels that are too high (over 300) will come down automatically as liver health is improved, as the thyroid level comes up, and as liver blockages are removed with cleanses.

As soon as you are well enough to do a liver cleanse, you may use this to improve a high cholesterol. Do not eat cholesterol-reduced foods nor take cholesterol-lowering drugs when recovering from cancer. Remember that high cholesterol and triglycerides are evidence that part of your metabolism is still working well. A too-low cholesterol will come up automatically as liver health improves.

The sugar, fat and cholesterol content of your blood tells you the state of your nutrition. Are you a well-fed specimen or barely getting by? Now, more than ever, you need to supply calories of the highest quality to accomplish the extra task of healing that your body has taken on.

Electrolytes

Sodium, potassium, and chloride are your electrolytes. Sodium and chloride together make up familiar table salt. As you eat it, daily, in foods, you must excrete it in exactly the same amount so that your blood level will stay the same—near the middle of the range. Excreting just the right amount is the job of the kidneys and adrenal glands. When sodium and chloride levels are too low, the kidneys and adrenal glands are letting too much escape into the urine. You must assist these organs in particular.

Five supplements are especially helpful for the adrenals when electrolytes are too low (below the range): vitamin B$_6$ (500 mg a day), magnesium oxide (600 mg with each meal), folic acid (50 mg a day), pantothenic acid (3 teaspoons a day), vitamin C (10 gm or two teaspoons a day).

Other supplements most useful for the kidneys at this time are lysine (5 gm a day), and cysteine (3 gm a day). Altogether, these can help you avoid the need for IV therapy with steroids, albumin, and saline. But if the problem persists or is even worsening, clinical assistance must be found.

Low levels of sodium and chloride contribute to fatigue. Yet eating salt does not raise these levels and would be quite detrimental. Tumor cells and other sick cells have become "waterlogged" with sodium and chloride. These elements must be coaxed out with potassium.

Potassium chloride is tissue or cell salt. When it is too low, you may feel fatigue, as with low sodium. Your tissues are constantly lapping up the potassium in your blood for the internal use of the cells. This would lower your blood level quickly if you did not replenish it by eating.

The healthy level for potassium as I have observed is 4.5 to 4.7. All cancer patients have a severe deficit of potassium which takes weeks to bring up to normal. The potassium level of your blood does not rise quickly. Most persons, even those who consider themselves healthy, have levels that are too low! The cause is not known, although I suspect vanadium may play a role by substituting itself for potassium. For cancer patients, it is very important to raise your potassium level to the maximum, 4.7. This is to stimulate respiration, namely, oxygen utilization by the cells. Potassium was one of the first nutrients found to stimulate oxygen utilization by tissues. At the same time it coaxes sodium and chloride to come out of cells and reside in the blood again, raising the electrolyte levels.

Often the chloride level is adequate, while the potassium level is too low. For this reason we do not supplement with potassium chloride but rather with potassium gluconate. This avoids raising the chloride level. If your potassium level is very low (under 3.5), you will need three teaspoons daily of potassium gluconate. Use one teaspoon with each meal, stirring it into food, or as "salt." (One teaspoon potassium gluconate supplies 480 mg potassium.) If your level is 3.6 to 4.0, you will need ½ teaspoon, three times daily. If your level is 4.1 to 4.4, you will need ¼ tsp. three times daily. Your tissues will gradually load up on this precious nutrient. Foods known to be high in potassium, such as bananas are not enough to raise the potassium level.

Whenever you are on a potassium supplement for more than a few weeks you must get a follow-up blood test. When a level of 4.7 is reached, you must stop the supplement, and rely on wholesome foods for further supplies. If you cannot schedule a blood test in this time frame you must stop taking potassium after three weeks just in case it is high enough.

Persons with a potassium level that is too high, such as 4.8 or higher, have a thyroid problem (not caused by taking potassium). Naturally, we would not supplement potassium when it is already high. Without enough thyroid hormones the tissues cannot lap it up; this lets it accumulate in the blood while the tissues are starving for it. Thyroid problems are mainly caused by dental toxins. High potassium levels (over five) can cause symptoms such as slow heart rate.

As you do the dental clean-up the thyroid recovers quickly, and now the tissues eagerly lap up more potassium from the blood stream. This can cause a sudden drop from too high to too low levels. Another blood test is necessary to see if you now need to supplement potassium. You cannot rely on your doctor to be aware of these subtle relationships. You must notice them yourself on follow up blood tests.

Your blood salt content determines your blood pressure to some extent. Salt holds water; it was meant to hold water in your arteries and veins. If your salt level drops too low, you cannot hold the water in your blood vessels. Water will escape into your tissues because the blood vessel walls are porous. As the fluid escapes into your tissues they become water-logged (edematous) and your blood pressure must drop, causing fatigue. Most of this escaped fluid can be drawn back into the blood vessels when the salt level rises again, but the bigger amounts cannot. Extra potassium in the diet helps to absorb edema.

A diuretic is sometimes used to <u>force</u> extra excretion through the kidneys so that an extra pulling force is felt at the location of edema. If you already have edema, help it drain by bandaging it in the morning, elevating it, as well as using supplements for the adrenals and kidneys. Now, more than ever, drink the kidney herb tea, increasing it to three cups a day after a few days. (Be sure to start slowly, though.) Hydrochloric acid drops (taken with meals) and cysteine are both diuretics, as is ozonated water. But you may still need an additional diuretic such as *spironolactone*, our natural diuretic (100 mg, two a day), or a drug variety.

When electrolyte levels are too high, this is nearly always evidence of dehydration. You need to drink more <u>water</u>. Do not confuse water with beverages. To help the kidneys excrete salt and other wastes, they need plain water to dilute all the wastes they must process. One liter/quart a day, plain cold tap water, besides other beverages, is a good rule to follow for rehydration. If rehydration is needed immediately, drinking water does not suffice; it must be given by IV. Prolonged diarrhea can result in such an emergency, and requires clinical help.

Calcium and Phosphate

These are considered together because they make up our bones and are regulated together by the parathyroid and thyroid glands.

Four little parathyroid glands the size of peas are nestled in the thyroid gland; they make *parathyroid hormone* (PTH). The thyroid gland makes thyroid hormones, such as thyroxine (T_4), but also *calcitonin*.

These two glands together control calcium and phosphate levels in the blood and whether your bones will become harder and healthier or will dissolve and become fragile.

The Syncrometer easily detects PTH in the parathyroid gland when nothing disturbs it. But when copper, cobalt, vanadium, the malonates, urethane, bacteria, or synthetic dyes are present in the gland, PTH disappears. This causes the calcium level to drop.

The Syncrometer detects calcitonin in the thyroid gland when it is healthy. But when these same toxins are present, calcitonin disappears and the calcium level rises. All this happens in days, not weeks.

Having two organs that regulate something in the blood and having them situated so close together that they actually touch each other shows us the wisdom of Mother Nature. We see the same principle at work in the kidneys and adrenal glands. They can stay closely coordinated. Toxins usually saturate the smaller organ first; the larger one has more reserves.

The parathyroids, being smaller glands, are injured more easily by dental toxins, so the calcium level drops first; PTH will test negative on the Syncrometer. As the toxins increase, they begin to affect the thyroid, eventually injuring it substantially. Now calcitonin is negative also and calcium rises too high. Bone is being dissolved as the calcium level rises. Dissolving bones release their phosphates too. Now both calcium and phosphate are too high.

A calcium level over 9.7 is too high even though it is well within the "normal" range. And a phosphorus level over 3.9 is too high also; it reflects bone dissolution. (Growing children are an exception, their phosphate levels should be higher.)

A calcium level below nine indicates a toxin in the parathyroid gland. Cancer patients may have endured ten years of such a low calcium level before serious disease sets in. Taking in more calcium in the diet helps a little, but does not correct the problem. Taking vitamin D helps a little, too, but must be carefully limited and frequently has lead pollution.

When the calcium is lowered by a parathyroid problem and at the same time raised by a thyroid problem, both problems together result in a level that may appear perfect, when actually serious disease is in progress. The calcium level in the blood test is therefore another "masked" value.

The disease process is unmasked as you begin to remove the toxins. If the parathyroids are cleaned up first, the calcium level elevates. If the thyroid cleans up first, the calcium level drops. Hurry, to clear both of them from toxins so no extremes result. Your body corrects itself very swiftly. Your calcium level may drop from a life-threatening 16.0 to10.0 in five days as the dental toxins, copper, cobalt, vanadium, germanium, food malonates, urethane from plastics, dyes, and bacteria leave the thyroid. Similarly, a life-threatening low of 6.8 can rise to 7.5 in five days by doing the same clean-ups.

Calcium levels higher than 15.0 may begin to cause mental confusion. Calcium may precipitate (settle) in the kidneys; this could become irreversible damage although the kidney herb recipe may still reverse this.

We have brought down a level as high as 19.0 safely, due to lightning-speed attention. Tooth extractions of all artificially-filled teeth, in a single sweep, on the day of arrival can bring the calcium level down several points the same day, to begin the recovery. Levels below 7.0 must have the same emergency procedure: tooth extraction will gain a few points in twenty-four hours, to bring you back into the extremely low, but surviving, patient group. The correct level is 9.1 to 9.6.

A relatively new class of drugs, the diphosphonates, can be used to block bone dissolution so that calcium levels are forced to drop. This may be life-saving and provide you with the window of time needed to detoxify your thyroid gland. A popular brand, *Clodronate*, is available in Mexico (and *Aredia* in the United States). Giving calcitonin is also useful for short periods. But ultimately neither medication can save you unless the thyroid and parathyroids are helped.

Phosphorus levels that are below three indicate a need for vitamin D. The correct level is 3.0 to 3.9 mg/dl. As your kidney health improves this will improve also. For this reason, we prefer to wait a week to see if it has corrected itself before giving a vitamin D supplement; there is always the risk of pollution to consider, especially with lead.

Besides vitamin D, vitamin C also plays a role in bone health. But when vitamin C is oxidized, it cannot participate, leading to scurvy, in which your bones (notably teeth) soften. Oxidation of vitamin C is common, due to the oxidizing action of phenol made by *Streptococcus* and due to the prevalence of *Ascaris* infection.

Textbooks may point out that calcium levels are tied to total protein levels so they go up and down together. And correcting one may help the other somewhat. But never wait too long for a textbook prediction to come true. Help both.

Total protein (T.p.)

The liver makes our two main blood proteins, **albumin** and **globulin**. One of their functions is to give your blood osmotic force so water will stay in the blood vessels rather than seep into the tissues (similar to the action of salt). Albumin is more effective and is, therefore, more important. But there is more than one kind of globulin, and they are also your antibodies, so have additional importance. The total of albumin plus all your globulin is called total protein (T.p.). It should reach a value of about seven; 7.5 is better. This assures good osmotic strength.

I have not been able to determine the healthy range or critical levels of albumin and globulin with accuracy. The amount of albumin, in particular, is so essential for life itself, that only an extremely careful study could decide the optimum level or irreversible terminal level. It is best to scramble with utmost haste to raise an albumin level that has fallen below 3.5. Cobalt and vanadium are the chief culprits in disturbing the albumin and globulin levels, and again, emergency dental care to extract toxic teeth is the only life-saving measure. It was reported in 1967 that vanadium can cut the albumin to globulin ratio in half[115] yet that fact seems to have gone unnoticed in Western medicine.

Unfortunately, eating more protein does not significantly raise T.p. You must improve your liver by removing cobalt and vanadium from it.

When albumin goes up, globulin is expected to go down, to keep the T.p. fairly constant. But if globulin goes up due to a mutation, and albumin does not go down, the T.p. can rise too high. Stopping the mutations is a much faster route to lowering T.p. than chemotherapy.

Another force pulling the albumin up or down is the calcium level. Yet all these legitimate forces and relationships can go astray. If albumin is mortally low, you cannot wait. Clinical help is advised. IVs of albumin and calcium are needed.

Albumin, as injectable, in 8.0 or 12.5 gram bottles, should be given without delay. Two bottles are needed if albumin levels are below three. Each albumin bottle should be sterilized to kill bacteria and *Ascaris* eggs by adding ½ cc of ethyl (grain) alcohol through the stopper, then shaken for ten seconds to prevent precipitation. Filtering alone does not remove the Coxsackie viruses that accompany *Ascaris* eggs. Many bottles also contain traces of benzene, isopropyl alcohol, copper, cobalt, and vanadium and malonic acid (from antiseptic contamination, no doubt). We customarily discard about twenty-five percent of all bottles for such reasons. You must weigh the need for IVs against the risk of these toxins being present.

Getting a few days of injected calcium and albumin can save your life and give you just enough time to do your dental extractions, parasite killing, new diet, new lifestyle, and supplement routine. Encourage your caregiver to use this time wisely for you.

Injections of calcium by IV should also be accompanied by magnesium to keep them in balance. Additionally about 25 grams (one entire bottle) of vitamin C should be given to bal-

---

[115] Roshchin, I.V., *Toxicology of Vanadium Compounds Used in Modern Industry*, Hygiene and Sanitation, v. 32, 1967, pp. 345-52.

ance pH and keep everything in solution. (These, too, must be sterilized with ½ ml ethyl alcohol and filtered). Whether the basic IV is chosen to be dextrose or salt (saline) depends on your blood test results. If your sodium and chloride level are also low, choose saline. If not, choose dextrose. If both are low, choose saline and add concentrated glucose. The IV bottle will be automatically sterilized when the injectable is added containing the alcohol. But if none has been added, then ½ ml alcohol should be added to the bottle itself.

Twenty-four hours after teeth are extracted, the relief is felt by the thyroid and parathyroid gland, as well as the liver, allowing albumin, globulin and calcium to correct themselves.

When <u>albumin</u> is too high (greater than 5), the same toxins are responsible, cobalt, vanadium, and dyes. Even when T.p. reaches twelve or higher, you can still recover by doing immediate dental extractions and filling removal. But time now matters to the minute. And there is nothing to lose—but life.

To sum up, cobalt and vanadium are what cause albumin and globulin to be too high or too low. These come from <u>both</u> plastic and metal tooth restorations.

Lactic dehydrogenase (LDH)

Hard exercise causes your muscles to make **lactic acid**, which is what makes you feel stiff next day. Your lactic acid was made from pyruvic acid because your Krebs cycle in the muscles couldn't keep up with the pyruvate you were making while exercising (see page 99). The enzyme that can interconvert lactic and pyruvic acid is LDH. Excess lactic acid can be used up by the liver while the muscles recover. Because LDH levels closely parallel lactic acid levels, labs can test for LDH instead of lactic acid. The test for LDH is much simpler, therefore, universally used to <u>infer</u> lactic acid levels.

We are taught that when an organ is metabolizing poorly the Krebs cycle also can't keep up with the pyruvic acid made by glycolysis. Soon the pyruvate is piled up. Again, LDH is produced so that a batch of lactic acid can be made out of the pyru-vate—just until your liver or organ can catch up with burning the excess pyruvate again. But if your liver is not functioning well so the "catch up" is never reached, the lactic acid will build up higher and higher; a blood test now shows rising LDH. This is rare in healthy persons, but quite common in cancer sufferers because a tumor plays the part of the crippled organ that me-tabolizes poorly.

So it is thought that there are two large problems already in existence when the LDH is slightly elevated. A crippled organ (or tumor), and an injured liver. But I don't agree. How a small tumor, often the size of a walnut, or even several of these could fill the bloodstream with lactic acid makes no sense at all. Espe-cially considering how efficient the liver typically is at remov-ing it. Liver enzymes are often not even elevated in liver cancer!

These uncomfortable facts are not discussed openly, ever, by professionals. Although every oncologist has seen the rising LDH in many cancer patients, discussions of it are as scarce as if it were a big secret! As if to say, Why ask questions that can't be answered?

The Syncrometer has found the correct answer, at last. There are two reasons why the LDH goes up, not just one. A mutation that directly raises the enzyme LDH occurs when the azo dye Sudan Black B is present in the cell. Azo dyes are known to be highly mutagenic.[116] All cancer patients with ele-vated LDH show this dye in abundance. It has been bioaccu-mulated because the body could not detoxify it nor could the immune system (WBCs) carry it away. WBCs belonging to the tumorous organ do not carry away the dye due to their inability to "eat" it, an immune dysfunction due to ferritin-coating of their outside surfaces and due to inability to move about prop-erly due to calcium deposits that keep them stiffened up. When we restore their immunity by removing ferritin and the calcium deposits (caused by lanthanide elements), the WBCs promptly

---

[116] Chung, K.T., *The Significance of Azo-reduction in the Mutagenesis and Carcinogenesis of Azo Dyes*, Mutation Research, v. 114, 1983, pp. 269-81.

show the presence of Sudan Black B dye. They are now finding it and eating it. But to our dismay, it causes the same mutation in them! Now their LDH levels go way up; it is spewed into the blood stream now, where they are traveling, where it can affect other organs and, of course, where it can be detected in the blood test. Any organ that dares to pick up some of this LDH will have its Krebs cycle suddenly curtailed since the pyruvate is now being changed to lactic acid.

So you can expect the LDH levels to go up at first as immunity improves! Symptoms are worsened. We must hurry. The affected WBCs must be helped with selenite supplementation to unload their toxic cargo in the kidneys and bladder for excretion.

The second cause of LDH elevation is indirect. When cells have lanthanide elements within them, a family of <u>nucleoside</u> analogs appear called <u>dideoxy</u> nucleosides. How this happens is not known, but that nucleoside analogs cause lactic acid elevation is well known.[117] It is the side-effect of drugs used for AIDS patients. Raising lactic acid would inevitably raise LDH. This needs further study.

By removing lanthanides with lightning speed (dental work followed by magnet therapy) as well as excess ferritin, the LDH drops without first rising and can be expected to drop 100 points in just five days, sometimes faster.

Remember that a normal LDH doesn't mean you are cancer free. Not all cancer sufferers have an elevated LDH. But once it begins to rise in a cancer sufferer, it spells doom because other enzymes are mutated too; all body tissues will soon be dysfunctional. Hurry to get the dyes (dental plastic, etc.) out of your body! And avoid eating both dyes and lanthanides, as discussed in *Food Rules*.

When the LDH is very high, over five hundred, all the dye treatments should be maximized. Normally, we reduce dyes with coenzyme Q10 and vitamin B_2. But if the LDH is over one thousand and all your treatments are not bringing it down in the

---

[117] *Positively Aware*, Jan/Feb 1999, p.31.

first five day period, you could be given a shot of *benzoquinone* oxidizer ("BQ", see *Recipes*) a clinical procedure originated by Dr. W. Koch. Even values as high as three thousand can be brought down with a shot of this oxidizer.

BQ treatment can be given several times, on alternate days. More will not help. It buys a week of precious time to accomplish dental work, deparasitizing, etc.

Thyroid supplementation is increased to maximum tolerated (four grains or more) to accelerate the LDH drop.

We use a cut-off point of 160 U/L for LDH if the laboratory uses a range up to 240. (But remember, not all laboratories use identical procedures, so if the range on your blood test goes up to 480, you would double 160 to get 320 for your acceptable limit.) This limit of 160 is arbitrarily chosen. A value well below 160, such as 120 to 130, may be better.

Occasionally, LDH values are much too <u>low</u>, below 100. This causes intense fatigue. I believe this is due to <u>cobalt</u> inhibition of glycolysis. Large amounts of oxidized cobalt are produced by *Ascaris* as they consume your vitamin B_{12}.

Alkaline Phosphatase (Alk phos)

This is an enzyme that moves calcium in and out of bones. The only time it should be above the normal range is if you are still a young, growing person.

High levels in cancer cases may implicate lungs as well as bones. Yet sometimes neither is involved! And sometimes they are involved without raising the alkaline phosphatase! This enzyme behaves as mysteriously as LDH. And for good reason! Its elevation is also due to an azo dye. When it is elevated, it, too, can be used as a tumor marker, to guide the way to cure. Its healthy level is 75 to 85 u/l.

One common azo dye is known to raise alkaline phosphatase levels, dimethylaminoazobenzene (DAB).[118,119] DAB is present as a pollutant (or as an intentional colorant) of the most common of all antiseptics, chlorine bleach. Use of this bleach contaminates all manufactured products where bleach is used, so traces of DAB are left in them. Wherever the Syncrometer detects DAB, it also detects sodium hypochlorite (common bleach). All cases of elevated alkaline phosphatase seen had DAB distributed widely in their tissues and built up in the fat tissues. I believe this dye induces a mutation that causes the alkaline phosphatase to be produced in excess. In fact, DAB and Sudan Black B frequently occur together, in which case both LDH and alk phos are elevated. Because white blood cells (if they are competent), busily eat up this dye, they are severely affected themselves. Their excess alk phos seeps out into the bloodstream, thus reaching the bones where the greatest harm is done.

Once you have too much alk phos, this calcium enzyme can start dissolving your bones, creating lesions typical of bone cancer. For this reason, I disagree with current thinking that might state "his prostate cancer metastasized to the bone." I would say "the same dye, DAB, that caused elevated alk phos in his prostate, has reached the bones, and is now causing the same mutation there, so bones are now under attack."

Even alk phos values as high as one thousand can be reduced by stopping all use of manufactured products and decontaminating your fruits and vegetables according to the Food Rules. But the accumulated dye does not leave the body quickly. It has become "bio-concentrated," like Sudan Black B, in your body fat and within your tumors. From here it trickles steadily to liver, spleen, and bone. For this reason, the 21 Day

---

[118] Mellors, R.C., Kanematsu, S., *Alkaline Phosphatase Activity and Basophilia in Hepatic Cells Following Administration of Butter Yellow to Rats*, Proc. Soc. Exptl. Biol. Med., v. 67, 1948, pp. 242-46.

[119] Pearson, B., Novikoff, A.B, Morrione, T.G., *The Histochemical Localization of Alkaline Phosphatase during carcinogenesis in Rats Fed p-Dimethylaminoazobenzene*, Cancer Research, v. 10, 1950, pp. 557-64.

Program has large doses of coenzyme Q10, vitamin B$_2$, and ozonated oil (another dye destroyer), for several weeks.

Total Iron (Serum)

Iron is transported on transferrin in the serum. Serum is the liquid part of the blood (not the blood cells).

The ideal blood level of iron is 100 ug/dL but values as low as seventy-five are acceptable. Even values as low as fifty will allow hemoglobin to be made so red blood cells can be born in the bone marrow. But below this, body systems begin to fail.

A hallmark of advanced cancer is low iron levels so hemoglobin and RBCs cannot be made.

Although the serum iron level may be low in cancer patients, this does not mean there is a real shortage of iron. It is merely piled up in a useless mound of ferritin or of ferric phosphate. Some of it can be retrieved in ferrous form as soon as vitamin C appears on the scene. (Only the ferrous form is utilizable.) Vitamin C in its reduced form (as well as cysteine) can convert ferritin back to usable iron. But reduced vitamin C is absent in the presence of *Ascaris* parasites and all iron that is eaten in food or as a supplement merely adds to the pile of "wrong form" iron. It is probably not advisable to add to this pile by eating any more. What counts is getting rid of *Ascaris*, so vitamin C can be in its reduced form but then, of course, there is plenty of iron available without supplementing.

There are reasons for being cautious with iron supplementation: 1) bacteria need it too; 2) oxidized or metallic iron could behave like any other metal and induce mutations; and 3) high ferritin (iron in storage) levels lower immunity.[120] Bacteria are likely to grab some of it for themselves especially while lactoferrin and transferrin levels are still low. These iron transport-

---

[120] Cardier, J.E., Romano, E., Soyano, A., *T Lymphocytes Subsets In Experimental Iron Overload*, Immunopharmacology and Immunotoxicology, v. 19(1), 1997, pp. 75-87.

ers keep it away from bacteria. For all these reasons, only a very small dose of iron is given as a supplement.

Part of the process of iron retrieval from ferritin is controlled by the enzyme *FMN*. The Syncrometer detects FMN in ginger. It seems advisable to eat ginger when iron is very low. (And both cysteine and vitamin C, of course.)

When levels drop below 20 and the RBC is near transfusion level and lanthanides have already been removed, we supplement with a capsule of 300 mg ferrous gluconate (33 mg of iron) given for 5 days only.

In general, however, you can expect your iron level to normalize by itself, as you clear up other problems.

Hemoglobin (HGB)

HGB is the molecule that carries oxygen to your tissues from your lungs. Red blood cells (RBCs) contain hemoglobin, so levels of HGB and RBCs tend to rise and fall together. An HGB level that is too low may need to be rectified with a transfusion *even if RBCs are adequate* and vice versa.

Carbon Dioxide

Low carbon dioxide implies you may be huffing and puffing, even from mere walking, thereby expelling it too fast. It is needed as an acid/base regulator. It might be better to be on oxygen. High carbon dioxide reflects an acid buildup. Reduce sulfur and HCl; and add sodium and potassium. High bicarbonate (trapped carbon dioxide) may indicate too alkaline a blood serum.

How Important Are Blood Tests?

Blood test values are never accepted as "absolute truth." The lab could make a mistake; something unusual could have happened; or a mysterious effect could be at work. Interpreting blood tests is still an art, hardly a science. For this reason blood tests are repeated before they are given great weight. And certain tests are given much more weight than others, for instance, the RBC, T.b, creatinine, albumin. Life depends on these and there is little room for variation.

Still, the time of day, whether you have eaten recently, or exercised, affect some results more than others. It is wise to wait for three or four blood tests before being too alarmed about most other blood test results.

Since labs use different tests and ranges, it is obviously wise to stick to the same lab for easy comparisons.

You Won't Die From Cancer

Rarely does a cancer sufferer die from their tumors. Long before a tumor presses too hard on a critical organ, something else will go amok. This is what cancer sufferers die from, **in my experience:**

Cancer Symptom	Result	Actual Cause of Death	Inci- dence
Tumor pressing on a vital organ	Tumors can block airways, arteries, bile ducts, put pressure on the brain, and so forth.	Cancer	25%
Anemia	When your red blood corpuscles and hemoglobin become so low that even transfusions can't keep up, your organs become starved for oxygen.	Heart failure.	50%
Uremia	High BUN levels damage kidneys (they can't excrete urea or creatinine). Ammonia levels rise.	The ammonia poisons your body.	20%
Hypercalcemia	Calcium levels over 16 can cause confusion, disorientation, and other mental symptoms. Researchers speculate the calcium is precipitating in your organs, particularly your kidneys. Any level over	Kidney failure.	10%

	17 can be fatal.		
Hypoprotein-emia	Low albumin permits edema (water retention). As it becomes severe, your blood pressure drops, damaging the heart.	Organs don't get oxygen, among other things.	10%
Hyperprotein-emia	High albumin and high globulin (T.p. levels over 10) cause problems, but the mechanism isn't clear.	A level over 16 can be fatal.	10%
Hyponatremia	When sodium and chloride fall too low, your blood pressure falls too low also.	Heart failure.	10%
Liver failure	High liver enzymes (SGOT, SGPT, GGT) reflect dying liver cells.	Coma.	10%
Jaundice	When the bilirubin levels reach 2, you may start to see a yellowish tint in the whites of the eyes. At higher levels the skin becomes yellow and at 30 you need it removed mechanically before you go into a coma.	The bilirubin poisons your body.	5%
Pneumonia	Lung cancer sufferers often accumulate water in their lungs. How tumors could cause this is considered a mystery, but I find maleic anhydride is the culprit.	Asphyxiation.	5%
Hypothrombo-cytemia	If you don't have enough platelets, you can't stop bleeding internally or exter-nally. Low blood pressure results.	Heart failure, among other things.	1%

The percentages obviously add up to more than 100%. That is because they often overlap.

Of course classical thinking is that cancer is responsible for all the symptoms described above, so the cause of death in all these cases is "cancer." But that is because oncologists don't have evidence that cancer can be cured. They feel once a cancer patient, always a cancer patient. My evidence suggests the opposite: there are two separate battles, tumors, and the toxins responsible for them. I have seen many people conquer their tumors, only to succumb to some aspect of toxicity. That doesn't mean cancer won. That just means cancer toxins are capable of doing a lot of damage to your body. Damage that doesn't magically go away like your tumors will.

You can win both battles.

Reading Your X-rays

How would you like to be a radiologist? Not for a moment am I suggesting I can give you a medical school course in one chapter, but I want to emphasize that there are many things you can learn from your X-ray that don't need great expertise to understand!

X-rays, computerized tomography (CT or "cat") scans, magnetic resonance images (MRIs), and ultrasounds all come as "negatives" to begin with. For this book those negatives were printed. A print reverses the light and dark areas. For instance, bones on negatives appear light, but on prints appear dark.

I am assuming you can obtain your negatives to take home. Because they are precious, your doctor is justifiably reluctant to give them to you, even on loan. Some radiologists are equipped to make duplicates. Ask your doctor to refer you to one.

Tape your negatives to a window that lets in bright light to give you good visibility. Get your bearings first: top, bottom, left, right. Some scans include a diagram to show you where in the body the pictures were taken. If you have numerous negatives choose a few that show the problem most clearly; they may have already been marked by the radiologist. Use these markings to help you understand your problem. Most problems are easy to recognize if they are large. Small problems should be pointed out to you by your health provider. It is not necessary to learn the names of anatomical parts to recognize that they are not normal!

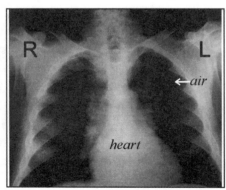

Fig. 34 Chest X-ray, front view

243

The front view of a chest X-ray shows the lungs as dark areas on the negative. The dark area is actually air. The larger the dark area, the better your lungs are. On the left side, marked L on the negative, a slanting edge marks the heart. It reaches to the middle and upward. A bulge above the heart shows where the aorta arches backward. The trachea, esophagus, aorta, and large abdominal vein all pass along the middle, between the lungs, called the

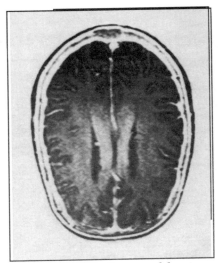

Fig. 37 CT of normal brain

mediastinum. They cannot be distinguished in such a view. Nor could a tumor be seen here. For this reason a side view is taken also. On each side of the midline, bright spots are seen, along

finger-like spokes. These are lymph nodes lining the tracheoles. They should not be enlarged or extremely dense (white on the print).

A CT scan of the lungs takes numerous pictures of imaginary "slices" made across the body. Each slice, or cross section, is pictured in a frame. Frames

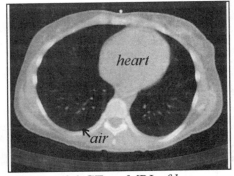

Fig. 36 CT or MRI of lungs

taken very close together (a few millimeters) will be able to spot things that are only a few mm in size. Frames taken far apart will miss things that are smaller than this spacing. The spacing is stated on the negative. The dark areas are the lungs, white specks are the tracheoles with their lymph nodes. The heart is in the middle. Cross sections of ribs surround the lungs.

The brain as seen from the top by CT or MRI looks like the meat of a walnut. The two halves are separated by a straight line. The center line should not be pushed to either side. Pressure due to fluid buildup, edema, is the usual cause of displacement of the centerline. The edema could result from an active tumor. The tumor itself is identifiable as an extra dense region that is not shaped as normal brain tissue should be; the shape is compared to the opposite side that is normal and healthy. A plain X-ray, of the skull, not shown, can often show a large brain problem, too, and is much less expensive.

The liver is best viewed by ultrasound. Ultrasound uses sound waves instead of radiation, is also non-invasive, and inexpensive. Like a CT, ultrasound produces a number of frames. The large right lobe should appear smooth in texture (have an even density). There should not be specially dense regions as seen in liver cancer. The gallbladder will be viewed on some frames.

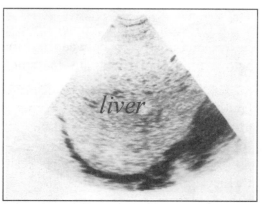

Fig. 38 Ultrasound of liver, right lobe

The left lobe of the liver is much smaller. The pancreas and spleen may be viewed on some frames.

Here is a CT scan of the liver. The texture should be smooth, without granules or dense areas. The dark mushroom shape is the spinal column.

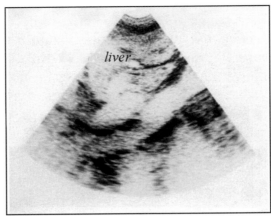

Fig. 39 Ultrasound of liver, left lobe

A CT scan of the abdomen shows numerous frames in a series of pictures taken between the liver above and the bladder below. Find your backbone, the spine, first. Notice the largest

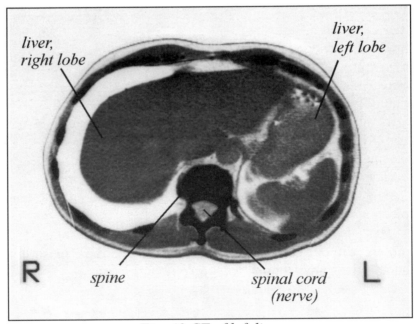

Fig. 40 CT of left liver

artery in your body, the abdominal aorta, just inside (above) the spinal column. The interior has loops of intestine. On each side

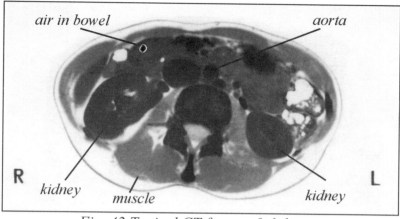

Fig. 42 Typical CT frame of abdomen

are cross sections of the kidneys. Although they may be of equal size in your body, one might be placed higher than the other so a cross section may make them appear dissimilar.

Note the CT scan shows the kidneys in relationship to the other organs, whether pushed aside by a tumor or edema fluid. Now compare the CT scan to an ultrasound of a single kidney.

The ultrasound shows their typical oblong shape, and ragged internal structure. It is a lot easier to see a mass in the ultrasound than CT. There should be no outlines of masses anywhere.

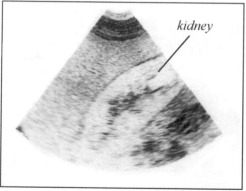

Fig. 41 Ultrasound of normal kidney

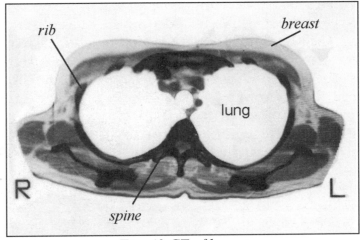

Fig. 43 CT of breast

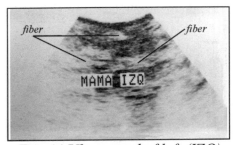

Fig. 44 Ultrasound of left (IZQ) breast

The CT scan of breast views cross sections that also show the lungs and rib cage. If the frames are closely spaced, a nodule can be found that may be missed on an ultrasound.

The ultrasound of breast shows typical white patches (dark on negative) where the tissue is more fibrous. The negative should not have intense dark areas of definite shape. A small amount of fibrous tissue is normal. Of course, large masses can also be felt or seen. But small masses may persist, though they can no longer be felt.

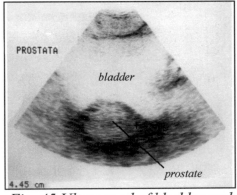

Fig. 45 Ultrasound of bladder and prostate

An ultrasound of the lower abdomen will include both bladder and prostate for men and bladder and uterus plus ovaries for women. The white area is the bladder. Beneath it is the roundish prostate gland. If the prostate becomes enlarged, it pushes against the bladder, indenting it with a "cookie bite" like appearance. The prostate gland should have a smooth external edge and a homogeneous internal appearance. The radiologist calculates its weight from its dimensions, often given on the ultrasound. Pictures taken at different angles will give different lengths and widths; such variations should be taken into consideration.

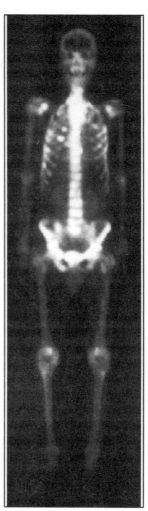

A bone scan views all the bones in your body, from the skull to your toes in one small picture.

An injection of radioactive technetium (an element) is given first, allowed to find its way to the bones (three hours) followed by imaging of your radiating bones! The regions where the technetium has accumulated will show up as intensely white "hot spots". These hot spots are cancerous bone lesions, to be distinguished by the radiologist from mere "inflammatory" or benign lesions.

You will be able to identify some of the hot spots yourself by matching them with your pain locations. You will also see hot spots that are not yet painful! Pain develops after these lesions become infected with bacteria. Bone lesions of any kind, malignant, benign, or inflammatory are soft areas, showing that calcium is not being deposited as fast as it is being dissolved. Even after you correct

Fig. 46 Bone scan

249

the problem, it is nearly impossible to <u>catch up</u> on the bone loss. There will always—or at least for years—be a region of low bone density at these locations. For this reason, a follow up X-ray or bone scan can never be expected to appear totally normal. But the hot spots will be gone and former lesions that were small can disappear, leaving only the evidence of former severe bone lesions.

Are You Ready For Your First Case?

Use your orientation to understand the scans in the case histories that come next. There will be pointers to help you. The more of these you look at, the easier it is to see things that should or should not be there.

The True Story of...

This is what actually happened to people using the methods taught in this book. They were not selected because they were all successful, indeed, some of the earliest ones were hampered by our lack of understanding. These true stories were selected simply on the basis of having confirming before-and-after evidence of what the treatment did for them. Naturally the names have been changed to ones randomly selected from a telephone book to protect the privacy of the patient. Furthermore, to include all the details in their file, including all the scans taken, would quadruple the size of this chapter, so I have just included relevant details and representative scans.

Nearly every case was diagnosed as "terminal." Yet most patients kept joy and hope in their hearts. Many gained a second life. Some did not. But each one taught a new lesson, sometimes at great cost, and for that reason the knowledge in this book is priceless. This is your guide to survival.

1	Katherine Morales	Bone Cancer

Katherine Morales, age seventy-eight, came September 21, for her bone cancer that had invaded her whole skeleton. She was in pain from top to toe, especially at the back of her head and neck and the bottom of her spine. She had recently been in poor health otherwise, too. She had shoulder, knee, and hip repaired and replaced, and now her digestion was bad and she coughed a lot. Katherine was on heart medicine (Verapamil). Her daughter, who came with her, could easily see the downward trend; her mother could only sit and had dropped below 90 lb. Katherine was anxious about herself, too. She felt a lump in her abdomen that she could not explain and her bowels had not moved for days.

Syncrometer® testing at the general body level showed ortho-phospho-tyrosine Positive at kidneys and bone, Negative at colon and liver. [*Testing at the general body level selects those problems that are widespread and, therefore, of greater level of toxicity and significance. When a tissue slide is included in the circuit, only problems at this tissue are detected.*] She not only had bone cancer as found by her doctor at home, but also kidney cancer.

We ordered a bone scan and kidney scan, but she wanted to do all scans and tests at home where insurance was certain to cover the cost.

Other testing we did included isopropyl alcohol (Negative: cancer sufferers always test positive to this, but Katherine had already stopped using all items on the isopropyl alcohol list); lead and vanadium (Negative); asbestos (Positive: she must stop using her dryer); arsenic (Positive: she must clear all pesticide from her home); fiberglass (Negative). She was also clear of the solvents benzene and wood alcohol. Finally, we tested for bacteria: three salmonella varieties, *E. coli*, three shigella varieties, and *Staphylococcus aureus* were all Negative. This was a pleasant surprise. I had usually found Staph responsible for bone pain–which she had! It would originate in a rotten tooth or old jaw-bone infection (cavitation). But Katherine's situation was different. She wore complete dentures. *Staphylococcus* could certainly be hiding in a cavitation and we would do a careful inspection. But any dental problem would be minimal. Would this give her a special chance to survive? She reminded me of my very special elderly house-mate who had died recently. Both were very frail and bowed with bone loss. Both had thick files in their doctor's offices for broken bones and sprains. But my companion, even at age ninety-seven, was pain-free and pill-free. Could I at least help Katherine out of chronic pain?

Katherine was to start taking the kidney herbs, kill parasites regularly, zap daily, and take two teas she could make herself at home. One was mullein herb for her cough. The other was burdock root to improve her constipation. She would also take 1 tablespoon of moose elm (also called slippery elm) made into a cup of half and half. And sodium alginate made up as ½ teaspoon added to 1 cup of boiling water. This would find its way through the toughest blockage in her intestine. She would be started on IVs and 2 vials containing rhodizonic acid daily.

All this could have overwhelmed Katherine, but her daughter took on the tasks eagerly. Katherine exuded the sweetness of the very elderly as she said goodbye. Did she really believe there would be a "Mexican miracle" for her? I gazed after her with wishful thoughts.

Three days later, not much had been accomplished. Nor had her bowels moved. But her digestion seemed better.

In another three days, much had occurred. She had begun to have bowel action the previous day; the alginate had found its way through. The abdominal scan had been done and revealed no tumors. The bone scan revealed "hot spots" of cancer from top to toe. Hardly a bone was free of lesions. No wonder she had pains everywhere.

Her blood test results are given at the end of her story, page 257. They showed the typical low blood sugar (66!) of cancer patients; she would soon be emaciated, not just tiny, frail and thin. Her BUN (4!) and creatinine were much too low, showing there was a block in their formation. She would soon be toxic with ammonia, unable to turn it into urea (BUN). Her LDH was completely normal though, as were all her liver tests showing that hair dye,

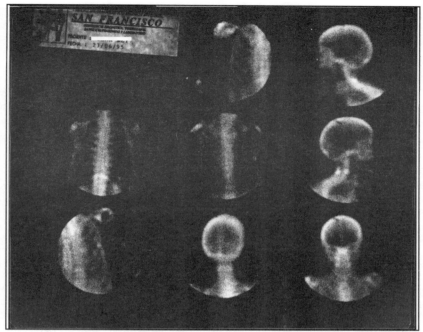

Hot spots on skull, neck, spine, rib, etc. (shoulder is prosthesis).
Part of original bone scan

food dyes, and lanthanides were not the main problem. Only the alk phos was somewhat elevated [*due to the dye, DAB*] though not at all runaway. But albumin, her precious liver protein, was too low and iron was frighteningly low (35!). She must get away from copper water pipes immediately. They promised they would find a new apartment at once. Her potassium was much too low (2.8!), too, probably causing her extreme fatigue.

Her first supplements included one quart milk daily for better nutrition and extra calories, plus magnesium oxide, boron, manganese, and vitamin D. All these were for bone building and bone hardening. The calcium would come from the milk.

Note: instructions in the current 21 Day Program can be different from those given a few years ago.

Also included was hawthorn berry, and coenzyme Q10. These two would eventually replace her heart medicine by supplying what the heart really needed. [*The reader is cautioned not to do this at home without medical supervision.*]

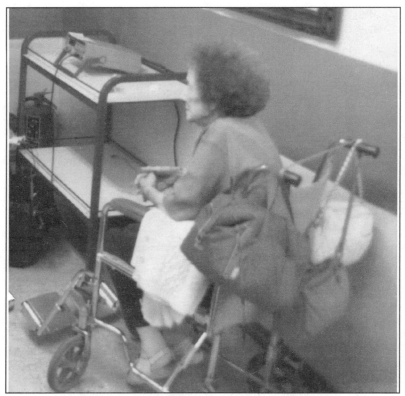

"Katherine" in the IV and zapper room

Next was a recipe of herbs to build bones, consisting of burdock, mullein, boneset, comfrey. I reassured her that any toxicity from these was mere hearsay. If she had any side effects, please let us know. There were none.

Her "Rhodakem" (proprietary form of rhodizonic acid; it costs about $3.00 per vial) was raised to 4 vials a day. There was nothing to lose by maximizing every treatment. Time was of the essence for her, while pain was not yet so intense that continuous painkiller was needed.

The following day she had her first IV. She began wheezing and coughing during the IV which couldn't be stopped. [*With hindsight, she probably got a dose of bacteria in her IV. We were unaware of the bacterial problem at that time and had not learned to sterilize the IVs with ethyl alcohol nor filter them.*]

The next day she arrived in the office, walking unassisted, but with her walker. She was much improved. Her pains were nearly all gone, only the lower back pain and neck pain persisted. Her bowels were functioning very well now. But she was still coughing from the day before. Testing showed she had picked up *E. coli* somehow [*the IV*]. She was given Echinacea and charcoal capsules for it. And "peroxy" water to drink (several drops of food grade hydrogen peroxide in her water).

Four days later, she was still keeping all her gains. She was doing well and could be gone a week now.

It was October 12, a week later. She had moved back to her own home to see if she could take care of herself. She was able to walk a bit without her walker. She was coughing less and could stop the herbs. Her IV series was complete. She was started on 1) hydrochloric acid drops with each meal and 2) Clodronate capsules.

In another week, October 19, she was still in her own home. She was walking in her home without a walker. Her cough was much better, but not gone. She was still on 4 rhodizonate vials daily, hydrochloric acid drops, and Clodronate. Her vitamin D dosage was decreased to one drop (50,000 IU) on alternate days.

The next week, October 26, she arrived with a lot of digestive problems again; nausea, and this time had lost weight. She was down to 82 lb. Her cough was gone, though, and the lump in her abdomen was gone. The pain at her lower back was gone. But *E. coli* could not be vanquished, it was very positive. She would soon be bedridden at this rate. She was given six vials of rhodizonate to take twice a day, chlorophyll, Lactobacillus culture (tested for other bad bacteria), moose elm, and scheduled again for a daily IV of glucose, vitamin C, and glycyrrhizin. [*At this time we had not yet learned the simpler remedy of turmeric and fennel for E. coli.*]

Three days later, she related that she had felt immediately better after the first six vials (of rhodizonate) and had gone down to four after that. She had gotten nauseous during the IV and had to stop it. We started her on thioctic acid.

The next week, November 2, she had gained weight (1 lb.!). The Clodronate was nauseating her, though, so it was stopped. Instead she was given a calcium carbonate supplement plus magnesium oxide (2 a day), to be taken with meals along with her hydrochloric acid drops. She seemed well enough to do a liver cleanse.

Then she was gone for three weeks, and we were getting quite anxious. Was this long absence good or bad? We were delighted finally to see her arrive. She was "feeling very much better" in her own words. She had done a liver cleanse and gotten about 400 medium to small stones out. She felt stronger, was able to read again. Nausea was much better. Appetite was up. Being able to read again meant a lot to her, she said.

The next three weeks we allowed ourselves to hope for Katherine's recovery. Indeed, she walked in December 14 stating that she felt fine, was doing more and more walking, and getting stronger. She had done her second liver cleanse and got a lot of stones again, including one large one. Her nausea was gone now, and she was eating well. There was no coughing. She was zapping daily. All bacteria tested Negative. The bowel was functioning perfectly. Her pulse was 68; there were no missed heart beats. So she was taken off Verapamil and left only on hawthorn berry capsules, one 3 times a day plus coenzyme Q10. She would have her pulse taken daily to see if this switch was satisfactory.

Three weeks after that, January 9, Katherine came in with purpuric (purple) spots on her arms. Her left hip also showed a "bruise mark" and was painful. She was taken off molasses and syrup sweeteners she was using—they contain sorghum molds that cause blood vessels to break, causing the purpura. She should make herself marmalade as a sweetener, using honey. This would provide bioflavonoids to strengthen her blood vessels. A supplement of bioflavonoids was added for a month. Otherwise, she was getting stronger. She had gained more weight back. A new blood test was scheduled. Next day we reviewed it together. Her blood sugar level was now much better. She was making urea well (BUN up to 13) though creatinine was still too low. Most significant was the further drop in alk phos, this represented the improvement in her bone cancer.

The entire staff was elated for her, as well as her daughter. Her liver could make enough albumin again so she was not in danger of developing edema followed by kidney and heart failure. Her uric acid was normal, but calcium was too high (10.3). She could go off her calcium supplement and reduce vitamin D drops to one a week. Her iron level was normal.

Katherine had seen her medical doctor recently, who had released her. We could also release her this time, free of pain, free of drugs, but still on a few supplements.

Three months later, she came in for a peculiar head problem. She had pain again, at the back of her neck. Notice how extremely "hot" the bone lesions at the top of her spine were initially. This implicates bacteria—the most likely bacteria were food bacteria since she had full dentures ruling out rotten teeth. Indeed, she tested Positive for *Salmonella* and *Shigella*. She was put on a Bowel Program including Lugol's, four times a day, turmeric, fennel, and digestive enzymes with each meal for one month. In one week she was much better, all bacteria tested Negative and she could stop the program. Only freon tested Positive now. It had filled her diaphragm. She would start drinking ozonated water and make a recipe of kidney herbs for herself besides changing her refrigerator.

In June she moved to a new apartment. Immediately she began coughing a lot. She was full of fiberglass. Dust tests led to the furnace room, where there was also arsenic. She received a benzoquinone shot (½ dose). Later that month she was well again.

Katherine Morales	10/26	1/9 next year
RBC	4.7	4.75
WBC	9,800	9,800
glucose	66	81
BUN	4 (5-20)	13 (5-20)
creatinine	0.8 (.8-1.4)	0.7 (.8-1.4)
AST (SGOT)	18	18
ALT (SGPT)	17	15
LDH	137	111
GGT	18	20
T.b.	0.4	0.5
alk phos	117 (39-117)	94 (39-117)
T.p.	6.7	6.8
albumin	3.8 (3.9-5.1)	4.5 (3.9-5.1)
globulin	2.9	2.3
uric acid	7.5 (2.5-6.8)	3.1 (2.5-6.8)
calcium	9.6 (8.5-10.4)	10.3 (8.5-10.4)
phosphorus	3.5	3.7
iron	35	74
sodium	137	141
potassium	2.8 (3.3-5.6) verified	3.9
chloride	97	102
triglycerides	119	175
cholesterol	233	280

Time passed. We did not see her. We grew anxious and called her daughter. Katherine was doing fine; she was taking care of herself and her husband at home. She was not using a cane or walker and was not in pain. She had purchased a special three-wheel walker for outdoor jaunts. Shark cartilage was recommended as a maintenance supplement.

The calendar rolled on. It would be three years before we saw her again (page 513).

NOTE: ranges shown in parentheses are laboratory "normal" ranges and are included only when they are notably different from laboratory ranges cited earlier (because laboratories differ). **To remind yourself what I consider a "healthy" range, please tear out the chart on page 207 and use it as a bookmark.** "Verified" means the lab knew the result was at an extreme and repeated the test.

2	Michelle Symanski	Liver Cancer

Michelle Symanski came to Mexico after she was told by United States surgeons that she had inoperable liver cancer. She was only twenty-three years old and had two very young children. She was wearing a pain patch (morphine).

One look at her liver scan explains this. She had tumors, including one very large one, making up all of the right side. But the left side (not shown) had a small portion that was uniform and smooth, without granules. This probably was the functioning part that was keeping her alive.

Due to my intense emotional distress over this young mother, I called in a brilliant alternative doctor (Dr. M). He in turn called in a brilliant allopathic doctor (Dr. V). Seldom do we all join forces. Dr. V pronounced that nothing could be done that would not add needless misery to the weeks or months remaining for her. But he would run a special catheter right into her liver so we could conveniently administer any treatment.

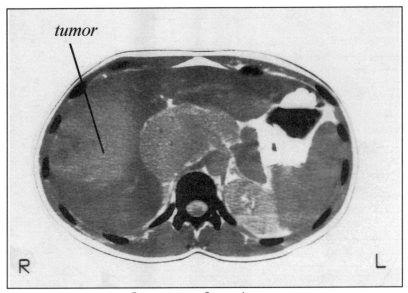

tumor

Liver scan from August

She was very pale, thin, small framed, but still vivacious.

Our electronic testing showed ortho-phospho-tyrosine, isopropyl alcohol, *Fasciolopsis buskii*, asbestos, fiberglass, aluminum were Positive. Mercury, lead, cadmium, arsenic, formaldehyde, and eight common food bacteria were Negative.

She was to stop using her clothes dryer or hair dryer to eliminate asbestos. She would bring in dust samples from home to track down the fiberglass source. She had less than the average number of toxins in her home.

She was to start the parasite killing program, zap daily, and go off everything on the isopropyl alcohol list. She seemed to be in a panic and agreed eagerly. She was to start the kidney herb recipe.

Her IVs would be formulated to contain glycyrrhizin, DMSO, B-vitamins, vitamin C, and laetrile beginning at once.

She felt better immediately, the same day, and skipped next day's treatment. The day after, she arrived quite fatigued. Although ortho-phospho-tyrosine and *Fasciolopsis* were now Negative, she was still Positive for isopropyl alcohol. She had gone back to using regular shampoo and drinking bottled water. She was helped to make borax shampoo and persuaded to stop bottled water.

Three days later Michelle was Negative for asbestos, fiberglass, and isopropyl alcohol. She felt well and had brought her children. She was started on Lugol's iodine, though, (6 drops, 4 times a day in water) to eliminate a Salmonella invasion.

Eight days later (she was missing her daily IVs and check ups), she arrived still Negative to toxins. Her swollen liver had gone down along with her abdominal pain.

She missed appointments another two weeks and had been seen shopping with her children. She was coaxed to come back. She had a new pain across the abdomen and was coughing. She only stayed long enough for one IV treatment even though appointments, IVs, and supplements were given free of charge, out of compassion for her tragic circumstances.

Another three weeks went by without communication. Then she arrived very depressed. Yet her energy was up, her health obviously better, and all her pain gone. Her coughing had stopped. A scan was scheduled. But it was skipped.

A month later, November, she had gained 20 lb., and had not yet done her scan. We were overjoyed to see her and quickly helped her get to the radiologist. The scan showed the large liver tumor had mostly disappeared, leaving only fragments. Notice how the texture of the entire liver was much improved, appearing more regular and smooth than her first scan.

She continued to miss treatments for another month, in spite of our

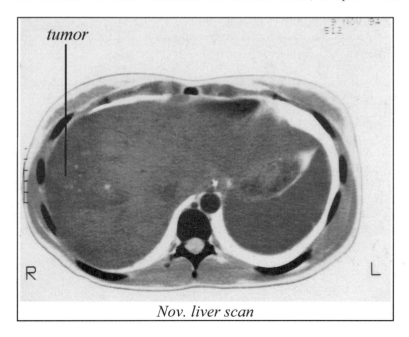

Nov. liver scan

anxious calls to her home.

When she appeared she was feeling very bad again. She had received conventional chemotherapy in the meantime. I could hardly persuade her to even come in for testing; she was just visiting somebody.

Ortho-phospho-tyrosine, isopropyl alcohol, aflatoxin and cobalt were Positive. She had her original problem back. She was crying and angry. She said she stopped zapping, used no parasite herbs, and had been using regular body products again. She had a new boyfriend and didn't want to appear "abnormal" to him. But she promised me personally to zap again and go back to her disciplined life style.

Michelle Syman-ski	April
BUN	9
AST (SGOT)	147
ALT (SGPT)	96
LDH	771
GGT	354
T.b.	2.4
alk phos	498
albumin	3.4 (3.9-5.1)
uric acid	2.8
Calcium	8.8
Iron	101
bands	5%
other tests	good

From time to time somebody reported she had been seen with her children. One report sighted her in a bar at night. Christmas passed and we heard she was seemingly well.

Four months later, she arrived extremely ill. She did not come to see me, but I obtained a copy of her blood test results. She was terminal.

Soon after this we got the news, Michelle died.

Summary: If we had a chance to do it all over, losing another $5,000.00 worth of IV supplies, besides supplements, we would gladly do it. She had a right to live life, free of chains. She had a right to appear "normal" to a young man of her choosing, whatever the place and time. We turned our grief inward. Society and government had let her down.

3	Julie Cote	Brain Cancer

Kevin and Julie Cote had been told in no uncertain terms by their friends at home that they must seek out our clinic at once.

Three weeks ago Julie had a five-day headache for no reason and suddenly lost her memory. She couldn't remember having had guests for supper the previous day.

An MRI of the brain done by her doctor at home showed a mass the size of a nickel in the right occipital lobe. It had an irregular shape, appearing white on the print. Her doctor thought it might represent a newly reactivated cancer since it couldn't all have grown so suddenly.

When she arrived on February 14, her husband did the communicating for her and steadied her along to and from her chair. She had numbness in the tongue, lips, cheek, and left hand. (Remember, the right side of the brain controls the left side of the body.) This made speech difficult; her vision was blurred and she felt dizzy and lost her balance easily. She also had chronic headache. Such symptoms can be a sign of an active tumor.

Her initial test results with the Syncrometer were Positive for orthophospho-tyrosine, *Fasciolopsis*, isopropyl alcohol, aflatoxin, lead, cadmium (from copper and galvanized water pipes), mercury (from amalgam fillings), *Salmonella typhimurium*. This systemic salmonella infection was probably what caused her dizziness; it may even have been responsible for activating her tumor. She was given 6 drops of Lugol's iodine in ½ glass of water before leaving the office, to begin killing *Salmonella*. She was to take the iodine dose 4 times a day, after meals and bedtime. She was instructed in taking the parasite-killing program and avoiding items on the isopropyl alcohol list as given in the book, *The Cure For All Cancers*.

She was shown how to use our zapper, daily. A blood test was done. Her diet was to be free of grocery-store bread and all nuts to get rid of aflatoxin.

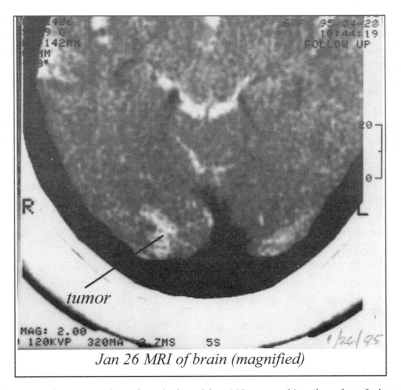

Jan 26 MRI of brain (magnified)

She was given capsules of methylene blue (65 mg each) to be taken 3 times a day and told to anticipate having blue urine. Methylene blue is a very old and relatively nontoxic dye. It acts as a reversible oxidizing and reducing agent, picking up electrons from brain cells that need oxidation, then giving them up again to neighboring chemicals. In this way, the brain's metabolism is helped.

They sat quietly absorbing their instructions on diet, changed life style habits, the need for a copper-free water source, and all the supplements to take. They were overwhelmed. I feared they would not accomplish their tasks. I decided to use the intravenous route for supplements instead. Unless we could correct the mental impairment very quickly, the damage would become irreversible. Or at least, take much longer to reverse than the three weeks they had come for. It was a fortunate decision since they did not return the next day. Even the day after that, they had not managed to begin anything. But they had found copper-free lodging.

On February 17, we reviewed her blood test results together. They were discouragingly poor. Both BUN and creatinine were too low, showing that the excretion path for ammonia was blocked and her muscles were not being fed with creatine. Her liver enzymes were somewhat high, and the GGT extremely high. This probably reflected aflatoxin damage as also seen in the rising total bilirubin. Unless this could be reversed right now, it would continue to rise beyond our capability to correct it. She would soon be jaundiced. The alk phos was extremely high also, suggesting lung or intestine or bone would soon be involved, besides brain.

The uric acid level was too low, revealing the lack of glutamine; glutamine is especially important to the brain. [*A failing Krebs cycle could explain the lacking glutamine since it is made from glutamic acid. At that time we were not aware that low uric acid also implicates clostridium bacteria somewhere.*] She was supplemented with glutamine.

Her iron level was much too low (38), revealing a toxic copper [*and germanium*] burden, no doubt in her amalgams. A good sign, though, were her triglycerides and cholesterol. Although they were indicated to be high by the lab, we knew it to be a good prognostic sign. She needed one. The LDH was satisfactorily low [*showing that her liver could still detoxify Sudan Black dye*].

The remainder of the test results were quite good. She announced that her urine was blue, as it should be, but that the liver and kidney herb recipes had not yet been started. Nor had dental work been scheduled–she needed amalgams removed.

I implored them to comply to perfection and let nothing stand in the way. They seemed blithely unaware that disaster was imminent, though perhaps still avoidable, as it is for the camper whose tent is pitched within inches of a cliff.

Her isopropyl test was Negative, showing she was making the right product choices. She had been given three IVs and was scheduled to continue these daily. In fact, I added several items to her IV schedule. (All IV bags and the injectables to be added to them were first tested for pollution with copper, cobalt, vanadium, isopropyl alcohol, benzene, and methyl alcohol.) To no avail. I did not see them for eight days.

When they arrived, Julie walked briskly, unassisted into the room and took over the communication for herself. She said they had done everything they were told. Eight missed appointments did not seem noteworthy. She was quite aware of her improvements, was sleeping better, and no longer dizzy. She was back to her old self and was doing the

Julie Cote	2/16	2/24
RBC	4.6	4.85
WBC	7.8	7.8
glucose	141	86
BUN	4 (5-20) L	11 (5-20)
creatinine	0.7 (.8-1.4)L	
AST (SGOT)	56 (1-50) H	30
ALT (SGPT)	80 (1-50) H	31
LDH	151 (94-250)	203
GGT	1075 (0-57) verified	20
T.b.	2.6 (0.1-1.2) H	0.3
alk phos	733 (39-117) H verified	80
T.p.	7.0	7.6
albumin	3.8 (3.9-5.1)	4.5
globulin	3.2	3.1
uric acid	2.0 (2.5-6.8) verified	3.2 (3.6-7.7)
Calcium	8.9	9.1
Phosphorus	3.6	3.1
Iron	38	81
Sodium	136	139
Potassium	4.2	3.7
Chloride	99	102
triglycerides	202	151
cholesterol	364	259

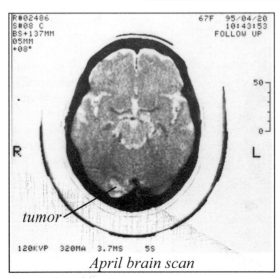

April brain scan

housekeeping again. What pleased her most was being able to read again; she had sorely missed this while she was ill.

A new blood test was scheduled, February 24. Her BUN and creatinine were now normal. All the liver enzymes were down to normal, the GGT was 20! The T.b. was back down from 2.6 to a healthy 0.3. And the alk phos was perfect at 80. The improvements were phenomenal. But they didn't know this, since, again, they did not return the next day to review it. Day after day, they did not return.

We had a private celebration over her good fortune, even while we scolded over her missed appointments. We called the area motels and RV parks, trying to locate them. Weeks later we found them...back home in their own country! We gave them the good news about Julie's blood test but they knew it already and were not very interested. They knew it from Julie's return to health! We also wanted to see a follow-up CT scan.

She sent us her follow-up CT done in April. Another was done in November, and then in November of the following year. The mass seemed to have shrunk very slightly, or at least it had not enlarged. The pressure it had been exerting on surrounding brain tissue was evidently relieved. She had no symptoms remaining whatever, although the tumor was not gone. Possibly, more vigorous treatment could have shrunk it, but the cost was prohibitive for them. And they chose to risk stopping and leaving well enough alone. Perhaps it was a wise choice, after all.

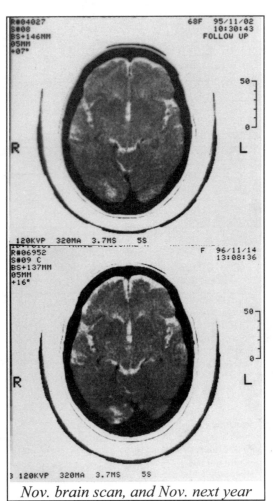

Nov. brain scan, and Nov. next year

Summary: Julie got fantastic improvement in ten days. What had she done? Her file does not state she got amalgams removed, but clearly her copper was gone since her iron level came up. She had taken Lugol's, certain supplements (not listed), methylene blue, and the kidney herbs. She sent us follow-up CT scans for a year and a half; then stopped that, too. Two years after the last scan she was reached by telephone. She was happy and well.

| 4 | Jason McGowan | Pancreatic and Liver Cancer |

Jason McGowan, a middle-age father of several children, was first diagnosed with irritable bowel syndrome at home. He was on antibiotics for a severe "flu" that wouldn't go away soon after that. A GI series of X-rays showed nothing, but an ultrasound of the liver revealed some spots. Then a CT scan was done. It showed a 5 x 7 cm tumor in the pancreas. This is equivalent to 2 x 3 in., the size of a tangerine. Plus several small masses in the liver, considered to be metastases from the pancreatic tumor. He did not

want to biopsy any of them since he knew this was terminal illness. He refused clinical treatment and headed for Mexico.

It was March 17. He arrived full of vanadium, gold, freon, isopropyl alcohol, three varieties of salmonella, one shigella, and *Staphylococcus aureus*. The vanadium came from his oil-heated home; he said you could smell the oil as you entered. The gold came from the crowns in his dental ware; gold has a preference for the pancreas. Salmonella and shigella are filth bacteria, colonizing the bowel of animals and spreading to human food via fertilizer and dirt. Staphylococcus comes from teeth, in the form of an abscess or cavitation.

He was started on Lugol's iodine, the parasite killing program, and

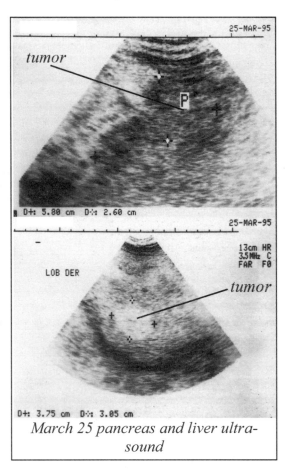

March 25 pancreas and liver ultrasound

zapping. He was helped to avoid isopropyl alcohol containing products. He was scheduled for dental work to replace metal and started on the kidney herb recipe. A consulting physician was asked to be in charge of the IV program. He would receive daily, vitamin C, vitamin B complex, glycyrrhizin,

Wobe Mugos digestive enzymes, and as much pain killer as needed of a non-morphine variety.

A blood test was ordered and it showed that tumor activity was not great, the LDH was only 179. Liver enzymes were very high, especially the GGT, a function of the liver that is also sensitive to aflatoxin and synthetic dyes. His RBC was too high as expected for vanadium toxicity.

By the third day, he was free of isopropyl alcohol, gold buildup, and the malignancy. Only shrinking the tumors and regaining health remained. He was monitored with the Syncrometer each day for solvents and bacteria. In spite of starting on ozonated water and liver herbs, he still had freon in his pancreas ten days later.

But on the eighth day, a new ultrasound of liver and pancreas showed a remarkable improvement. The pancreatic tumor that had been 7 x 5 cm was now only 5.8 x 2.6 cm. He was off to a good start. The largest of the various liver tumors was 3.75 x 3.05 cm in the right lobe ("LOB DER").

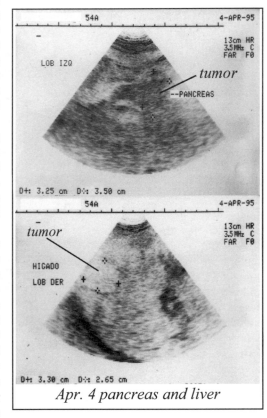

He was still getting chills every night and pain at both sides, over the right liver and over the pancreas. Coffee enemas to reduce pain were recommended daily.

The freon refused to leave him; it was found to be present in his room so he moved to a room without an air conditioner. On the fourteenth day, he was still feeling very bad, dizzy all the time. He could not shake his systemic salmonella... not until it was found polluting his water pitcher! He was changed to a glass jar instead of the

Apr. 4 pancreas and liver

plastic pitcher beside his bed. [*Drinking water from a standing source is never advisable.*]

Two days later, after the last metal was out of his teeth, [*we were replacing amalgam with composite at that time*] he was feeling, strangely, much better. The pain over his pancreas was gone, but it remained over the right side (liver). A new blood test and ultrasound were ordered.

In spite of his obvious improvement—he was eating now in the dining room, taking short walks and socializing—his blood test results were worse [to be expected as tumors drain, but dismaying at that time].

At the time I did not know the relationship between bilirubin and aflatoxin. In our joy at seeing him eat, I could not advise against the pancakes and maple syrup he always had for breakfast. He was somehow getting a lot of aflatoxin or food dye [actually, from his tumors]. All the liver enzymes, especially GGT, were elevated (870). His RBC was not yet correct, due to persisting vanadium in his teeth. [*The dental plastic problem is apparent soon after the amalgam has been changed to composite; it too contains vanadium.*] Creatinine was much too low.

He felt fine, though. His pain-free periods were quite long, although pain still disturbed his sleep. Best of all, his ultrasound of the pancreas showed further shrinkage of his tumor to 3.25 x 3.5 cm. The largest of the liver tumors was now only 3.3 x 2.65 cm.

All this good news led him to one conclusion: that he could go home for Easter with his family. As much as he argued that he could, I argued that he couldn't. He agreed to stay one more week and repeat the blood test and ultrasound. During this time, several toxicities were inexorably at work. He was continuing to eat aflatoxined food (moldy grain), driving his liver

Apr. 12 pancreas and liver

enzymes and bilirubin up. Malonate inhibited the Krebs cycle and possibly the urea synthesis cycle. But other things were improving; vanadium was leaving his red blood cells (RBC) and globulin was declining.

His new ultrasounds (April 12) carried the day for him. The largest liver tumor now measured only 2.15 cm long. And no actual tumor was seen in the pancreas; only some irregular morphology, reminiscent of tumor. This was all he needed to board the next plane home. In spite of intensive last minute pleadings by all the doctors: "A successful start deserves a successful ending," "When you've got a good thing going, don't stop," "Don't get in the way of a lucky streak," he didn't hear.

I never expected him back. I expected his oil-filled house to push his liver to exhaustion, land him in the hospital at home from which never to emerge. But I was wrong. He called to say he was in trouble and would hurry back.

Three weeks from the time he left he returned, quite jaundiced now, in pain and with no appetite. He was full of vanadium again (fuel oil). We checked into surgery as a way to relieve obstructions of the bile ducts, even though we knew there would be no obstruction found. The liver was simply failing to conjugate (detoxify) the bilirubin. Bilirubin was saturating his body, turning him yellow.

He was returned to the IVs and supplements that had worked magic for him the first time. Besides this, he got a BQ shot (1 ug) in the hip in antici-pation of a higher LDH level. He was sent out for serum cleansing, using a device that pumps out the blood, centrifuges out the bilirubin and lets the cleaned blood return. After this, his complexion was much less yellow and he felt better.

But his blood test revealed the truth; he was in beginning kidney failure, both BUN and creatinine rising.

Presumably the saturating bilirubin [*or the methyl malonate from new plastic teeth*] was halting kidney function. This would allow albumin to es-cape through the kidney, so that the "total protein" would not be high enough to keep the blood plasma in the blood vessels.

Seepage of plasma into the tissues would let the ankles swell first, then the rest of his body, never to be regained. By now, he was aware of his pre-dicament; he quickly sought out other doctors; he was tried on various drugs and chemotherapies. I could not guess the real culprit was probably his new plastic teeth and the toxins that had drained from his tumors. I suggested calling his wife; she had said earlier she wanted her husband home for his last days.

Weak and yellow and on a handful of pills and continuous IVs, he elected to go to a hospital in another doctor's care. There was no opportunity to say goodbye or let him know that his wife had been calling. I obtained the next set of blood test results from his kind doctor at the new hospital.

It was his last. Final heroic efforts to save him can be seen in the low-ered BUN. He did not die of cancer or tumors or pancreatic failure in my estimation. He died of aflatoxin [*from opening tumors*] and dye in dental plastic which blocked conjugation of bilirubin, all made worse by copper, cobalt and malonates. But I did not understand all this until sometime later.

Summary: A lesson can be learned. We do not necessarily die of a tumorous condition. Jason's tumors were nearly gone. As long as the body can carry out its functions it can also put up with these obstructions. We die from <u>toxicities</u> that block these functions.

Jason McGowan	3/20	4/3	4/11	Easter Vac.	5/13	5/15
RBC	5.3	5.0	4.9		4.05	3.9
WBC	6,900	8,050	6,600		8,600	9,550
glucose	112	108	94		114	88
BUN	9	10	9		26	15
creatinine	.8	.7 (.7-1.4)	.8		3.9	.2 (.7-1.4) verified
AST (SGOT)	66	85	92		73	122
ALT(SGPT)	126	150	174		118	89
LDH	179	198	238		161	284
GGT	409	870	960		150	639
T.b.	.7	1.2	2.0		8.2	23.8 verified
alk phos	225	408	562		494	556
T.p.	7.5	7.1	7.2		5.2	4.7
albumin	4.3	4.1	4.4		3.0	2.8
globulin	3.2	3.0	2.8		2.2	1.9
uric acid	4.1	4.3	3.0		3.3	0.9
Calcium	9.2	9.0	9.2		8.9	8.1
Phosphorus	3.1	2.8	4.9		3.5	3.4
Iron	94	67	52		---	154
Sodium	138	137	136		142	131
Potassium	4.4	3.9	4.1		4.0	3.8
Chloride	102	100	97		100	94
triglycerides	119	114	119		201	113
cholesterol	270	260	251		212	120

5 Norman Shirkey   Prostate Cancer

Norman Shirkey, age seventy-nine, padded lightly into the office, following his determined caregiver. She was so determined to get him well, we were sure they would manage.

Norman's PSA was 105 (normal is 0.0-4.0 ng/ml), he was on a catheter, and was given six months by his doctor. This merely doubled her determination.

Norman had the following toxins in his prostate: freon, arsenic (pesticide), cobalt, and patulin (from common moldy fruit). He also had a dental infection: *Staphylococcus aureus*.

He was told to: (1) zap three times a day until well; (2) change his refrigerator to a non-CFC variety and do the freon-removal program; (3) clean the pesticide out of his house; (4) use no more detergent (to eliminate cobalt); (5) stop eating fruit except bananas and lemons (to eliminate patulin); (6) get his amalgams changed to composite and clean cavitations (to eliminate staphylococcus); (7) take vitamin C, vitamin B-complex, vitamin A, zinc; (8) get a benzoquinone (BQ) shot. But his finances did not allow regular visits or IVs. We begged him to persevere.

Two weeks later his cobalt was gone. He had ordered a new refrigerator. Arsenic was gone; patulin was gone; but salmonellas were now present in the prostate. He was given Lugol's to take for that. Also rhodizonic acid.

It wasn't working. At his next visit another two weeks later, his PSA was up to 130 ng/ml. He had a lot of pain around the ribs and lower back. He was asked to do a bone scan. He had his new refrigerator, and patulin was still Negative, so he could eat a few more fruits. *Rhizopus* (fungus) was growing in his prostate and Peyers patches (the lymph nodes of the intestine). [*We are able to grow fungus right inside our most hallowed organs, the lymph nodes.*] His latest blood test showed a low RBC. He was started on an IV containing potassium, magnesium, cesium, and B complex. He was in the middle of dental replacement. His next blood test showed exceptionally good results in spite of his poor condition. But the protein level was slightly high, and LDH also high. He was given another BQ shot. The outcome looked assured. But why was he worsening?

Another week later he had picked up patulin again. And mercury was still Positive even after amalgam removal. It was traced to his new pink denture; he was to replace it. He was given another IV. He was to continue rhodizonic acid, two a day.

He did not show up for his daily IVs, in spite of entreaties. In fact, he didn't return for two months. His friend gave explanations of a sort. When he arrived this time he was feeling very well. A blood test he brought with him showed: LDH 245 and PSA 167. The tumor was not shrinking. And deep inside, patulin fungus was again growing, as was *Aspergillus mycelium, conidia* and three other aspergillus varieties. There was mercury at the prostate; he was using cotton swabs daily. [*We did not understand the importance of leftover amalgam tattoos at that time.*] He was given cloves, cinnamon, L-G (homemade lysine-glutamate as described in *The Cure For HIV/AIDS*), wormwood, and bee pollen. This was our antifungal program at that time. He was given another BQ shot, to bring down the LDH. And two IVs of EDTA plus vitamin C.

Two weeks later, he appeared more bowed and shuffling than ever but still walked unassisted. Patulin was again at the prostate, as was insulin-like growth factor. Both *Fasciolopsis* eggs and *Fasciola* miracidia were thriving there, too. He was reminded to zap, and take the parasite herbs regularly. His caregiver was doing her level best.

Three weeks later, he had pain everywhere around the middle and in his spine. The catheter showed bloody urine. There was staphylococcus everywhere. And fibroblast growth factor in the liver. He was given 4 tsp. black walnut tincture extra strength in a quart of very warm water by enema plus 1 tsp. black walnut tincture extra strength by mouth. His PSA was 169. His LDH 274. His doctor at home, where the test was done, was calling him urgently for treatment. His RBC was 3.35.

In another three weeks his pain around the mid-abdomen was much worse. He still had not done all his dental work. The bone scan showed widespread bone cancer. Staphylococcus was still everywhere. He was to continue taking enemas.

Six days later he arrived in a wheelchair, just a wispy shadow of his former self. He said he was numb everywhere. His blood test results were RBC 3.74 (an increase!), LDH 268 (slight decrease), uric acid 2.4 for which he was given glutamine. He was given a BQ shot and an oral dose of DMSO (just half a dose). IVs were not helping him so were not recommended. He was given Lugol's again to be taken four times a day for salmonella everywhere. There was also staphylococcus everywhere due to uncompleted dental work. He was now too sick to sit in a dentist's chair. He was given magnesium, plus Cascara sagrada for constipation. And black walnut tincture extra strength was increased to 2 tsp. on alternate days.

He went home to die and I did not prevail upon him to do more. His whole treatment program had been "too little, too late." His caregiver quietly pushed him through the front door and we looked our last goodbye.

Eleven months later she reappeared by herself. I wanted to know about Norman's last days. She almost giggled as she spoke; Oh, Norman's fine, she said. He's living on a mountain top. I thought she meant as an angel in some religious sense. Oh yes! I said and listened on. She related that he wanted to die on a piece of family property—mountainous land—far from his city home. When he left our office he decided to live his last at this mountain retreat. He threw away his pills and potions, all his vitamins, special herbs, etc. But instead of dying he got stronger. He got out of the wheelchair, began to cook for himself, went for walks on trails and enjoyed each sunrise and sunset. He planned to stay there and not return for any more treatments.

Later, as I absorbed this "miracle" I wondered: Was it his toxic home that he was getting away from? Some food dye? A toxic supplement? Was it the enemas that helped? Was it the L-G and bee pollen? Was there magic in the mountain property? We'll never know. The truth still lies carefully hidden.

PS He didn't need his catheter any more either.

Summary: It was tempting, as an author or researcher, to omit this case history. It ridicules all our efforts as therapists. And perhaps other patients will try this and shorten their days. One cancer patient, who knew Norman, did choose Norman's abandon, went to a mountain retreat and lived on coconuts and other natural food. She died a few months later, emaciated and in pain. It is not easy or simple to abandon all civilization's foods and products. She kept her hair dye and eyebrow pencil, perhaps her vitamin C, and a few other select items. These may have been the traitors.

Norman Shirkey	6/20/ 95	6/23/ 95	9/25/ 95	10/17/ 95
RBC	3.78	4.0	3.35	3.74
WBC	5,000	7,000	5,200	4,200
PLT	244	-----	198	210
glucose		87	95	96
BUN		20	20	18
creatinine		0.9	1.1	0.9
AST (SGOT)		33	26	43
ALT (SGPT)		20	16	29
LDH		232	274	268
GGT		23	33	35
T.b.		1.0	0.9	1.0
alk phos		121	87	94
T.p.		8.1	7.2	6.9
albumin		4.5	4.0	4.6
globulin		3.6	3.2	2.3
uric acid		4.7	3.8	2.4
Calcium		9.1	9.5	9.6
Phosphorus		4.3	3.6	4.4
Iron		93	67	59
Sodium		138	136	133
Potassium		4.7	4.1	4.1
Chloride		103	99	95
triglycerides		124	105	141
cholesterol		214	195	187
PSA	130		169	

I decided to keep the story. It has more hidden wisdom than we can understand; at the very least, a terminally ill patient should leave the dwelling where the disease was acquired.

6   Brian Castro   Bone Cancer

Brian, age seventeen, was a tall, athletic looking teenager, who came with his parents for his bone cancer on July 14. They could stay at the clinic only four days. Three weeks earlier, his right arm began hurting and a bump arose on his forearm about half way up to the elbow. His whole arm and hand were painful and he couldn't move his thumb back. X-rays showed the bone tumor on the ulna.

Earlier in the Spring (March), Brian had become very tired. He slept most of the time (16-18 hours a day), the rest of the day he was dizzy and felt cold. [*Dizziness is usually due to Salmonella; feeling cold could be due to anything abnormal in the thyroid.*] His blood pressure was low and he was pale. He had a dog. His mouth contained amalgam.

A visit to the doctor at that time, March 9, got him a blood test and a diagnosis of Epstein-Barre virus. There was nothing to do but "outgrow" it. He did not have enough energy to attend school and if he tried to play, he felt as if he would faint. But looking at the blood test of March 9, we see a number of metabolic problems. They could not all have arisen in the previous year. He must have been suffering from certain parasites and pollutants for many years, perhaps from age four when he had Kawasaki disease.

The RBC was too high, showing cobalt and vanadium toxicity. And creatinine, which is muscle-related, was much too low. No wonder he was tired. Creatinine is made from creatine, the muscle energy factor. Creatine is made by the body from arginine and glycine and also requires methionine. Was he

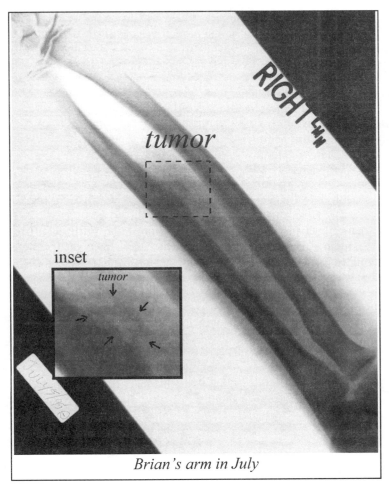

Brian's arm in July

not getting enough of these amino acids or was a parasite inhibiting their formation?

273

Most notable is the high alkaline phosphatase. This is the bone enzyme. It is normal to be high when your bones are growing, and Brian had grown 6 inches during the past year, but still, 378 is too high. (It's more than twice the highest normal value of 150.) Was Brian's growth spurt a causative factor, an effect, or just a coincidence with his bone cancer?

The T4 indicates thyroid function. It's very low, and would contribute to Brian's lethargy.

They had brought an X-ray of Brian's arm. The growing lump was easy to see. The doctor had given an ominous prognosis: it was better to amputate than try to treat; this variety of cancer was lethal in children. The doctor immediately arranged for the surgery—there was to be no waiting. That was July 5. On July 6 his family started him on our parasite killing recipe, using the book as guide. On July 10, another visit to his doctor brought only dire predictions if the surgery were not carried out quickly. Three days later they flew in to see us.

These were Brian's initial test results using the Syncrometer: isopropyl alcohol Positive. He was referred to the isopropyl alcohol list in *The Cure For All Cancers*; he agreed to be meticulous about compliance. Wood alcohol Positive. Ortho-phospho-tyrosine Negative. Evidently he had killed the flukes and their stages already with the parasite program.

Copper, mercury, *Mucor* (fungus), freon were all Positive at bone. Where was it coming from? Household water tests for copper were Positive in the bathroom. A home air test (dust sample) was Positive for freon in living room and Brian's bedroom.

The parents planned to immediately move the refrigerator outdoors while finding a new non-freon replacement. They would change the copper water pipes immediately also. Brian's dental amalgams would be changed to plastic. [*At that time we did not know that dental plastic could also be polluted with copper, cobalt, vanadium, malonates, dye, and urethane, all with cancer promoting action.*]

His instructions were: (1) continue the parasite killing program according to the book recipe and to zap daily. (2) Drink 2-3 glasses of ozonated water daily to remove freon, and take ¾ cup kidney cleanse recipe daily (½ dose). (3) Take benzoquinone orally for three days to kill *Mucor* fungus. They would make a homeopathic dilution of it (one part per million) and give Brian ¼ tsp. of the final solution. To make a 1 ppm solution they would first put ¼ tsp. powder into a glass quart jar of solvent-free, copper-free water obtained from a busy laundromat's cold faucet. The jar would be closed and shaken a few times. It dissolves quickly. Then ¼ tsp. of this brown-colored solution would be placed into another quart jar to be filled with water also. The final solution should not be more than 10 minutes old before Brian drank the ¼ tsp. liquid.

His food supplementation was calcium, from 3 to 4 glasses of 2% milk in plastic carton daily, correctly treated, magnesium oxide, manganese, boron, zinc, chromium, selenium, vitamin A, vitamin B complex, vitamin C.

Three days later, Brian was tested again. His arm was now free of pain, the lump was down. New tests showed solvents Negative; *Mucor* Negative; copper still Positive at bone and parathyroid; mercury Positive at bone and parathyroid; freon still Positive at bone and parathyroid. Dental work had not been done yet.

The blood test (July 14) showed considerable improvement from the one done in March, especially in alk phos, creatinine level, and thyroid function (T_4). They had accomplished this themselves before arriving.

They left for home, returning a month later. Brian's arm pain had not returned; the lump was visibly smaller, nearly normal-feeling. His new Syncrometer tests showed: isopropyl and wood alcohol Negative; copper Positive at bone and parathyroid; mercury Positive at bone; *Penicillium* spores (fungus) Positive at bone; *Mucor* and yeast fungi Negative at bone; freon Positive at bone and parathyroid.

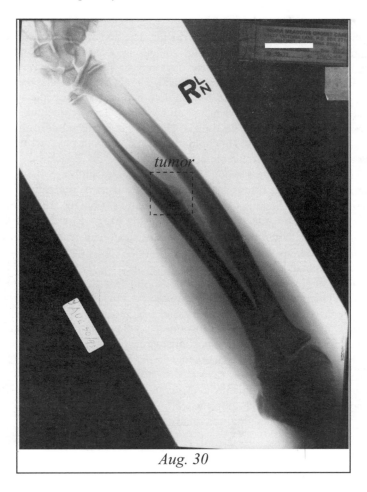

Aug. 30

275

A dust test from home was negative for freon; they had moved the refrigerator outdoors (but it takes six weeks before freon is removed from the body by drinking ozonated water).

His household water continued to be Positive for copper; the plumbing had not yet been done. His new instructions were to take thioctic acid, cysteine, taurine, methionine (I would have liked to give these sooner, but did not have the opportunity), and to continue with his old instructions, taking another single dose of benzoquinone to kill remaining fungus.

By August 25, all his amalgam fillings were replaced with composites. Final Syncrometer testing showed: *Penicillium* spores Negative at bone, mercury Negative at bone.

A new item was added to his supplement list, L-G (a lysine-glutamate compound). He next appeared on October 23. His arm still showed a slight swelling where the lump had been.

They informed me that a second X-ray had been taken August 30, showing that the top part of the tumor was gone; the base was still there, maybe even larger, according to his doctor. The doctor now advised to "keep doing whatever it is we are doing, something seems to be working" and scheduled another X-ray for thirty days hence. The third X-ray was taken October 4. The tumor had decreased in size again and texture appeared more bone-like; nevertheless, the doctor referred them to an orthopedic surgeon.

Brian was no longer exhausted all the time. He was sleeping only 9-10 hours a night and did not need naps. He was attending school full-time and kept up with schoolwork. He could attend P.E. without physical limitations. He seemed to be back to his old healthy self.

Their regular doctor appointment had been on October 9, the doctor had compared all three X-rays stating he "didn't usually see tumors do this, didn't usually see them get smaller, they usually get bigger. This is unusual." An MRI had been ordered. It showed that the base was not larger than the first X-ray had shown it to be. Nevertheless, the doctor recommended a total surgical bone biopsy in order to see it himself. The parents decided to "wait and see" instead.

Here they were, now, on October 23, doing their "waiting and seeing." Isopropyl alcohol Positive; *Fasciola* miracidia Positive at bone; *Fasciolopsis* eggs Positive at parathyroids. They had become way too relaxed about all Brian's instructions; he was consuming cold cereals and soda pop (they contain traces of isopropyl alcohol antiseptic).

He was to continue the maintenance parasite program once a week and give away his dog. He was reminded to boil all dairy products, avoid aflatoxins, stay away from salad bars (*Salmonella*, etc.), consume no cold cereal, or bottled water, no soda pop, no corn chips, no popcorn, no nuts, and no raisins (mold) until his ulna was totally normal again.

The next visit to his doctor, in November, brought them his fourth X-ray. This time the doctor said "Well, this is the best X-ray yet. Keep up the good work. The blood work looks real good. Let's do this again in five weeks and see what it looks like then." Gone was the recommendation to do surgery.

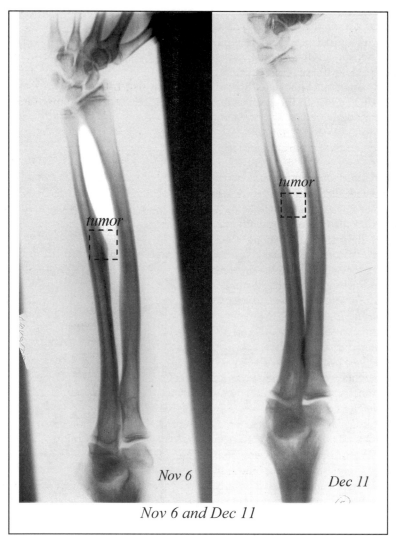

Nov 6 and Dec 11

The fifth X-ray was taken December 11. The tumor was still present but getting smaller, in fact, almost gone. The doctor was delighted, exclaiming it was "like a ferocious beast had attacked but then decided to run away. This is hard to understand," he said, "it looks great. I want to see it again in three months." A blood test done by his doctor was dated December 27.

The RBC is too high, due to cobalt and vanadium from left over tattoos [*or possibly from the recent dental composites installed*]. The WBC is now too low, implicating toxins in the bone marrow. The LDH is correct now; so is the alkaline phosphatase for the first time (note range change for alk phos); this indicates normal bone health. The albumin was normal now, as was iron. Urine tests (not shown) had normalized also.

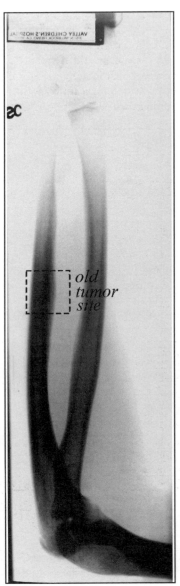

We didn't actually see Brian and his family again till February 28 of the next year. He had lost 15 lb. and was fatigued a lot. He had malonic acid in the bone, bone marrow and liver. [*At that time we did not suspect a food source, nor the dental plastic source.*] We assumed he had picked up a tapeworm stage again. This time we used coenzyme Q10 in 4 massive doses of 3,000 mg taken four days apart. He was also given glutathione. This should help normalize bone metabolism after the malonic acid attack.

Our Syncrometer tests showed: vanadium Positive; cobalt Positive. [*The sources for these were not suspected to be right in his own mouth. Now we know he must remove the composites as well and even make a dedicated search for tattoos before he can be free of their toxicity.*] The parents were encouraged to learn the Syncrometer technique so they could follow his progress at home.

His last X-ray was taken on April 1: His doctor had come into the room and said, "Well, it's all gone now. That was a strange thing, but there's nothing to worry about now. He must have injured it or something because it's not there anymore. It looks like normal healthy bone. I don't know what that was. It was sure strange, but you don't need to come back. Whatever that was, it's gone now."

Brian's parents were meticulous about writing down what the doctors said,

April 1, next year

both now and before, so they were just a tiny bit chagrined. After all, two radiologists knew exactly "what it was," and two other doctors agreed. They "knew it needed immediate surgery"; amputation, in fact.

But joy outweighed chagrin, as it should.

Summary: Of course, we know that the last quote, "it's gone now", should be changed to "it's gone for now." He will need to remove plastic and leftover metal in his mouth. He will need to clear *Ascaris* and tapeworm parasites from his body repeatedly. He will need to keep his distance from animals (pets). And to lead a health-conscious life. Maybe his early Kawasaki disease should tip him off to his special needs. Maybe he'll grow into a tough, robust athlete in spite of everything. We wish him his heart's desires. In exchange for a little caution! His parents, though, deserve A-1 grades for pulling their teenager through this experience, with arm intact.

Brian Castro	3/9	7/14	12/27
RBC	5.39 (4.6-6.2)	4.85 (4.36-5.73)	5.31 (4.3-5.9)
WBC	6.1	6.35	4.1
PLT	246		213
glucose	119	95	94
BUN	11	13	17
creatinine	0.3 (.9-1.4)	0.9	1.0
AST (SGOT)	19	26	16
ALT (SGPT)	10	25	12
LDH	193 (130-280)	186 (91-250)	122 (90-225)
GGT		14	11
T.b.	0.6	0.5	0.7
alk phos	378 (20-150)	245 (39-117)	219 (150-450)
T.p.	7.8	7.2	6.9
albumin	5.2 (3.9-5.1)	5.0	4.6 (3.5-5.0)
globulin	2.6	2.2	2.3
uric acid	6.3	4.6	3.5
Calcium	9.7	8.8	10 (8.5-10.5)
Phosphorus	6.0 (3.5-5.5)	5.6 (2.5-5.5)	4.6
Iron		58	112
Sodium	142	137	152
Potassium	4.2	4.0	3.8
Chloride	109	108	105
triglycerides	142	73	129
cholesterol	173	226	189
T4	5.5 (4.5-11.5)	8.2	6.7

7	Jamie Humbert	Liver Cancer

Jamie Humbert, only fifty-nine, came with her daughter in high hopes of becoming cured of her liver cancer. They had already had conventional therapy, followed by alternative therapies in Mexico. But one look at her blood test revealed the ominous fact that her LDH was much too high (3415!).

[*When Jamie arrived I had no reason to doubt the clinical explanation for elevated LDH, which is cancer plus liver failure, as explained on page 234.*] Why was it so high? I soon found that there is a mysterious lack of information on reducing LDH in the scientific literature. [*Which I now think reflects the hopeless nature of the problem as perceived by scientists.*] Nor was there any conventional medicine or treatment to reduce LDH. [*My unconventional treatment, benzoquinone ("BQ"), was not yet discovered. Jamie would turn out to be the first person to try benzoquinone to see if it would reduce LDH.*] Clearly it <u>was</u> partly due to a failing liver because the other liver enzymes were much too high, also. [*But I had not yet discovered that Sudan Black B and lanthanides cause LDH elevation.*]

Although Jamie was in a wheelchair, nothing else on her blood test was particularly bad, except the creatinine level. It was much too low. Either it was being lost with the urine or its production was blocked. [*At the time, I did not know of the great shortages of amino acids cancer sufferers have, some of which are required to make creatinine.*] But a low level of creatinine or BUN is not considered serious, clinically. What was obvious, clinically, was that she would die of liver failure. But just as obvious was the fact that one <u>need not die</u> of an LDH over 3000! She was in good spirits and eager to begin something. She could eat and digest, was not in much pain though terribly fatigued.

The tumor in her liver was "only" the size of a baseball, but there were ominous signs of brain involvement: her left arm was becoming useless. I ordered a brain scan and ultrasound of liver. There was also a tumor in the pancreas.

She was started on the parasite killing program, but only a 2 tsp. dose. She was given numerous IVs and zapped, though I knew it would not save her. She was full of mercury, although all amalgam had been replaced at an earlier time. She was full of vanadium [*but its significance as a mutagen was not known then; nor did I suspect the plastic in her dental restorations*]. Vanadium was coming from the refrigerator and gas line to her motel room. There was no environmentally safe room for her yet.

After ten days, though, her nausea and vomiting had stopped and the tumor in her pancreas had shrunk to half its size. But seizures were increasing in spite of medication to block them.

Still, she had gotten through ten unbelievable, unprecedented days. Would she survive? Could she? Her daughter was determined.

Our hopes were dashed at the next blood test. The whole liver picture was worse and the LDH was now an unbelievable 5119 and the GGT over 500. [*Today I know that opening the tumors releases the toxins that cause this.*]

We had transferred Jamie to a hospital ten days before this second blood test, but defeatism was not in our nature, even there. The doctors were encouraged to test and treat up to the very end. The hospital water contained no copper which was the basis of my choice of hospital. Of course, it was still coming from the plastic dentalware [and tumors].

Jamie's daughter was allowed and encouraged to do her mother's cooking, feed her, and do personal chores. She was also getting three IVs a day, containing amino acids, fat emulsion, besides numerous vitamins and minerals. She was not in pain. Each day, her daughter coaxed a cup of "high-calorie food" down her; she did not resist.

Suddenly, May 1, Jamie got better. She talked on the telephone and took a shower—standing by herself! They were both jubilant and Oh! so hopeful. Would the miracle happen? The next day she did a blood test. Hopes were dashed again. LDH had set a new record, 5350. Yet Jamie was definitely better in a number of ways. This could not simply be due to that small drop in the transaminases, SGOT and SGPT.

On May 2, when the blood test showed no improvement, a special preparation of benzoquinone was made for her. The concept was taken from Dr. William Koch. I had been reading his books to the wee hours of the night. Librarians helped locate these long-lost monographs at obscure libraries. Dr. Koch discovered half a dozen highly oxidizing compounds that could safely be given to cancer patients. He cautioned against giving too much or too often. He described one of these as benzoquinone, a familiar compound, which in a minute dose of 1 ml of a 1 ppm solution could miraculously "cure" a bedridden, terminally ill cancer patient. He had pictures of "recoveries" to prove it. I gave it to myself several times first. After I noticed no ill effects, staff volunteers took the shot. It seemed safe, and was, after all, in a homeopathic dose. We gave it to Jamie.

The next five days she got better and better. She stayed out of bed and wanted food. She stopped vomiting and hiccuping. Her family arrived, too, seemingly to applaud her gains.

But on May 8, Jamie had no insomnia and was sleepy through the day. The next day was no better, in fact, worse. We did a blood test to find the cause, but it was too late. Jamie was slipping away. Her family surrounded her as she lay in a coma in bed. Voices were lifted in song. She left at 6 p.m. on May 10.

The blood test results were available at 8 p.m. LDH was an incredible 338(!) and the other liver statistics showed similar improvement. But if that wasn't the problem, what was? Perhaps you have already spotted it: high calcium levels. Simple hypercalcemia, plus a rising bilirubin.

Neither I nor the other doctors suspected it, and it would have been correctable if we had just ordered the blood tests a day earlier. And what if Jamie had gotten the BQ shot a day earlier? It was not to be. The family was more than kind and gracious and forgiving. She did not die in pain or on morphine. Was it the benzoquinone shot that worked the miracle? Or everything else?

Summary: It is never possible to know the true cause of death. For Jamie, it wasn't heart failure (the test for this, creatine kinase, Ck, was done), nor kidney failure, nor even the expected liver failure. Thank you, Jamie and family, for your truly spiritual contribution to this book. You taught us that LDH over 5000 isn't hopeless. You taught us how to fight it. You taught us not to cower in fear of it. When the next patient handed us a similar challenge, we could begin where Jamie left off. And Jamie got five weeks of extended life when only one was expected.

Jamie Humbert	4/13	4/18	4/27	5/2	5/9
RBC	4.5	4.53			
WBC	6.3	5.4			
PLT		251			
glucose	99		83	146	110
BUN	8 (7-25)		6 (5-20)	6	25
creatinine	0.4 (.7-1.4)		0.6 (.8-1.4)	0.6	0.9
AST (SGOT)	260		381	353	52
ALT (SGPT)	147		206	129	130
LDH	3415		5119	5350	338
GGT	158		523	747	140
T.b.	0.3		0.4	0.5	8.5
alk phos	122		231	295	143
T.p.	6.7		6.0	6.0	5.8
Albumin	3.6		3.4	3.5	3.0
globulin	3.1		2.6	2.5	2.8
uric acid	6.2		4.1	4.0	4.3
Calcium	9.1		8.8	9.1	13.8
Phosphorus	4.0		4.1	3.8	3.9
Iron	68		62	48	
Sodium	142		139	134	133
Potassium	4.3		4.8	4.5	3.7
Chloride	105		104	106	93
triglycerides	158		180	115	170
cholesterol	262		291	257	291
Ck					62

8	Anthony Stephens	Cancer of the Parotid Gland

Anthony Stephens, sixty-nine, had a lump that measured 1½ x 1½ in., outer dimensions, on the right side of his face, at the angle of the jaw just in front of the ear lobe. It was a tumor of the parotid gland, one of our salivary glands. At first it was thought to be a dental abscess. But an oral surgeon thought it was a tumor and referred him back to his doctor. Such tumors are notorious for growing right back after they are removed. His MRI dated September 5, shows it clearly.

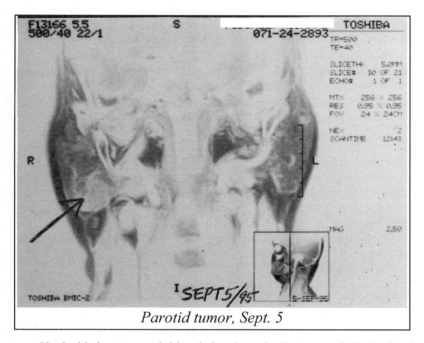

Parotid tumor, Sept. 5

He decided not to get it biopsied and surgically removed. So by the time he arrived, he had already been on the parasite killing, isopropyl alcohol-free regimen for seven weeks. He was also on the "macrobiotic diet." And, indeed, when he arrived in Mexico he tested Negative for isopropyl alcohol and ortho-phospho-tyrosine (malignancy). But why didn't the tumor shrink during these weeks? The answer will be clearer as we follow his progress.

He arrived on October 2. His toxin test was done the first day after arrival. Promptness in testing for home toxins is essential because toxins disappear from the body quickly, in days! It showed the following at the "whole body": Negative for isopropyl alcohol, wood alcohol, benzene, xylene, arsenic, aluminum, asbestos, nickel, cobalt, thallium and patulin. Copper was Negative in general, but Positive when I checked the parotid. Toxins present were cadmium, formaldehyde, lead, beryllium, mercury, and CFCs. The pathogen picture was worse. Negative for two species of salmonella, but Positive for *Salmonella typhimurium*, one shigella, staphylococcus, and *E. coli*. In addition he was tested for seven common fungus varieties; he was Positive for five, including *Aspergillus*, in his parotid gland.

He was also Positive for fibroblast growth factor (FGF) and fibronectin at the parotid, made by *Fasciola* stages (not *Fasciolopsis*) and bacteria.

We started with an intensive bacteria killing program in the intestine. He was given Lugol's iodine to take 4 times a day to kill salmonella, as well as the Bowel Program. And, of course, he would continue with the parasite program, both herbal and zapping.

He was given cysteine, taurine, and methionine to detoxify formaldehyde buildup. He was started on the freon removal program. And instructed to reduce bacterial and fungal growth in the intestine with a series of daily enemas. It consisted of 1 quart very warm water with 4 tsp. black walnut tincture extra strength added. At the same time, he would take 1 tsp. by mouth in water. This would kill the parasites hidden in the intestinal contents.

His blood test showed very little damage yet, either from the tumor or from the toxins causing the tumor.

His blood sugar was much too low (62), and T.p. was too high. This was the beginning evidence for cobalt and vanadium toxicity. Even tiny amounts of these, not even detected at the initial "whole body" test would, nevertheless, seek out the vital organs.

Tumors of the mouth and throat can be very swift and so disfiguring! It was reassuring to see his triglycerides and cholesterol high enough to see him safely through this ordeal.

Anthony was meticulous with his total program even while away for the next twelve days. Upon his return, the parotid tumor was already shrinking and actually draining on the inside. He had not started dental work yet! Just killing bacteria, parasites, and fungus evidently was enough. He could stop the enema routine and simply take the parasite herbs once a week.

Again he had to leave, this time for four weeks, returning November 15. The parotid tumor could no longer be seen. His cheek was flat. Most of the dental metal was out—but not all of it—and replaced with plastic. He was Negative, now, for *Staphylococcus aureus*, dental bacteria. He tested Negative consistently for isopropyl alcohol, benzene, and wood alcohol. He received no IV therapy or extra supplements. Evidently, getting rid of bacteria in his mouth and reducing them in the intestine had empowered his immune system to clean it all up again.

Three weeks later he returned again to relate how he had passed a tape worm of the long variety common in horses and cattle. It was after taking Rascal, a popular anti-tapeworm herbal mixture. We immediately tried to "mop up" after it with 8 tsp. of black walnut tincture extra strength since the scolex can be very hard to kill. This was followed by 3 niacinamide tablets, (500 mg each) then another dose of 8 tsp. black walnut tincture extra strength followed by zapping. We feared the scolex was still present somewhere. He then left for three months, taking his new lifestyle with him.

On March 6 of the next year he returned for a follow-up. His face looked perfectly normal, but malonic acid was Positive at the parotid gland. By now we were using coenzyme Q10 to kill buried tapeworm stages; he required 5 grams. He was also given glutathione for one week. After this he felt noticeably better, although he had not felt ill before. Malonate was now Negative at the parotid gland. He left for home.

284

By September, we were aware of the presence of malonic and maleic acids in dental plastic. We let him know he was at risk from his new plastic fillings. He hurried back in October. His toxin test now showed he had not only malonic acid buildup, but benzene, isopropyl alcohol, wood alcohol, *E. coli*, shigella, asbestos, cadmium, cobalt, mercury, vanadium, and aflatoxin! But staphylococcus and clostridium were missing due to his earlier dental cleanup; this probably saved him from a recurrence of his parotid tumor. He arrived October 10, still with a perfectly smooth contour to his face.

He had 17 plastic fillings in his mouth to be tested. Three of these were Positive for copper, cobalt, vanadium, and malonates. [*We did not suspect carcinogenic dyes yet.*] We determined this by filing each tooth with an emery board, then testing the emery board electronically. His blood test of October 10 reflects the new toxins in his mouth, carried for one year.

The red blood cell level is now higher than before switching to plastic, showing that his body is now deprived of oxygen due to cobalt and vanadium toxicity. He was also making too many white blood cells (11,800). Calcium had begun to drop due to toxins in the parathyroid gland. And the phosphorus level was now too low. The iron level was also dropping.

His 3 toxic plastic fillings were replaced.

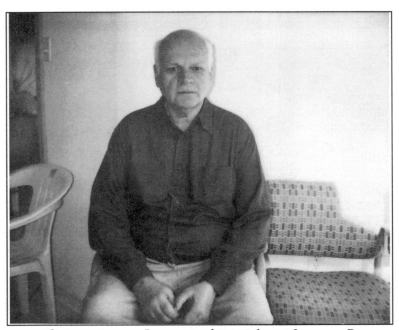

Oct. next year. Lump used to stick out 2 cm on R

Summary: Before leaving this time, he agreed to pose for our camera with his beautifully flat cheeks.

This may still not be the final step to be taken for Anthony, but he understands the power of nature and the feebleness of research or medicine and may act in time. We wish him well.

Post Script from Anthony, December 4.

"The next routine appointment with my regular, allopathic doctor produced this exchange: Dr.: 'Did you have surgery?' Anthony: 'No, I did not want surgery so I went offshore, alternative.' He dropped the subject and we moved on to other matters." We also received a letter a year later, and again almost a year after that reassuring us that there had been no recurrence.

Anthony Stephens	10/3	10/10 next year
RBC	4.4	5.32
WBC	9,000	11,800
PLT		293
glucose	62	89
BUN	20	15
creatinine	0.9	1.0
Sodium	143	138
Potassium	4.1	4.0
Chloride	105	105
Calcium	9.3	9.0
Phosphorus	4.3	2.6
T.p.	7.8	6.9
albumin	4.8	4.7
globulin	3.0	2.2
T.b.	0.7	0.6
alk phos	70	71
LDH	157	149
GGT	31	
AST (SGOT)	21	19
ALT (SGPT)	29	1.0
uric acid	5.5	4.4
Iron	97	69
triglycerides	178	212
cholesterol	272	224

9   Ronald Hartnett   Brain Cancer

"Little Ronald's" adventure with brain cancer taught us a lot about the brain.

It began at age eight, diagnosed as glioblastoma multiforme/astrocytoma. We saw him first at age nine. He was now in Stage IV. He had already gone through six surgeries to remove the tumor, but each time it grew back. He also had received intense chemotherapy and six weeks of radiation. The family had decided not to do another surgery this time for the new growth. Ronald was extremely weak; nothing had worked. He was on Decadron, 4 mg a day, to prevent brain swelling. He was also on Tegretol for sei-zures.

He arrived in a wheelchair, unable to hold his head up or raise his arm. He was not interested in talking or listening or being tested. His face was tearful as were our hearts.

His initial toxin test showed isopropyl alcohol, asbestos, copper, cobalt, freon, formaldehyde, *Salmonella*, *Staphylococcus*, Positive. Mysteriously, mercury was also Positive yet he had no tooth fillings. We traced the mer-cury to an everyday personal product. This did not surprise us because most paper products like toilet paper, paper towels, Q-tips, sanitary napkins, tam-pons, paper diapers test Positive to mercury on the Syncrometer! Perhaps this is due to using mercuric chloride as a sterilizing agent. It may be illegal in the USA to sterilize with mercury for the environment's sake, but it is not illegal in other countries where such products are made. Or perhaps mercury is used in the wood pulp industry because in addition to paper products, toothpicks often test Positive to mercury. Ronald was to avoid all use of pa-per sanitary products. Next, the copper plumbing had to go. They agreed at once. This was probably the decisive step that would save him. Their refrig-erator was quickly changed to a new non-freon model. Detergent use was stopped (cobalt). All foam cushions were taken out of the house (formaldehyde). A dose of 6 drops of Lugol's in ½ glass of water was poured down him; he gulped without struggle. Where did the *Staphylococcus* come from since no dental work had ever been done? Was his immunity so low his own skin bacteria would invade him?

After a blood test, he was given 1 tsp. black walnut tincture extra strength in water. He was to take this daily at bedtime followed by zapping. He was to start the freon removal program and continue for six to eight weeks. They would come back in four days.

He returned in his wheelchair, holding his head up now; he listened to me and watched things around him, could hold his hand out for testing.

His blood test was reviewed. The LDH showed evidence of tumor activ-ity, as did the high alk phos [*both the result of azo dyes acting on the liver*]. The high GGT showed a liver problem possibly from his medication or a food dye. The high calcium (10.1) showed a thyroid problem. The extremely low iron (8.0) reflected on the underlying cancer problem: copper [*and ger-manium*] toxicity. The effect of cobalt, too, could already be seen in a very slightly elevated RBC.

At this second visit, Syncrometer testing showed isopropyl, *Salmonella dysenteriae*, *Staphylococcus aureus*, Negative. The family was doing its part. The remaining six bacteria in our standard "food bacteria" test were also Negative. Five cancer antigens tested Negative; three growth factors tested Negative.

Copper was Negative at cerebrum (brain) and parathyroids, but still Positive at live. They were in the middle of changing water pipes; had carried his drinking water home from our clinic at last visit. He was started on thioctic acid. Since he couldn't swallow a capsule, it had to be stirred into pure honey. He took it, although it tastes dreadful.

Formaldehyde was still Positive. He was started on taurine and cysteine to detoxify this. The clothes drier had not yet been tested for asbestos release.

He was started on methylene blue powder, 65 mg, one capsule daily. It would turn the urine blue. The purpose for the methylene blue is, theoretically, to bridge the gap in his brain's respiratory metabolism. Since metabolism is extremely hampered in a tumor, many normal chemicals are missing or in over abundance. It was thought, from the 1920's on, that a "magic bullet" might be found that could substitute for the missing items. Various compounds were tried. Although some were quite successful in some kinds of cancer, they were not successful for all cancers at all times. So they were abandoned along with the concept. This is like abandoning the concept of a locomotive (an early Ford engine) because it couldn't immediately go up a hill at 30 mph. Methylene blue is exceedingly safe; not much is needed. I use it for all brain cancer cases.

The October 4 MRI has many views (frames) pictured on the negative. I chose the view that was numbered 141. This number is shown on the index picture to be a slice that just grazes the top of the white areas. This

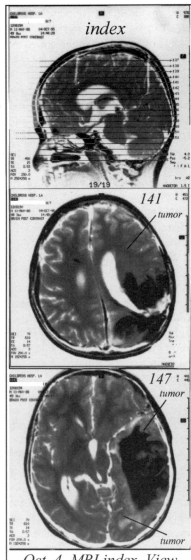

Oct. 4. MRI index. View 141 shows large tumor pushing midline off center. View 147 shows depth of tumor.

frame shows the midline quite bent out of its normal straight line. The dark region on the side and extending down to the edge is the gigantic tumor (plus black empty space left by surgery). Fluid from the tumor (edema) has no place to go and, therefore, creates pressure that pushes the brain aside. Another slice, at 147, shows how very extensive (deep) this tumor is.

Here are further notes taken from his file:

November 24, it is four days later. He is keeping his improved status. Still in wheelchair but talking, wanting to give me a gift. Testing showed: benzene, isopropyl alcohol, wood alcohol Negative. Copper Negative at parathyroids and liver (plumbing job at home completed). Formaldehyde and eight food bacteria Negative.

November 27, he is deteriorated, sleeping and crying all the time. I suspected something toxic was back in his brain. Tests were done on his saliva since he could not hold out his hand for testing.

Isopropyl alcohol Positive. He had used regular soap in the bathroom while visiting friends. We then tested for the entire set of 35 tapeworm slides. Three were positive: *Dipylidium caninum* composite, *Taenia pisiformis* composite, *Hymenolepis dim.* Composite. The "composite" slides actually contain pieces of intact tapeworm, without the scolex. Somewhere in his body, he had three intact tapeworms! We administered 8 tsp. black walnut tincture extra strength which he took without rebelling.

December 4, it has been a week. Ronald walked into my office; doesn't need a wheelchair. He is doing much better. No headaches. Has more energy all day until 6 p.m. Better mood. Test results: benzene, isopropyl, wood alcohol and the three tapeworm composite slides all Negative. Evidently the tapeworms were killed by the 8 tsp. dose of black walnut tincture extra strength. He has not needed Decadron for one week and is not on Tylenol-codeine painkillers any more. They will return in one week; it is Saturday.

December 6, Monday. (He returned only two days later), several family members are with him. He is back in a wheelchair—semi comatose. Extreme setback started on Sunday. This may be his last day. He is quite still. Family and staff are poised for action. Or will we give up? I had decided much earlier not to subject him to IV therapy. The pain and hassle of needles coming out of position or trying to immobilize his arm and the constant disciplining seemed to be not worth the expected benefit. His days were all too few. But now I turned the question over afresh. Should we do life-support? A saliva sample had been taken and rushed to the testers. A dose of black walnut tincture extra strength, 8 tsp. was carefully poured down his throat, just in case some tapeworm remnants were responsible. His throat bubbled as he gasped for air.

The saliva sample tested Positive for benzene. They had allowed him to eat dessert (on benzene list) two days ago to celebrate his great improvement then. He was told to take vitamin B$_2$, 900 mg/day for 1 week.

I noticed a family member pouring another dose of 8 tsp. BWTES into his mouth, cradling his head and carefully avoiding choking. This was his second dose. Someone had misinterpreted my instructions which were a single dose. And someone zapped him.

Later, I was notified that they were getting ready to wheel him out. I arose to say goodbye to the family at the exit door and to take that last-goodbye-look at little Ronald.

Before I could get up, <u>he</u> came running into my office door. His face was animated. He was caught and set back in the wheelchair. What had happened? Was it the zapping? Was it the 16 tsp.?

He was suddenly well enough to sit for testing! We lost no time. The entire tapeworm set of 35 slides was to be tested at nine brain locations or as long as he could sit. This extensive search turned up at least one of six different tapeworms (or stages) at seven brain locations! Two brain locations, optic chiasma and astrocytes were Negative to everything I tested.

Location	Tapeworm Found
spinal cord/cervical region	*Hymenolepis nana* eggs, *Diphyllobothrium latum* eggs
optic chiasma	none
astrocytes	none
medulla	*Diphyllobothrium latum* scolex
pineal body	*Hymenolepis diminuta*, *Taenia solium* eggs
choroid plexus	*Hymenolepis nana* eggs
post central gyrus	*Dipylidium caninum* scolex
basal ganglion	*Taenia pisiformis* composite, *Taenia solium* cysticercus, *Dipylidium caninum* scolex
dura mater	*Taenia solium* cysticercus, *Taenia pisiformis* composite

Evidently, tapeworm stages had been accumulating in the brain and were not so easily vanquished, not even by a dose of 8 tsp. black walnut tincture extra strength. But he had gotten <u>two</u> doses about ½ hour apart. Would that be effective enough? This slate of tapeworm stages was a formidable one. Success was dubious at best and probably too late.

We said goodbye, but it wouldn't be the last one.

December 8, it is two days later; a phone call (he must still be alive!). His mother will be bringing him in. He walked in. He is very well. Is playing at home. Hadn't played for a very long time. His mother thinks he is feeling better from deep inside. Test results: benzene, isopropyl, wood alcohol Negative. Malonic acid Positive.

At this time we had just learned that wherever a tapeworm was to be found, malonic acid could also be found. In fact, about $^2/_3$ of all the tapeworm slides themselves were actually Positive for malonic acid! So merely testing for malonic acid would be a quick way of finding tapeworms. Of course, we would miss many. But if the test was Positive, we could expect a tapeworm there without going through the 35-slide test. The exact tapeworm could be identified later, if feasible. Right now, Ronald was still Positive for tapeworm, according to this interpretation.

He laughed and he spoke. The staff enjoyed seeing every movement of his. He was dosed with black walnut tincture extra strength again.

December 15, improvement is maintained. Patulin and copper Negative at cerebrum. Malonate Negative at cerebrum. Were the tapeworms really all dead or gone from his brain?

Meanwhile, our new tapeworm killing program was shaping up. We found coenzyme Q10 could kill tapeworms, but the dose was not yet set. Ronald was started on Q10, 500 mg, two a day, and continued on black walnut tincture extra strength, one tsp. a day, plus niacinamide. He could be off cloves since they burned him. And wormwood was down to one dose a week.

His mother had cut his Tegretol dose in half since he was having no seizures. He was to start on some vitamin C—but we had recently found it to be contaminated with selenium (metallic selenium is very toxic). We could not trust it. Ronald must wait till a new brand of vitamin C was found.

December 18, he is very well, brought me and staff Christmas gifts. He is an affectionate child. Still on 200 mg Tegretol but no Decadron for three weeks. Before this he needed it daily. He continues on methylene blue, one a day, and Q10 250 mg, one a day.

December 29, he got through Christmas without one slip-up on forbidden sweets. His benzene test was Negative. His mother was complimented. They brought his new MRI done at home two days ago. We compared it with his Oc-

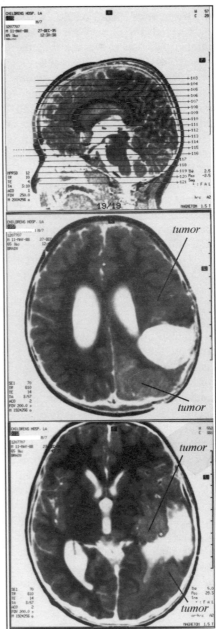

Dec. 27. MRI index. Frame 107. Frame 112.

291

tober 4 MRI. The improvement was astounding. There was 1) no midline shift and 2) no swelling.

To compare MRI results, we must look at exactly the same place. We must search for the slice that just grazes the top of the putamen foramen, number 107. Now we see that the vertical dividing line between the two brain hemispheres is quite straightened. There is still considerable tumor at the bottom right and side, but decidedly less than before. And a lower slice also shows definite improvement.

Ronald's mother said he had not had any regressions; they were as vigilant as on day one with him. To the staff he seemed lively, walking moderately well, and very alert with hugs and kisses and gifts for all.

His mother stated that Ronald's doctor wants to give him gene therapy, experimentally.

He still cries in the night, most nights.

January 17, 1996, he has only cried in the night once since last visit. Malonate Positive at spinal cord cervical region, evidence for tapeworm again. But at least malonate was Negative at astrocytes, spinal cord, lumbar region. Benzene, isopropanol, methanol Negative. He was started on our new tapeworm treatment, Q10 3 gm, once a week in a single dose. If 3 grams of Q10 was definitive (kills them all), why would there be any need for another treatment? For some strange reason, all the malonate could disappear a few hours after the big dose of Q10, but reappear a few days later! Were they newly acquired? [*This seemed unlikely at the time. We were unaware that common raw vegetables are spattered with tapeworm eggs.*] I thought he was hatching eggs that

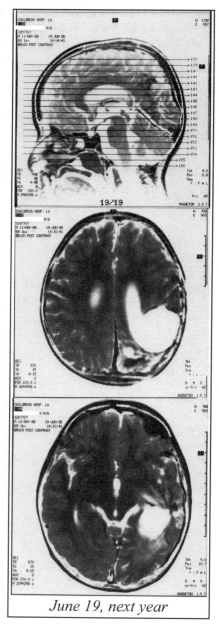

June 19, next year

had gone undetected before! Many things were possible; we couldn't take any chances so we killed them over and over.

January 26, malonate was Negative for the first time throughout his brain, testing at about two dozen locations. And his mother needed to get back to work. Ronald could be taken care of by a family member. The staff and I were very anxious about this new arrangement.

February 21, a month has passed. Ronald is doing well. Malonate, isopropyl, benzene, methanol are all Negative. They are watching him closely at home.

March 5, no symptoms. No crying at night. Sleep is good. Continue methylene blue. Test results: glutathione (reduced) Negative at cerebrum, glutathione (oxidized) Positive at cerebrum. There is obvious lack of reducing power. There is some interference with glutathione metabolism.

I focused on the cerebrum and found mercury, thallium, D-malic acid Positive, while cobalt, copper were Negative. D-malic acid does not belong in the human body. There was still a parasite.

We started him on a supplement of glutathione, reduced, 100 mg three times a day, and this time again identified paper towels as a source of mercury and thallium for him. They agreed to discuss this with his "sitter". These would use up his precious glutathione.

March 11, March 28, and April 30, doing fine. Still his affectionate self.

July 27, doing very well. He has been evaluated and is ready to go to school in fall.

Ronald Hartnett	11/16/95
RBC	4.82
WBC	7300
PLT	275
glucose	85
BUN	12
creatinine	0.7
AST (SGOT)	6
ALT (SGPT)	9
LDH	189
GGT	83
T.b.	0.4
alk phos	156
T.p.	7.3
albumin	4.9
globulin	2.4
uric acid	5.4
Calcium	10.1
Phosphorus	4.9
Iron	8.0
Sodium	137
Potassium	4
Chloride	105
triglycerides	101
cholesterol	261

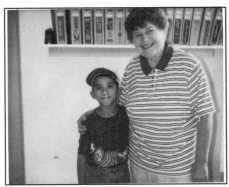

July 27, "Ronald" with the author

Mother brought latest MRI, done June 19. Slice number 142 shows a midline that is straight; there is no evidence of pressure or edema. Slice 148 shows more normal structure, too.

The mother was ecstatic and little Ronald beamed: "They had made me

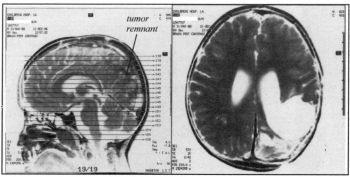

Dec. 11. MRI index. Frame 142.

a copy of the MRI for my very own" and Ronald presented me with it. Ronald wanted a picture taken.

December (his last visit). I did not see Ronald myself. His mother brought in a duplicate of his latest MRI and a good report from his regular doctor. Considerable healing can be seen on the index which has the side view. The former disturbance is now closer to the edge. Slice 142 looks even more normal than six months ago.

Autumn of the following year and Christmas of the next two years: a telephone call from his family related that he was doing fine at school.

Summary: 1) Was it the absence of metal or plastic in his teeth that gave Ronald his chance to survive? 2) Was it the absence of IV therapy that improved his chances? 3) Was it the methylene blue? Should I be using it for other cancers, too? 4) Was it that lucky mistake with the double dose of black walnut tincture extra strength that saved his life? One thing is certain: his family gets top grades for changing water pipes promptly, for getting all the supplements down him, for never giving up.

10	Jennifer Pinney	Breast Cancer

Jennifer Pinney, a young mural artist of considerable note, offered the clinic some of her paintings in exchange for service. Two months earlier she had discovered a rather large lump in her right breast. It was 3 inches in diameter right under the center. She had already been on the herbal parasite program for five weeks when she arrived so she was free of malignancy (ortho-phospho-tyrosine), but still tested Positive for isopropyl alcohol, which would prevent the tumor from shrinking. She was also Positive for asbestos, copper, cobalt, PCB, patulin, arsenic, chlorine, mercury, thallium, *Staphylococcus aureus*. These were "whole body" tests with no tissue slide in the circuit, reflecting on her rather high "systemic" levels of these toxins.

There were numerous bacteria in the breast, too. She was switched to the new parasite program, which uses 2 tsp. of black walnut tincture extra strength instead of the earlier "drop" recipe she had started herself on. She was to begin zapping, also. And stop wearing a regular bra (only the athletic variety) to improve lymphatic drainage under the breasts.

She was to go off the isopropyl alcohol list, stop using pesticide and bleach, change her refrigerator to a non-freon variety, and start the freon removal program even though freon tested Negative on her "whole body" test. My experience had been that we always found it present at the tumor site, even when it is absent in the systemic test. She said that three air conditioner failures had occurred in the past summer, implying that freon had escaped into her air space and she breathed it up. She believed that her water pipes at home were plastic, not copper, but she would bring in a water sample next time she arrived for follow up.

She was to stop using detergent or washing soda (which now also has cobalt) and arrange for removal of metal from her teeth. She was to use Lugol's iodine daily to prevent salmonella species from getting into the breast, although they did not show up at the "whole body" test.

A blood test was scheduled, but she could not wait for the results. Work necessitated her return; she stated she had only come to assess our capability of curing her cancer. Her ultrasound of breast did not get done. The blood test results were back next day. A single glance reveals the toxic effect of either cobalt or vanadium, the RBC is much too high; a check of the initial toxin test (above) revealed cobalt was Positive. And the WBC was also much too high showing an intense bacterial infection somewhere. Albumin was elevated, another cobalt effect. LDH was somewhat elevated showing liver toxicity [actually Sudan Black dye].

Also, there was a toxin in the thyroid, allowing the calcium to be too high; this could be due to cobalt, copper, or any other toxic substance. Creatinine was much too low, implying poor ability to make this compound or a high excretion rate, both typical of cancer.

Liver function tests (AST, ALT, GGT) were good, as was alkaline phosphatase. Uric acid was probably "masked", hiding the true disturbances.

The potassium level was too high, implying inability of the tissue cells to absorb it. This usually reflects on the thyroid, which we already see is malfunctioning (high calcium), but it could also mean that malonic acid is directly or indirectly inhibiting potassium uptake by the potassium pumps of cells.

So the tumorous process was, indeed, underway. How would she stop it, all by herself, without our guidance in a distant place? We underestimated her determination.

Two months later she returned with a much smaller lump. She had achieved a lot on her own. But she wanted it all gone. This time she was willing to stay three weeks. An ultrasound showed a tumor, 3.6 x 3.0 x 2.1 cm (3.0 was the depth).

It was palpable, meaning you could feel it quite easily. In fact, the radiologist thought it was merely a cyst now and could be drained. Jennifer declined.

She was now Positive for Salmonella—she had run out of Lugol's and was unable to get it locally. She was also Positive for formaldehyde, zirconium, aflatoxin, copper, and

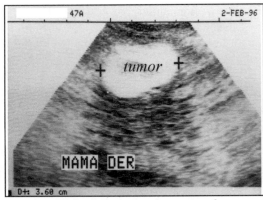

Feb. 2 Breast ultrasound

patulin. Her patulin was particularly high, so that tumor necrosis factor (TNF) the body's own tumor shrinker, was missing. Copper was especially high, too. She was started immediately on an EDTA IV to pull it out, together with DMSO, vitamin C, and magnesium. She also had benzene toxicity for which she was given vitamin B_2. It was easy to see why the tumor could not shrink further.

A new blood test was done. A glance at the RBC shows she is still toxic with either cobalt or vanadium. We will compare the two tests, item by item.

Jennifer Pinney	11/27	2/1	Results
RBC	5.05	5.09	No change. Probably still cobalt as before.
WBC	12,100	7,600	Many fewer bacteria, since tumor is smaller.
BUN	10.0	9.0	Urea formation is further inhibited.
creatinine	0.6	0.7	Still too low
AST	28	19	All liver enzymes (AST, ALT, GGT) are improved.
ALT	33	16	
GGT	11	9.0	
LDH	202	135	Liver is healthier, can metabolize lactic acid now. [Sudan Black B is gone.]
alk phos	62	59	Same as above.
albumin	5.2	4.7	This is now normal in spite of continued cobalt toxicity.
uric acid	3.2	1.5	There is a severe lack of glutamine (*as well as ongoing Clostridium infection and purine shortage*)
calcium	10.4 (8.4-10.4)	8.5	The problem has shifted from the thyroid to the parathyroids, resulting in too low calcium.
iron	92	119	Perfect each time. Not being affected by copper or germanium yet.
potassium	5.0	4.3	It has returned to normal. Thyroid is function-

			ing better. There is less inhibition of the potassium pumps.

She was given glutamine as a supplement. Also calcium and hydrochloric acid, 10 drops of a 5% solution at meals twice a day. She was started on glutathione 500 mg., three times a day and coenzyme Q10, 3 gm every fourth day for a total of 5 doses. This would give her oxidizing power to kill pathogens, burn up their poisonous amines, and help accelerate the Krebs respiration cycle.

She was also taken off fruit in her diet to quickly eliminate patulin. It was gone in a few days and now her TNF tested Positive. She could begin shrinking her own tumor. She began to do her dental work.

In two weeks all toxins were testing Negative. Her breast lump was smaller to touch. She was no longer feeling twinges going to the breast. Only *Staphylococcus* and *Shigella* continued to test Positive at the breast and parathyroids.

A new blood test (Feb. 7), reflected on the removal of heavy metals; the RBC was finally normal.

But the LDH had risen just enough (over 160) to suggest a tiny bit of tumor activity again. What was happening? What was new? Dental work! [*We were not aware how the new plastic dentalware could put azo dye right back into her mouth permanently. And cobalt, vanadium, malonic acid, and copper, too.*] Would all her gains by avoiding toxins be lost in a sudden introduction of them by dental work? Kidney function continued to be hindered and albumin was again too high. But the calcium had come up, so I knew the parathyroids were now functioning better.

By the next week, she was still in the middle of dental work. The entire breast had now visibly shrunk and looked perfectly normal. Her IVs were stopped and a new blood test done (Feb. 13). The LDH was, gratifyingly, back down and liver enzymes, too. But albumin was not yet normal; was there still some old cobalt in bits of forgotten amalgam [*or was it new cobalt freshly put in her mouth*]?

She was given evening primrose oil and a selenium supplement. Salmonella continued to plague her. So she stopped using all dairy products. Then she accidentally picked up isopropyl alcohol and benzene during a weekend visit to friends. They appeared again in the breast. The breast was twinging, too, to tell her so. But patulin was not back so she continued to produce TNF and continued shrinking the tumor.

The third week was ending. A blood test and ultrasound were ordered.

The blood test was too beautiful to read without emotion as it was compared to her first one. Tumor activity (LDH) was even below the level of security. Albumin, and calcium were normal, as was potassium and the RBC. Only the low BUN and creatinine told the secret of malonate toxicity while low uric acid told of *Clostridium* infection.

The ultrasound showed what we felt and knew to be true. The breast was softer, less fibrous. The size of the tumor was down to 3.05 x 2.15 cm; it was obviously benign now to the radiologist's eye.

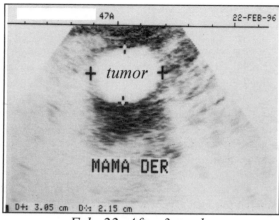

Raw flaxseed was added to her diet before going home. She could soak it for five minutes to make it chewy rather than hard. This would substitute for evening primrose oil which would always be processed.

Feb. 22. After 3 weeks

Summary: Has she kept her new state of health or will the new dental plastic sabotage her gains? We got her murals, they decorate our walls with inspiration and joy.

Jennifer Pinney	11/27	2/1	2/7	2/13	2/20
RBC	5.05	5.09	4.53	4.38	4.36
WBC	12100	7600	8700	7400	7700
PLT	331	395	315	319	280
glucose	95	135	90	94	78
BUN	10.0	9.0	10.0	10.0	7
creatinine	0.6	0.7	0.8	0.7	0.7
AST (SGOT)	28	19	26	24	18
ALT (SGPT)	33	16	28	18	16
LDH	202	135	169	132	121
GGT	11	9.0	17	7	12
T.b.	0.6	0.5	0.6	0.6	0.6
alk phos	62	59	83	62	70
T.p.	7.5	6.7	7.2	7.1	6.9
albumin	5.2	4.7	5.4	5.0	4.8
globulin	2.3	2.0	1.8	2.1	2.1
uric acid	3.2	1.5 (2.5-6.1)	2.2	2.9	2.7
Calcium	10.4	8.5	9.6	9.3	9.5
Phosphorus	4.9	3.9	3.9	4.5	3.5
Iron	92	119	103	75	91
Sodium	138	133	135	141	138
Potassium	5.0	4.3	4.6	4.4	4.6
Chloride	104	98	106	105	102
triglycerides	98	13	45	57	48
cholesterol	215	153	---	196	161

| 11 | Irene Bambrough | Liver Cancer |

Irene Bambrough, sixty-two, was the perfect example of a lucky patient. Her liver cancer had been diagnosed in August 1995, so she had put herself on the drop-routine for the BWT parasite program and the kidney herb recipe. She left her home in a northern climate to stay with a friend in Arizona who had plastic water pipes. (This is probably what saved her life.) When she arrived at our clinic from Arizona, her initial toxin test was already Negative for isopropyl alcohol, CFC's, and copper, though she still had copper at the liver. She was off to a good start, but was still Positive for fiberglass, aluminum, arsenic, cadmium, thallium, patulin, aflatoxin (very high), and salmonella bacteria.

She wore full dentures. (This is probably what saved her life again.)

On the day she arrived, November 24, she was given these instructions: (1) change her metal glasses frames to solid plastic—no metal, and washed carefully before wearing them. (2) Use no hygiene products from the drugstore, such as bandaids, cotton swabs. These have mercury and thallium residues. [*At that time we did not suspect leftover bits of amalgam in her jawbone as a source of mercury and thallium or other metals; in retrospect, such tattoos were the probable source of her thallium.*] (3) Take Lugol's for *Salmonella*, four times a day as written in the cancer program. (4) Take black walnut tincture extra strength, 2 tsp. daily in a ½ glass of water; (sip it) for 4 days. Then zap. Also, take 7 cloves and 7 wormwood capsules the first day. (5) Get a blood test. (6) Get an ultrasound of the liver.

She didn't return for four days. We had planned to outline our cancer program to her and really get her started on her second day. Was she just not taking this seriously?

On November 28, she returned. She had accomplished everything without help! We reviewed her blood test. Besides her anemia and her extremely high white blood cell count (15,800), her liver enzymes were too high, especially the GGT. Her LDH was somewhat elevated indicating tumor activity, as was the alkaline phosphatase [both due to dyes]. Her triglycerides and cholesterol were rather low, showing she was losing her good nutritional status. Calcium was ominously high at 10.5, showing there was a problem in her thyroid gland. The high potassium level was further evidence.

Indeed, she had been born with a cyst on her thyroid gland and had part of it removed. She also had radium treatment for it. Now she was on Synthroid tablets daily. (Her third piece of luck was that her thyroid tablets were not polluted with isopropyl alcohol.) She was started on the freon removal program. She was given coenzyme Q10 to kill tapeworm cysts or other stages that inhabit every tumor. The plan was to search for surviving tapeworm stages the next day. She was also given silymarin tablets to improve her liver function. She was scheduled for three IVs a day, containing glycyrrhizin, laetrile, and vitamin C (50 gm daily).

The next day, the surviving tapeworm stages in the liver were searched for from a set of 33 slides. She still had: *Taenia solium* cysticercus, *Taenia solium* eggs, *Diphyllobothrium erinacea*, *Moniezia expansa* eggs, and *Taenia solium* scolex.

Evidently coenzyme Q10 was not effective, at least not at this dose. We decided to go back to our previous tapeworm treatment, a big dose of black walnut tincture extra strength. She was given 8 tsp. in water, sipped in ½ hour, and another 8 tsp. two hours later.

The next day, November 30, she was tested for tapeworm stages again. Four out of the five tested Negative now (the fifth, *Taenia solium* cysticercus was omitted in the test; this slide was temporarily mislaid). She had also gotten rid of her aflatoxin by avoiding all grains in her diet and eating no nuts.

She missed more days—precious IV days. Arriving on December 4 she was tested again; all tapeworm stages were still Negative. Aflatoxin was still Negative. Even copper was now gone from her liver, although no EDTA was used in her IV to chelate it out.

We discussed her liver ultrasound done on November 27. It was abysmally bad. There were tumors strewn about like trash on a windy day. There was no way to count them. Yet she smiled blithely as we spoke about them. The radiologist simply described them as "multiple liver metastases." Only two were measured in each lobe. Why couldn't she take our program more seriously? It would be a certain fatality. Should I send her to a different cancer doctor, one who would frighten her with threats and vivid descriptions of what it's like to die of cancer? Tubes everywhere, pain in spite of morphine, a distended belly, no appetite, etc. I decided against it,

Nov. 27 ultrasound of R and L liver lobes

for a few more days. Other doctors would manage to keep her more dutifully getting her IVs, but the same IVs would be polluted with isopropyl alcohol and *E. coli*—the risk seemed greater than the benefit.

On December 5, she was feeling exceptionally well. She tested Negative for pyruvate at the liver, indicating the pile-up was gone. Malonic acid was Positive, though, and very high at the liver. The question immediately arose: how could she have malonic acid in her liver when no more tapeworm stages existed?

I concluded [*wrongly*] that she must still have a tapeworm stage, but not a variety I had tested for. She was given another two sets of black walnut tincture extra strength, 8 tsp. each, one hour apart. (This was her fourth piece of good luck; in our ignorance we maximized her treatment, instead of minimizing it.) Then she zapped. She was perfectly cheerful about this, without a snippet of a complaint about the taste or the cost. With equal cheerfulness, she announced she was leaving in a few days for home!

Leaving for home with a liver full of ticking bombs? It seemed the height of folly. We scheduled her final ultrasound, but did not manage to do a last blood test, at least not then.

She was back on December 8, ultrasound in hand, and an impish grin on her face. She couldn't interpret the negative herself, but the radiologist had told her there were no tumors!

We quickly taped the negatives onto the windows for all of us to review. There was nothing that could be identified as a tumor. The texture was bad. Possibly a CT scan of the liver would have shown more detail. But the overriding truth was she had made tremendous improvements in the past two weeks and would survive. She could count on living again. How did it happen? She had missed most of her IVs, and taken very few supplements. [*Nor did she observe a*

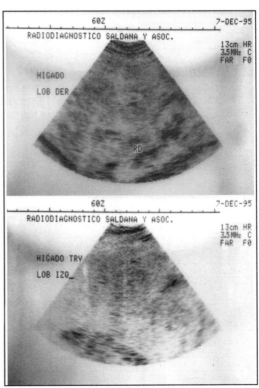

Dec. 7 R and L liver lobes with no tumors

301

malonate-free diet because we didn't know there was malonic acid in food at that time.]

She left for home, to be with her family for Christmas. She promised to come back in January. We felt she was squandering all her gains.

But her husband had a new refrigerator for her for Christmas, all fiberglass was sealed up tightly, the water pipes had been changed—it was a case of true love.

We had wished her a Merry Christmas in wonderment. On January 24 she returned, quite lively and energetic looking. Could she really be that well? She tested Positive for benzene this time…maybe she had allowed herself some lotion or soap she got for Christmas. And *Salmonella* was plaguing her again, but cadmium was her only heavy metal now. Was it her pink dentures or her galvanized plumbing? Patulin and aflatoxin were again Positive. But all in all her results were much better than before.

A new blood test rewarded her for her family's efforts. The RBC and WBC were now perfect! The liver enzymes had improved! But LDH had crept up to 238. Did this reflect new tumor activity or the burden on the liver from opening tumors [releasing their Sudan Black and lanthanides]? The tell tale sign of aflatoxin was present in the bilirubin. It too, had just passed the 1.0 mark. We carefully warned her about moldy food. The calcium level had dropped, iron had risen, and potassium was normal again.

And she was obviously much better nourished, judging by the triglycerides and cholesterol. But we had mislaid her file and had nothing to compare her results with as we reviewed her blood test. We couldn't make a strong case for her staying longer for more treatment. And she was off again to care for her home and family. She had made a success story out of an imminent tragedy.

Summary: A year later, a beautiful Christmas card arrived. Was it from her bereaved family? It was in her handwriting, signed by her. She said she was entirely well and wished us all the very best.

Did she have a fifth piece of luck? What was it? That we lost her file? Or she just didn't like malonic acid foods and nobody

Irene Bambrough	11/27	1/24
RBC	3.96	4.64
WBC	15,800	6,300
PLT	166	188
glucose	83	102
BUN	16	13
creatinine	0.7	0.1
AST (SGOT)	65	55
ALT (SGPT)	59	50
LDH	209	238
GGT	409	332
T.b.	0.6	1.2
alk phos	120	129
T.p.	6.5	6.5
albumin	4.0	4.3
globulin	4.0	4.3
uric acid	3.6	3.4
Calcium	10.5	8.9
Phosphorus	3.2	2.8
Iron	70	82
Sodium	140	139
Potassium	5.3	4.7
Chloride	109	107
triglycerides	80	258
cholesterol	128	146

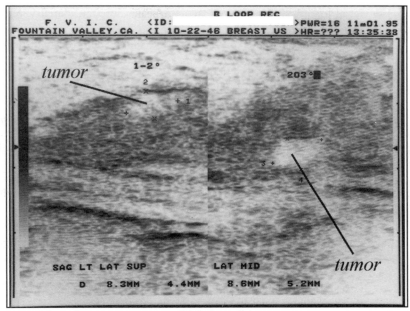

Nov. 1 mammogram. Oblong white areas are tumors

gave her chocolates and such for Christmas? I wished all cases were this easy.

12	Janelle Ford	Breast Cancer

Janelle Ford arrived with her therapist friend because of a Positive mammogram obtained four weeks earlier. She had brought the mammogram showing two small tumors, each just under 1 cm long. They had grown over the past year while "being carefully watched" by her doctor.

Now her doctor wanted to biopsy them, but her therapist wanted her to change her lifestyle drastically first, in accordance with the instructions in my earlier book, *The Cure For All Cancers*, to see if this would work. In fact, her friend had already started her zapping and taking the herbal recipe.

By the time she arrived, her ortho-phospho-tyrosine was already Negative (meaning no malignancy) but her isopropyl alcohol test was very Positive! She was evidently taking something or using some product that had it. This would allow the growth factor, human chorionic gonadotropin (hCG) to form [*as well as isopropylidene ascorbate and isopropylidene nucleic acids*[121]] which would certainly prevent the tumor from shrinking.

---

[121] Clark, H.R. *Syncrometer Biochemistry Laboratory Manual*, New Century Press, 1999.

303

Her initial toxin test also showed freon, asbestos, copper, mercury, *Salmonella*, *Shigella dysentery*, *Staphylococcus aureus* Positive.

Her first instructions were to go off all the supplements she had been taking. They could be polluted with isopropyl alcohol. She should learn to use the Syncrometer and test them herself later. Her therapist agreed to do this herself since she had given the advice to take them.

Continue the parasite program, complete with niacinamide, zap daily. Change her water pipes to PVC. Change her amalgam to composite [*at that time we were not aware of the hazards of dental plastic*]. Start the freon removal program, but first get a new non-freon refrigerator; also test the car dust for freon. Take turmeric and fennel to get rid of *Shigella*. Take Lugol's iodine, 6 drops in a half glass of water four times a day after meals and bedtime to eliminate *Salmonella*. Stop wearing a regular bra (athletic bra okay) to improve circulation of lymphatic fluid under the breast.

"Is that all?" she said. "Is that all I have to do to get rid of these, ugh...lumps. And I don't have to have that needle?" Her extreme anxiety was visible. But her therapist's determination to be successful was just as visible.

Janelle had also brought a blood test, done at the time of her mammogram. Nothing was abnormal, yet, except uric acid. It was much too low (2.5), showing a lack of glutamine. The enzyme, glutaminase, is stimulated by malonic acid and would decrease the level of glutamine. (Later we discovered the complete absence of purines, accompanying *Clostridium* infection, as well as absence of glutamic acid.) She was given glutamine, 500 mg, one a day for 5 days [*although our present choice is glutamic acid*].

She was eager to get all these things done and planned to come back in two months. When she came she brought a list of her accomplishments:

She was on the maintenance parasite program.

She had been on the kidney program four weeks.

She had zapped daily.

She had been on Lugol's for six days so far.

She was still on the freon program.

Electronic testing now found benzene, wood alcohol, isopropyl alcohol Negative. Tumor necrosis factor (TNF) was Positive (good!) at the breast. Malonic acid was Positive, and assumed to be due only to tapeworm stages, so she was given CoQ10. GSSG (oxidized glutathione) was Positive at the breast and GSH (reduced glutathione) was Negative. This is opposite to what it should be.

Copper was still Positive at the breast; this would certainly oxidize glutathione. She had not changed her copper water pipes yet, in the hope that a new device she had purchased to clean her water would take it out. It did not. She had not completed her dental work yet.

A month later, she followed up with a visit; she was bloated and uncomfortable. And she still had twinges of pain going to the breast. Testing showed *Salmonella typhimurium* Positive at the whole body. She was returned to taking Lugol's and the Bowel Program. On the bright side, malonic acid was Negative at the breast, and GSSG/GSH were Negative/Positive.

In another month the twinges in her breast were gone. She had recently been ill with a viral infection and was still quite short of breath when she arrived. Testing showed: benzene, isopropyl alcohol, wood alcohol, copper, mercury, thallium all Negative at the breast. Malonate Positive at the breast.

Noting malonate again, we gave her another large dose of CoQ10 (3 grams) to take daily for 7 days. [*Another regimen we tried in our effort to abolish tapeworm stages definitively. We didn't realize you could reinfect from raw vegetables.*] We also supplemented her diet with glutathione.

TNF was still positive. Were the tumors shrinking in spite of setbacks?

In May, seven months from her first visit, she arrived with her new ultrasounds of the breasts. She was beaming. Only one tumor remained and her

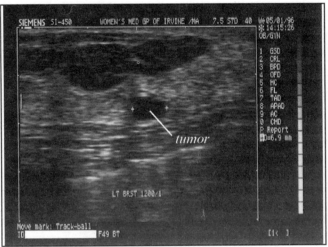

May 1, one small, benign tumor left

doctor considered it benign, not worthy of a biopsy anymore. The length was estimated at 6.9 mm (pea size) quite a bit smaller than earlier.

She still needed to replace copper water pipes and complete work on two teeth. She felt very well.

Four months later, she returned to get updated on our tapeworm program, since she had heard it had been changing. We were happy to announce that malonic acid also came from certain foods and dental plastic, as well as pollution, not solely from tapeworm stages. But she was too <u>pleased</u> to be annoyed that there was more to do and certain foods to be avoided. Pleased with the new ultrasounds she was bringing. They showed there were <u>no</u> tumors at all in her breasts anywhere. Even the texture was much less fibrous though not yet normal.

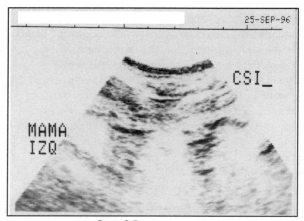

Sep 25, no tumors

Her toxin test showed malonic acid Positive, benzene, isopropyl alcohol, wood alcohol, all bacteria Negative. Freon was Negative (she had a new refrigerator). Asbestos was Positive (due to her new hair dryer?). I recommended that she use no dryer at all. Copper was Positive (she was still treating her water instead of changing pipes). Mercury was Positive (probably an amalgam tattoo). Aflatoxin was Positive—she should eat home baked bread and avoid peanuts.

She was feeling very well and had her new blood test results with her. Her uric acid was up to 3 now. Calcium was too low, showing a developing parathyroid problem. No doubt, her toxins were accumulating in her parathyroid glands; this reduces parathyroid hormone enough to test Negative with the Syncrometer, and keep calcium absorption very low. Calcium is also kept low by malonic acid, which simply chelates it away.

Janelle Ford	11/6/95	9/16/96
WBC		5,400
RBC		3.74 (3.9-5.2)
PLT		177
glucose	85	92
BUN	14 (8-25)	10 (7-25)
creatinine	1.25	1.0
AST (SGOT)	17	14
ALT (SGPT)	14	12
LDH	126	101
GGT	10	10
T.b.	0.2	0.5
alk phos	56	62
T.p.	7.2	6.9
albumin	4.3	3.9
globulin	2.9	3.0
uric acid	2.5 (2.7-6.5) mg%	3.0 (2.5-7.5)
Calcium	9.6	8.9
Phosphorus	3.7	2.7
Iron	76	108
Sodium	144	137
Potassium	4.0	4.1
Chlorine	104	107
triglycerides	255	127
cholesterol	197	199

Her albumin to globulin ratio had shifted slightly, so that albumin was just a bit too low (to accompany the low calcium) and globulin too high, an effect of cobalt toxicity. Both effects had been discovered to be due to plastic dentalware that same fall.

Her LDH continued to be very low, in fact, too low (101), a toxic effect of cobalt, I believe. Her RBC was also too low, definitely anemic.

We were now able to inform her that both malonate and cobalt could come from her new dental plastic. It should be removed. Her last two amalgams should not be replaced till safe plastic was found for her. [*Waiting could be disastrous, too, so I now recommend extraction.*]

As before, she took the news without resentment. Her expectations had been more than fulfilled. Her breasts belonged to her again. She planned to rid herself of toxic plastic, too. Truly, an exemplary patient. Her therapist, with her through it all, smiled with satisfaction.

Summary: Janelle was fortunate to have a therapist, someone who really cared about her welfare.

Certainly the "wait and see while we carefully watch" policy of clinical doctors is better than nothing. But it is as irrational as waiting and seeing if crocodiles will bite while you swim in their territory. In a disease partly caused by mutations, the mutagens should at least be searched for and eliminated during the "wait and see" period.

13	Albert Mikalauskas	Liver Cancer

Albert and Pamela Mikalauskas came from Israel for his liver cancer in November. Four years ago he had surgery for a colon tumor. He was presently on a pacemaker and was afraid to zap. He had been on the parasite program for four months already, but he was still full of isopropyl alcohol. They were quite shocked and disappointed to think it was lurking in the vitamins and other supplements he was taking [*and coming from Clostridium bacteria*]; they had brought quite a large bag of them. But they didn't pine over them, or over the money lost, they just threw them out. They were happy to hear that liver cancer is not necessarily difficult to clear up. Their heritage served them well in meeting adversity without a whine. Perhaps he also reminded me of my own father who died of liver cancer at age sixty-two. The appearance of a slightly built man, sallow and chronically ill tugged at my memory every time he arrived. He was on diuretics and heart medicine. The CT scan he brought (not shown) showed the entire liver full of tumors except part of the left lobe. This was sustaining him.

He had large purpuric patches on hands and forearms (purple patches where blood vessels had broken). He was tested for sorghum mold and found Positive so he was taken off brown sugar and any other sweet except honey.

His initial toxin test showed he was full of freon, besides nickel, aluminum, copper, cobalt, and mercury. He also had aflatoxin, *E. coli*, *Salmonella*, and *Staphylococcus*. He was started on the freon removal program, Lugol's, and supplements of assorted minerals (zinc, manganese, molybdenum, selenium, chromium, boron) in a daily small dose. He would continue the parasite program and add niacinamide daily.

His starting IVs contained cesium chloride, glycyrrhizin, laetrile, vitamin C. Cesium is used in liver cancer on the assumption that it pulls excess sodium out of tumor cells and surrounding tissues. Glycyrrhizin, too, is specially useful for liver cancer; it is licorice extract.

His blood test showed nothing presently life threatening, although the liver enzymes were clearly elevated. The iron level was very low (33), yet his bone marrow was still making RBCs as needed.

To pull the copper out of him quickly, two 3 gm doses of EDTA were added to his IVs the next day. At the same time cesium and glycyrrhizin were doubled. He was sent to the dentist to exchange amalgam for plastic.

He was started on coenzyme Q10 and silymarin tablets. But all this got his stomach churning constantly, interfering with his food intake. The cesium dose was cut in half again, which relieved his stomach.

A week later, there was clearly a worsening of the blood test. His bilirubin was over 1. He was eating some high-aflatoxin food [*a liver tumor opened*]. It affected nearly all the other liver enzyme tests, too, raising AST, ALT, and LDH. This would be very serious in a matter of days. The aflatoxin was found in the bread brought from home; they were still eating it because it looked and tasted good. Aflatoxin was also found in some white rice they had purchased from a bulk bin. He was taken off all grains, including bread and rice, as well as nuts. Only oatmeal and corn on the cob were allowed.

In spite of this setback, a new ultrasound (not shown) indicated the masses were of lower density in his liver than before.

To get the LDH down, a BQ shot was given on alternate days. His IV was changed to include 50 gm vitamin C, plus calcium and vitamin B complex.

Next day, his dental work was complete; his energy was much better; and he had very little stomach distress, so he could eat well. He was given 10 drops of hydrochloric acid (5%) to put in his beverage, once a day at dinner time.

A week later, *Echinococcus granulosis* (tapeworm larval cyst) was found at his liver; no other tapeworm stages. But *Fasciolopsis* stages were also present. His dose of black walnut tincture extra strength was raised to 8 tsp. to make sure all bowel parasite stages would be killed. Two days after this, he could sleep without a sleeping pill for the first time. And a new blood test showed improvement. The bilirubin was nearly back to normal (1.1); the LDH had dropped sharply; liver enzymes were much better and calcium was back up. A new ultrasound of liver (not shown) revealed further shrinkage of the right tumor masses.

By the third week, his purpuric spots were almost completely faded.

By the fourth week, his homesickness overwhelmed them. After a last blood test (Dec. 8), they flew home.

Many things had improved. His iron was coming up, so more RBCs could be made. But, obviously, he still had aflatoxin arriving at the liver. All liver enzymes were again elevated. The bilirubin was especially sinister. We could only pray that back home, their customary good habits would bring them all down again. At any rate, the tumors were softening and shrinking.

It lasted for three and a half months; then he was in trouble. His LDH was up. He quickly returned. This time with a friend, not his wife. It was just before Easter.

He appeared in rather good health. He was energetic. His insomnia had returned, but he had no other symptoms. However, the blood test showed there was no time to lose. A rising BUN signaled beginning kidney failure! Years of diuretics in the past had no doubt taken its toll on them. [*We did not suspect* Clostridium *or methyl malonate yet.*] He would have to go off his diuretics and substitute the kidney recipe. Double strength was recommended, sipped slowly throughout the day. He was started on glutathione, and coenzyme Q10 to abolish all malonic acid.

Aflatoxin was again Positive, this time at the kidney [*beginning to drain a new tumor*]. His bilirubin had edged up a bit. He was off grains and nuts again.

On the fourth day, Albert was in sudden distress in the night. He recognized it as his old congestive heart problem. He was waiting for me as I arrived at the clinic in the morning, breathless and with chest pain.

In a strange land, with a strangely behaving body, and strange recommendations made for it, it is easy to make a mistake. He had gone off his diuretic but had completely forgotten about the kidney herb recipe. Now he had not only kidney failure, but heart failure. We thought of his wife patiently waiting for him to arrive at home magically cured in Mexico a second time. We ran to the kitchen. Somebody was dispatched to the grocery store for an armful of fresh parsley. While he waited, he was given hawthorn berry and coenzyme Q10, also folic acid, B12, and magnesium oxide. In an hour, some strong herbal brew was ready. He was to sip throughout the day, in spite of discomfort in the bladder.

A new ultrasound of liver had been taken upon his arrival (March 21). The right lobe of liver showed a very large mass of tumor, seemingly made up of smaller tumors. The large size would make it difficult to measure accurately, since a slightly different angle could make the measurement quite different. The left lobe of liver also was one large tumor mass. Yet, there was enough functional liver outside these masses to carry out life's functions.

A day after the kidney herbs were started, a new blood test was done, dated March 26. It is tempting to believe the kidney recipe bailed him out. But the drop in bilirubin was more likely responsible. And down came all the liver enzymes. The drop in LDH would let more uric acid be excreted, an-

309

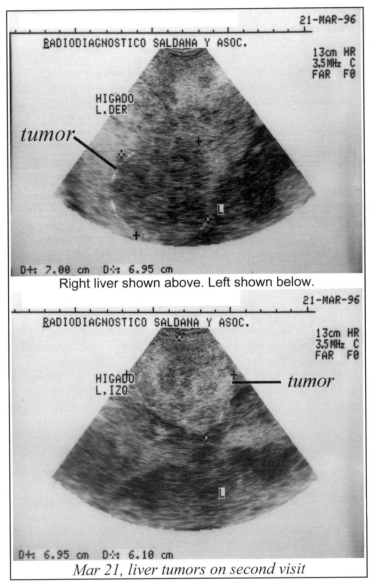

Right liver shown above. Left shown below.

Mar 21, liver tumors on second visit

other help for the kidneys and heart. The BUN was down again and kidney failure averted.

He was now given half a dose of spironolactone (the body's own diuretic) for a few days, twice a day to help the kidneys further.

Another blood test was done in two days because the previous test was simply too good to be believed. Was he really saved from kidney failure or heart failure or advancing jaundice? And another ultrasound of liver was

,scheduled. Yes, the bilirubin was <u>staying</u> low, liver enzymes were <u>staying</u> down, LDH slightly lower. And best of all the BUN and creatinine were those of a healthy man!

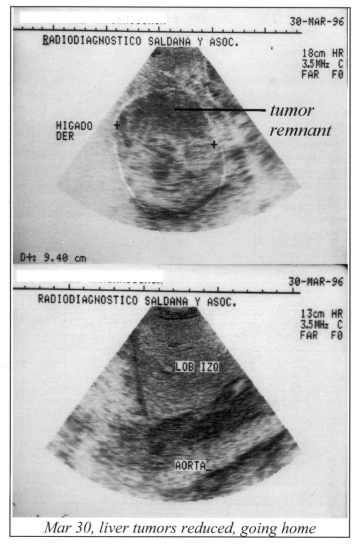

Mar 30, liver tumors reduced, going home

He could reduce the kidney herbs to half a daily dose. His breathlessness had disappeared completely, a minor chest pain persisted and procaine was added to his IV recipe. (Procaine doubles as pain reliever and benefactor to heart.) But home was even a better recipe. His wife and an ethnic holiday were waiting for him. He was homeward bound once more and once more very prematurely.

His final ultrasound (Mar. 30) showed the large tumor in the right lobe much less dense in its bottom half. The overall dimensions were greater, an effect of scattering of hard centers. The left lobe tumor was gone. It could not be found in three different frames. This lobe now looked quite smooth and healthy. To be certain, a CT scan should be done, but that could be done at home.

Summary: Albert deserved his good fortune; if only my father could have lived at a time when this treatment was known.

The chance that Albert could keep his gains at home would be very slim, though. His improvement was not solid enough. In fact, it had only just begun. But forces greater than the need to survive tug at us. Albert died at home a year later.

Albert Mikalauskas	11/13	11/21	11/28	12/8		3/21	3/26	3/28
RBC	4.53	4.08	4.05	4.52		4.3	3.63	4.09
WBC	10,400	10,100	9.8	7.8		10.6	9,000	10.4
PLT	139	191	255	180		181	161	185
BUN	---	15	16	13		27 (7-21)	16 (7-21)	15
creatinine	1.0	1.2	1.0	.9		1.2	.9	1.1
AST (SGOT)	109	158	77	171		48	39	41
ALT (SGPT)	84	165	87	182		25	20	22
LDH	265	528	310	343		431	329	315
GGT	171	114	103	130		147	115	112
T.b.	.8	1.8	1.1	1.2		1.3	.6	.7
alk phos	197	145	159	173		199	185	191
albumin	3.6	3.7	3.5	4.0		4.2	3.5	3.7
globulin	3.6	3.0	3.2	3.3		3.5	2.9	2.9
uric acid	8.4	3.8	---	4.0		10.2	5.8	6.4
Calcium	9.2	8.7	9.3	9.3		9.4	8.5	9.1
Iron	33		32	54		57	44	38
Potassium	4.2	3.5	3.4	3.8		3.3	4.0	4.8

14   Tammy Adsit   Bone Cancer

Tammy Adsit left her husband and children in England to find a cure for her bone cancer. She had already had a double mastectomy and had been on tamoxifen since then, but the cancer was now throughout her bones. A bone scan was done two days after she arrived (Dec. 22, page 317).

The white regions represent bone. There should be no intensification of white zones within bones nor fuzziness along bone edges. They represent lesions where bone is dissolving. Lesions or "hot spots" can be seen in the ribs on each side. The front view shows the breast bone is involved. The neck, skull, spine, and ribs showed massive cancer invasion, as did the pelvis and legs, not shown.

She had been on the parasite program and zapper for seven days upon arrival. She was already free of malignancy. The bones still had copper, freon, patulin, benzene, and two bacteria: *Shigella dysenteriae* and *Staphylococcus aureus*. [*Cobalt and vanadium were not tested because they were not yet suspected as routine carcinogens.*] Exchanging amalgam for composite in restored teeth and removing copper from the water supply were our first priorities. She was started on 3 IVs a day, obtaining EDTA, Clodronate, vitamin C, and magnesium. The EDTA would pull out copper; the Clodronate would stop bones from dissolving. A panoramic X-ray showed a number of infected teeth, besides. These would prove to be her undoing as our dentists at that time did everything in their power to "save" them, repair and restore them, in fact, do everything but extract them. She was also given vitamin B$_2$ to detoxify benzene, coenzyme Q10, the freon removal program, and Lugol's; of course she would continue the parasite program, stay off the benzene and isopropyl alcohol lists, and zap.

The next day she was free of copper and her *Staphylococcus* level was down, though still Positive in her bones. Her IV was changed to contain laetrile, instead of EDTA.

Her blood test results were still quite good. Only the LDH was slightly elevated, considering anything over 160 implies toxicity and tumor activity by our standards. [*The low RBC reflected bone marrow insufficiency, but the true cause, vanadium or cobalt toxicity, was not suspected.*]

In six days she was able to walk a few steps unassisted. A new blood test showed numerous improvements. Lower alk phos slowed down bone dissolution. Removing copper let the iron go up higher. Giving folic acid let the uric acid drop to a value below the range, exposing the serious shortage of glutamine (and glutamic acid) that existed. Potassium was now too low also, showing the body's ability to utilize it better. But the calcium rise unmasked a thyroid problem. The parathyroids had become well again (removing copper, freon, and patulin), so calcium absorption could occur. To heal bones, we need to further stop bone dissolution by means of calcitonin made in the thyroid. What could still be lurking in the thyroid gland? [*At this time we were unaware of the roles played by clostridium bacteria, malonic acid, and food dyes.*]

She was given glutamine. [*Later, we would give glutamic acid instead.*] Malonate was Positive, so she was given a massive dose of Co Q10 to kill tapeworm stages. [*Its origin in dental plastic and food was not known then.*]

In another six days she was pain-free except for her upper chest. Pain at the spine was gone and her walking was improving. Malonate was no longer present at the kidneys. Rhodizonic acid was added to her supplement list, taking one capsule (100 mg) 4 times a day. Also, hydrochloric acid (5%), 10 drops in beverage with each meal. Her next blood test showed two good changes: the LDH was dropping and uric acid rising. The lymphocyte level (not shown) was only 12%, though. The lymphocyte level should be at least 20%; 12% implicates a toxin in the bone marrow consistent with the dropping RBC and WBC. Her IVs were continued, the same as before, 3/day.

In another two days, she was more aware of the pain at the right rib. (She was still in the middle of dental replacement.) The dentist found an abscess under a wisdom tooth and pulled the tooth. This cleared the rib pain.

A new bone scan now showed a 50% reduction in lesions. Many small lesions could no longer be seen. We were overjoyed. Our herbal bone tea was now added to her regimen.

The next blood test done a few days later, Jan. 9, showed further small improvements. The lymphocytes were up to 29%. But what happened to the alk phos? Were tumor cells dying, letting their alk phos escape? [*The presence of carcinogenic dye (DAB) and its connection to elevated alk phos levels was not suspected until a year later. Her new dental plastic was no doubt supplying it.*]

A few days later she was suddenly in a lot of pain. Copper had accumulated again. Its source was found by the testers and removed by her; the new pain disappeared, then returned again. Finally, a few days later, another "bad" wisdom tooth was extracted and the extraction site thoroughly cleaned. She got immediate pain relief for her bones. She could go off all pain killers. She could walk now.

Her IVs were reduced to 2/day. She was given Clodronate to take by mouth instead of IV. Malonate was still positive at her joints, although tapeworm stages were Negative. The source was not known at the time.

The next blood test showed an extreme blood sugar drop, unexplained. Uric acid was down again. But calcium and alk phos had declined. The bones were healing. And potassium had come up.

She was still in a lot of newly created pain from recent dental work. The dentist had persuaded her to go on antibiotics and use <u>cold</u> water packs instead of <u>hot</u> as in our Dental Aftercare. The pain spread to her whole body and left side of skull again.

Bedridden now, she was too afraid to go off the antibiotics for fear of heart damage, in spite of our pleading.

A friend came to take Tammy to her home nearby for the total care she now needed.

Ten days later, she was brought back in a wheel chair, too ill to care about much. She wanted to go home to England while she could still appreciate her family a little longer. We feared if we released her, she would not even survive the trip home. We prevailed upon her to stay one more week. She agreed to go off antibiotics and let herself be hot packed instead, continually, all day long. She changed her departure time.

A week later she walked in the door unassisted. Her pain was nearly gone. Her mind was alert and her face smiled. She wanted her picture taken because "she was going home!" Half a dozen fellow patients jumped up to oblige her request.

Her new test results (Feb.6) showed great improvements. Her bone marrow had finally turned around and was now able to produce both red and white blood cells. There was still a toxin present, though [*we still did not suspect plastic teeth*]. The alk phos was up again. The LDH was its best ever. The calcium rise showed a toxin in the thyroid again. Albumin was slightly elevated to keep up with calcium. She also got a final bone scan, which showed great improvements as well. But not nearly enough to go home with. Yet, she missed her family. She promised to return if pain would return. And return it did.

Three and a half months later she arrived on two crutches, feeling well though, and having gained weight. Another large abscess in the lower jaw had been found by her dentist at home, but she was too fearful of the consequences to risk pulling it there (she would be put on antibiotics again to replace thorough cleaning of the socket).

Her first blood test showed a threatening BUN rise. This was top priority. It must be contained at once. The kidney herb recipe was started immediately. Alk phos was improved, but LDH had risen.

There was *Staphylococcus* and malonate in the bone marrow, while glutathione was absent.

Our new food list of malonate-free varieties was given to her. New supplements were also given, including taurine, cysteine, B_{12}, folic acid. And a solution of white iodine to irrigate her mouth frequently. We gave her new mineral supplements prepared from yeast varieties. They included molybdenum, manganese, chromium, zinc, as well as boron.

Her IVs now contained magnesium, vitamin C, Clodronate, DMSO, vitamin B complex and calcium.

Seven days later her blood test showed numerous improvements.

She was once more turning the corner with her bone cancer and bone marrow function; both RBC and WBC were coming up. LDH was going down again, a gift from the gods it seemed, as was alk phos.

But calcium was now too high. The BUN was down to normal, but the uric acid dropped too low. More glutamine was given. Potassium was doing well now. But iron had dropped. Was there copper somewhere? Indeed, copper was found in the bone marrow. Cobalt, too, was found there [*the source in the new dental plastic was not guessed*]. And *Staphylococcus*, again. Another rotten tooth was suspected. She was given 1 dose of EDTA to pull out copper and cobalt; they were both Negative next day.

She was getting better. She could visit the friends who had taken care of her earlier. She got her fourth rotten tooth extracted. This time she applied hot packs and did hot swishes all day from the time she got out of the dentist's chair. She merely smiled when the dentist gave her the antibiotic prescription and put it in her pocket.

We scheduled one more blood test (May 27). Calcium had come down.

With wellness came happiness. She wanted to go home again. Although healing was underway, we felt the chance of another abscess hiding in her jaw was quite good. It was not simply a matter of taking X-rays of teeth, spotting the infected teeth, and dealing with them. These abscesses were hidden. [*At that time I did not know about digital X-rays.*] She should stay till this possibility was cleared completely. But she was quite sure her dentist at home would do all the proper things. Our pleadings were in vain. She had one more bone scan done (June 2) to prove her point, it seemed. It was much improved. Bones are more distinct, less "fuzzy." Scan shows much less whiteness.

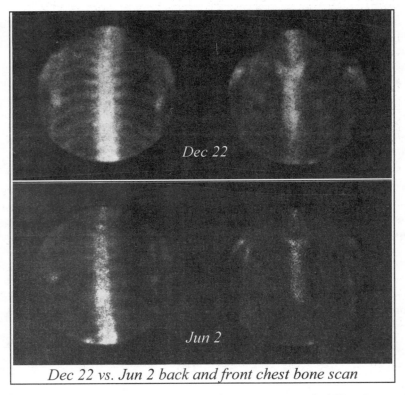

Dec 22 vs. Jun 2 back and front chest bone scan

She could walk without crutches. She was not on pain killer. It was the perfect time to continue, it seemed to us. But her children beckoned. And go she must, in true motherly fashion. Would she ever come back? She promised. But promises mean nothing to the great reaper.

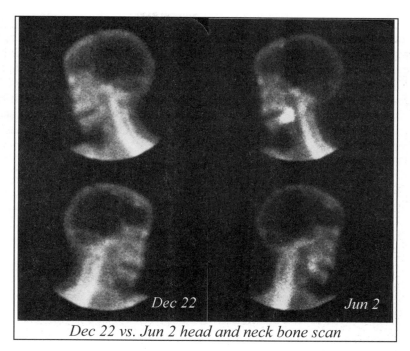

Dec 22

Jun 2

Dec 22 vs. Jun 2 head and neck bone scan

A few months later she was in deep trouble. Too sick to travel to her dentist. Too impoverished to travel back to us. It seemed likely to be just another abscessed tooth. But her friends and family interpreted her visits to our clinic as useless, since she didn't "really get well." What a toll such hasty and uninformed judgment can take. We heard no more.

Visit #1

Tammy Adsit	11/20	11/26	1/3	1/9	1/16	1/25	2/6
RBC	3.96	3.89	3.7	3.71	3.41	3.86	3.89
WBC	4,900	3,700	2,800	2,800	3,100	3,400	4,300
PLT	151	159	142	198	148	186	187
glucose	77	71	126	81	54	65	94
BUN	14	13	12	10 (7-21)	13	11	17
creatinine	0.8	0.8	1.1	1.0	1.0	0.9	1.0
AST (SGOT)	35	27	27	26	32	30	27
ALT (SGPT)	31	24	23	20	18	21	23
LDH	209	201	183	184	180	203	168
GGT	19	13	19	20	16	21	22
T.b.	0.5	0.5	0.6	0.5	0.4	0.5	0.5
alk phos	77	50	66	113	107	150	196
T.p.	7.2	7.1	7.0	7.0	6.6	7.5	7.8

albumin	4.3	4.9	4.8	4.7	4.0	4.8	5.0
globulin	2.9	2.2	2.2	2.3	2.6	2.7	2.8
uric acid	4.8 (2.5-7.5)	2.4 (2.5-6.1)	3.5 (2.5-6.1)	4.4 (2.5-7.5)	2.2	4.1	5.6
Calcium	9.4	10.3 (8.5-10.4)	10.4 (8.5-10.4)	10 (8.4-10.3)	9.6	10.1	10.1
Phosphorus	3	4.6	5.6	4.1	4.9	4.9	4.3
Iron	89	97	91	96	77	93	109
Sodium	140	142	137	140	142	144	144
Potassium	4.2	3.9	3.7	3.9	4.3	4.3	4.3
Chloride	104	100	107	98	96	107	104
triglycerides	109	93	60	73	---	101	58
cholesterol	147	151	161	148	---	156	193

Visit #2

Tammy Adsit	5/16	5/23	5/27
RBC	3.73	3.83	3.91
WBC	3,800	4,300	3,900
PLT	226	209	202
glucose	61	78	95
BUN	24	19	21
creatinine	1.0	0.8	1.1
AST (SGOT)	35	33	38
ALT (SGPT)	19	21	27
LDH	214	189	178
GGT	42	36	37
T.b.	0.6	0.3	0.5
alk phos	132	119	151
T.p.	7.8	7.6	7.9
albumin	4.7	4.9	4.6
globulin	3.1	2.7	3.3
uric acid	6.3	2.6	6.0
Calcium	10.0	12.1	10.8
Phosphorus	3.7	4.8	5.4
Iron	75	60	75
Sodium	143	148	140
Potassium	3.8	4.5	3.9
Chloride	102	107	102
triglycerides	81	96	67
cholesterol	205	198	207

Summary: In hindsight, we should have pulled all her teeth at once, upon arrival, as we do now instead of piecemeal and only at the brink of death. The newly developing problems were also due to plastic replacements for teeth. We would not make that mistake again, either. She should have and could have survived. If only we were given second chances.

| 15 | Sean Pokorny | Lung Cancer |

Sean Pokorny, fiftyish, came with his wife after he had lung surgery at home to remove a cancerous tumor. He had been through radiation and chemotherapy already, too. But now his original symptoms were coming back: a lot of back pain and a pitting edema of the legs plus swelling. That was how his cancer had struck him at the very beginning.

We found he was still positive for malignancy, but it was not in the lung, lymph nodes, stomach, or bone; it was at the kidneys.

His first tasks were to get off isopropyl alcohol sources, kill the intestinal fluke, get his plumbing changed at home, and do dental work.

His initial test showed aluminum, chlorine, cadmium, nickel, cobalt, patulin, and aflatoxin to be positive. Freon and copper were very high at the kidneys, not elsewhere. Malonic acid was at the kidneys, too.

He could stay three weeks, certainly enough time to learn preventive measures, so his cancer and tumors would never return. His lung cancer surgery was 1½ years ago; it had spread to the lymph nodes then. But we did not do a chest X-ray or bone scan at first. We requested an ultrasound of the kidney region instead.

While waiting for the blood test and ultrasound, he was started on IV therapy, receiving two a day. They contained EDTA to remove copper; laetrile; vitamin C, calcium, and magnesium. The freon removal program and dental work got off to an early start, too.

Two days later his blood test was reviewed with him. His RBC, WBC, and platelet count were all slightly elevated. [*At that time I was not aware that cobalt or vanadium toxicity could each raise the RBC. In this case, Sean had tested Positive to cobalt.*] The WBC is also elevated; suggesting a hidden infection somewhere, getting out of control. The elevated platelet count suggests minute bleeding. Lung tumors have a propensity for bleeding, but his lung cancer was in the past, or so we thought. At any rate, we needed to focus on the kidneys, because of severe edema, pain, and the current malignancy there. Tumors at other locations would be healing right along with the healing process going on at the kidneys.

The globulin was too high. [*But its link to vanadium toxicity was not suspected then. We thought it was just a normal, though mysterious, fluctuation of this liver protein product.*] The most relieving result was the LDH; according to this, there was little tumor activity when Sean arrived, December 27. Yet according to the elevated alk phos, there was considerable tumor activity. [*This discrepancy is easily understood now; he was full of DAB dye, not Sudan Black B.*] The low iron level was interpreted as a copper toxicity and should be easy to correct. His better than average cholesterol and triglycerides would help, too.

He was a model patient. Every recommendation was implemented immediately. Even his metal tooth fillings were removed by the end of day two.

He also got a fever, possibly from a general *Staphylococcus* release during dental work, but it was gone in a day.

By the fourth day, his edema was gone. TNF was already present, but his leg pain and back pain persisted. An ultrasound of the kidney area showed no tumors so, whether they had been there or not, he should be ready to leave on schedule, having acquired some new anti-cancer tactics.

By day seven he was feeling very well, but malonic acid was still positive [*malonic acid was not suspected in food or dental plastic, only in tapeworm stages*]. We gave him the definitive dose of Q10, 3½ gm. After this, he had no more fevers.

By January 8, his alk phos had dropped over 100 points, indicating tumor activity was way down. But iron had dropped, too, in fact, "out of sight". And, indeed, copper was found at both parathyroids and liver. Since his motel had all plastic pipes, the copper source was mysterious. [*We could not guess at that time that it might be put, along with cobalt, vanadium, and malonate derivatives right into his mouth in his plastic dentalware.*]

We supplied him with Iron Booster (chlorophyll product), 1 tbs. a day and quickly applied more EDTA by IV to pull out more copper. The Q10 had done its job and killed bacteria, along with tapeworm stages.

Notice that his calcium had swung from too low (8.9) to too high (10.3), shifting the problem from parathyroids to the thyroid. Immediately the toxin in the thyroid shut off calcitonin production, allowing bones to dissolve and flood his blood stream with both calcium and phosphate. We added Clodronate, a diphosphonate, to his IV to inhibit bone dissolution.

Meanwhile, the LDH had gone up, instead of down, implying new tumor activity. How could that be? Could it be happening in a <u>different</u> organ that was getting a new larger dose of malonic acid, cobalt, copper than before? We gave him a BQ shot to lower LDH.

By January 12, we stopped his IVs—he was simply too well. The next day a new blood test was done. Obviously, his bacteria were under control, wherever they had been, since the WBC was now normal.

Calcium, too, was returning, but was still too high along with phosphate. The albumin to globulin ratio was now correct. The liver enzymes ALT and GGT were very much better. Most important, the LDH was back down and the alk phos was down to normal too. If there were additional tumor sites, they must be fairly inactive.

Copper continued to plague us though and iron stayed low. This was in spite of taking iron pills, as well as Iron Booster liquid. He was due to leave in a few days. His mission was accomplished from his point of view: no tumors seen, blood test greatly improved, edema and swelling gone, pain down. He could walk normally, which he interpreted as beating the race against cancer. And his time and money were spent. They left for home.

But we knew there was a mysterious source of copper and also malonic acid, two vicious tumor growers.

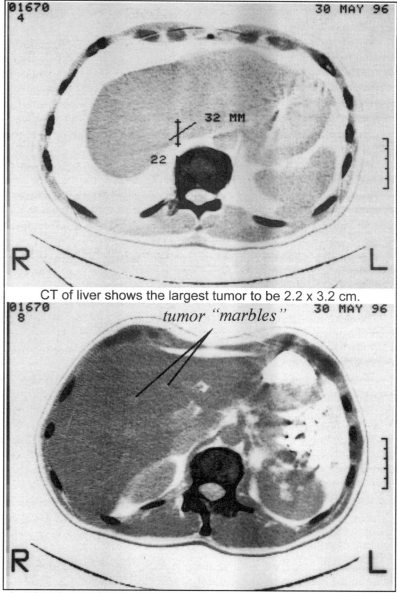

CT of liver shows the largest tumor to be 2.2 x 3.2 cm.

tumor "marbles"

Another level of the same scan shows numerous small "marbles" (tumors).

May 30, arriving with new liver tumors

Four months later, he came back. He was full of pain, full of isopropyl alcohol, full of cobalt and PCBs and fiberglass. This must have aggravated his lungs continually while he was home. Two *Shigella* varieties were growing in him. His copper level was quite high, again at the kidneys. And his low back pain required constant pain killing drugs. A CT scan of upper abdomen as well as lower abdomen was ordered and he was started on glutathione.

The lower scan showed normal kidneys. The surprise came from the upper scan. His liver had a half dozen small tumors, including one, not so small at 2.2 x 3.2 cm. This should be our top priority.

His new blood test (May 28) showed a general worsening. In fact, iron was so low, it could not even be detected. This was an emergency. He was put on iron pills, liquid "Iron Booster," and given iron shots again, on alternate days.

Our testing soon found one source of copper and cobalt. They were riding along as pollutants in his iron pills! [*We still did not suspect the dental plastic.*] To help the liver, we gave him silymarin, B_{12}, folic acid, and vitamin C.

His IV now included calcium, magnesium, vitamin C, glycyrrhizin and DMSO. The new blood test showed that alk phos was up slightly, not the LDH. The low LDH implied no tumor activity at all. While the alk phos implied some.

The very low iron, together with the elevated platelet count suggested minute bleeding, possibly in the lung. But, again, another organ took precedence. The lung would not be life threatening (unless it hemorrhaged), the liver would.

In five days, his pain level was down. He had been staying off malonate-containing food. He was on all the programs, parasite, kidney herbs...all of it.

We had decided to do weekly ultrasounds of the liver for him to follow his progress, since they were inexpensive, about $45.00. He brought in his first one June 4, at the end of his first week.

The ultrasound was Negative! No tumor could be seen. This was just too much good news. We planned to back this up with a CT scan in two more weeks. Could it really be true? Our hopes, fears, denials, determination were at a peak with suspense. The new blood test, June 5, told the same story. Something had allowed the serum iron to shoot up in a single snap. This is seldom seen from taking iron supplements.

And finally, for the first time, the platelet count was coming down. Did this mean the hidden bleeding had stopped? Kidney function was better too.

But why had the RBC gone higher, if the cobalt-polluted pills were stopped? This time it was due to vanadium. The source was not found [*in the dental plastic*]. He was again having some plastic put into his mouth. The vanadium toxicity can easily be spotted in the elevated globulin, too. [*Also note some newly encountered Sudan Black B dye can be detected by the LDH rise. And newly encountered inorganic copper or "bad" germanium caused the iron level to plummet again.*] He needed more glutamine—uric acid was still only 2.4.

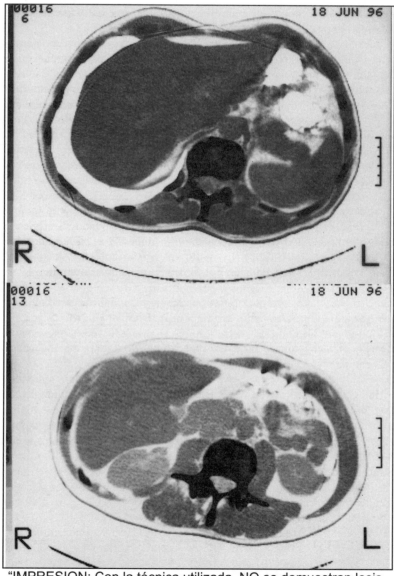

"IMPRESION: Con la técnica utilizada, NO se demuestran lesiones tumores secundarias." (With the technique employed, no metastases are seen.) Another slice reveals no "marbles", although texture is still poor.

June 18 right lobe CT of liver reveals no tumors

It was June 18, the "magic" date for repeating his liver scan. The pictures tell it better than the radiologists' words.

The liver tumors were gone, the nightmare of cancer about gone. Only a chronic, mysterious toxicity problem remained, the same as before: copper, cobalt, vanadium, and malonic derivatives.

Would Sean and his wife leave again before finding the source? Sometimes he would be Positive for mercury and thallium making his leg pain worse. This time his pain was not all conquered. staphylococcus bacteria would not leave. And he continued having dental plastic put into his mouth.

They were not thrilled about having his liver tumors vanish. They were too torn about staying or leaving. He was coughing a lot. His wife voted for staying. She thought he should have a chest X-ray. Sean thought he was "all done" again.

It was July 1. The blood test continued to show toxicity effects from vanadium, copper, and malonic acid. The LDH was back down, but alk phos was not. And the platelet count stayed high. His wife finally persuaded him to have a chest X-ray. On July 3, a chest X-ray revealed a <u>large lung tumor</u>! This could explain the numerous mysteries we had encountered. His wife was happy to find it and wanted to focus on it immediately. The tumor appeared fluffy and not too dense. It should not be difficult to dissolve. But Sean was crushed. He felt he had "put in his time" and wanted nothing so much as to leave.

Lung tumors have a propensity for producing pain and for bleeding. But we had gained experience with a new Chinese herb, Yunnan paiyao. It seemed to prevent bleeding or reduce it, often stopping it. We started him on this, fearful of using tumor shrinkers that would work too fast and cause more bleeding.

By now, he had two new crowns in his mouth, against recommendations. Had the dentist swayed him? He was coughing more, although not bringing up blood. Still, he felt demoralized. Perhaps all the new toxins placed in his mouth caused depression (copper often does that). He should have been hopping with excitement over his successes, not labeling the remaining task "failure." They decided to leave.

Summary: They went home with mixed feelings. Maybe all will be well, as it so often is. A lung tumor that isn't hemorrhaging is, after all, "the best kind". And, of course, it could be surgically removed. Maybe they did that. We wish them the best.

Sean Pokorny	12/27	1/8	1/13	5/28	6/5	6/12	6/26	7/1
RBC	4.93	4.82	4.83	4.91	5.1	4.76	4.44	4.08
WBC	11,900	9,200	7,300	8,100	12,000	8,600	13,300	8,800
PLT	461	407	432	516	394	471	459	487
BUN	12	12	11	24	14	18	18	14
creatinine	0.9	1.0	1.4	1.1	1.0	1.1	0.9	0.9

AST (SGOT)	26	19	18	17	22	16	33	38
ALT (SGPT)	41	26	16	18	16	30	19	21
LDH	181	246	178	154	163	190	185	143
GGT	41	26	25	36	31	39	36	37
T.b.	0.5	0.7	0.6	0.5	0.4	0.5	0.3	0.3
alk phos	321	181	87	151	150	159	164	169
T.p.	7.1	6.9	7.0	6.8	6.8	7.6	7.1	6.8
albumin	3.9	4.1	4.4	4.0	4.2	4.2	3.5	3.4
globulin	3.2	2.8	2.6	2.8	2.6	3.4	3.6	3.4
uric acid	5.1	4.3	3.5	4.2	0.2	2.4	5.0	5.2
Calcium	8.9	10.3	10.0	8.3	8.9	9.0	9.0	8.6
Phosphorus	2.9	4.5	4.7	4.2	4.5	5.1	3.8	3.9
Iron	39	12	20	0	76	13	42	43
Potassium	4.7	4.6	4.1	4.5	4.4	4.5	4.5	4.4
triglycerides	178	117	150	142	112	104	120	176
cholesterol	223	214	228	183	101	186	186	182

16   Betty Fries   Breast Cancer

Betty Fries, under fifty, seemed quite well and certainly desirous of living when she arrived with her teenage son from Australia. But she had been given 18 months to live; her previous breast cancer had gone to her liver where she now had five or more large tumors. The breast had been removed, there could be no recurrence there. It had all been a big success by clinical standards, but these standards would not let her survive.

She had already started the parasite program, but was still using isopropyl containing products.

Her initial test showed *Salmonella paratyphi*, copper, *Shigella dysenteriae*, cadmium, CFC's, mercury, asbestos, patulin (fruit mold toxin), nickel, aflatoxin (grain and nut mold toxin), all Positive. All of these were high enough to be detected systemically with the Syncrometer.

A blood test was done and ultrasound scheduled. Removal of amalgam was scheduled. She moved into a nearby Mexican "copper-free" motel. Her son started her on the freon removal program, Lugol's iodine, and three grams of coenzyme Q10 to kill tapeworm stages. She was given silymarin for the liver, in addition to the liver herbs in the freon program. She zapped daily. It was December 30, a Saturday afternoon.

The ultrasound arrived a few hours later; it showed the five masses in the right lobe to be about the size of small potatoes, while the left lobe had a similar tumor.

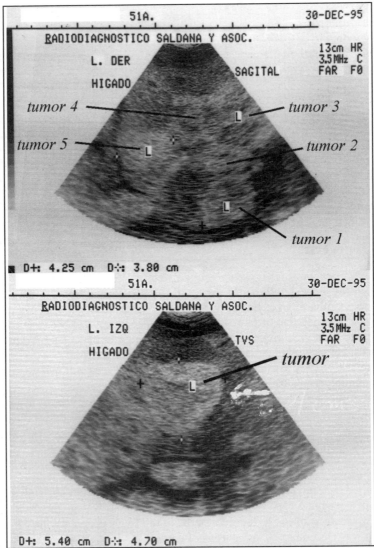

Right lobe (top) has 5 tumors, left lobe (bottom) has a large
one with white arrow drawn on negative by radiologist.
Dec 30 right and left lobe liver ultrasounds

There was no time to lose. She was started that same day on 3 IVs daily,
containing EDTA (metal chelator) to remove copper, glycyrrhizin for liver
support, vitamin C, and magnesium.

326

By the next day, she had gotten rid of isopropyl alcohol and was negative for ortho-phospho-tyrosine. The malignancy was gone. But would she survive with a liver full of tumors?

On Monday, her blood test results arrived. We feared the worst, and were pleasantly surprised. Not that a GGT of 794 did not send chills down our spine. But the LDH (tumor activity) was only 278, the alk phos only 156, and calcium quite correctable, too, at 10.0.

Electronic testing at the liver showed malonic acid and aflatoxin Positive, as well as cobalt. [*At this time, we did not know all the sources of malonic acid and cobalt.*]

By Monday, the copper was gone and her IVs were simply glycyrrhizin, vitamin C, and magnesium. Potassium was supplemented by making her table salt a mixture of sodium chloride and potassium chloride. [*Currently, we emphasize potassium supplementation much more.*]

She had developed insomnia. Testing showed it to be due to *E. coli.* Three days later, she still had it in spite of zapping, using Bowel Program herbs, and another big dose of Q10. We gave her hydrochloric acid (5%), 10 drops in beverage at mealtime, 3 times a day for several days, which cleared it. By January 5, patulin was negative, aflatoxin was negative, TNF was Positive.

On January 8, she was much improved; she had much more energy now; she had spent two hours on the beach; and she was not sleeping during the day anymore. She was in the middle of dental work. Her IVs were changed to include laetrile.

The following day a new blood test showed her RBC was down from 5.3 to 4.98. Had she lost her cobalt toxin? But her liver enzymes had climbed, not dropped, as we had hoped [*due to opening tumors*].

Surprisingly the alk phos was up, so bone or lung could be involved. Yet, she had no symptoms at these locations, and we did not investigate either; we had enough to cope with.

A new ultrasound on January 10 showed a passageway of normal liver tissue separating the tumors on the right side.

In spite of worsening liver tests, she continued to feel well, she was eating and sleeping. But the next blood test, on January 13, again did not bring good news. The RBC was back up, the WBC stayed too low [*more opening tumors*]. Liver enzymes continued to climb, but the GGT and alk phos were beginning to decline.

The dropping serum iron was the clue: it must be copper again, and cobalt besides. [*We never suspected her new dental plastic to be seeping copper, germanium and dyes. We found it in the water from her "copper-free" motel.*] She was requested to move and her son eagerly arranged it. Her IVs were changed again, adding cesium chloride (about 8 grams), and DMSO to the previous recipe.

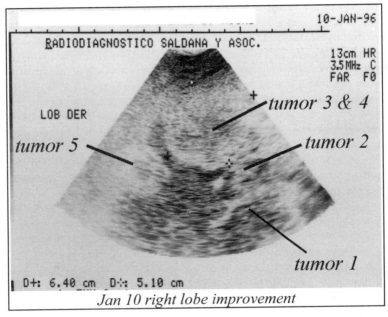

Jan 10 right lobe improvement

On January 18, a new blood test and ultrasound were done. The RBC (5.55) showed persisting cobalt toxicity; it was poisoning the bone marrow; we had not found her sources [*hidden* Ascaris *colonies*].

The copper problem had been improved by her move, and serum iron was rising again. The ultrasound showed great improvements. The largest mass in the left lobe measured 2.65 x 5.75; had a piece become severed?

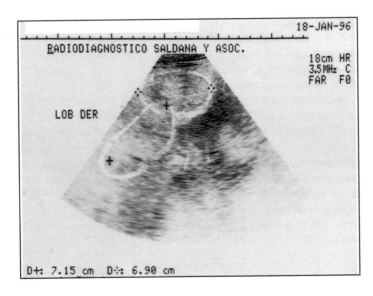

Was it breaking up? And the five tumors in the right lobe all looked smaller.

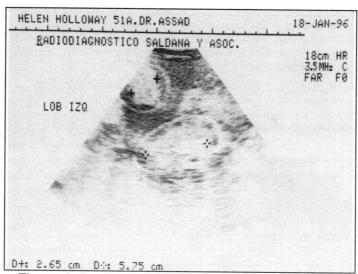

HELEN HOLLOWAY 51A.DR.ASSAD   18-JAN-96

RADIODIAGNOSTICO SALDANA Y ASOC.

18cm HR
3.5MHz C
FAR F0

LOB IZQ

D+: 2.65 cm   D-:- 5.75 cm

The encircling lines were drawn on the negative by our pathologist.

Jan 18 right and left lobe liver ultrasounds

In spite of all this good news, Betty was beginning to worsen [*toxicity from opened tumors*]; she could not go for walks and spent her daytime in bed. Her son had to coax her to eat every mouthful. What was wrong? We added thioctic acid to her regimen. Her son admitted that Betty had been taking supplements [*just what was needed to combat toxicity*] as directed for over a week already. She was failing rapidly. A nurse was sent to her residence to do a CBC. It had improved! RBC was 4.72, WBC was 4,600. (Remember, an RBC over 4.7 reflects a cobalt or vanadium toxicity):

Yet she continued to decline and had a fever. A saliva sample brought to us was positive for *Salmonella* and *E. coli*. All her foods were quickly tested. But I was sick myself for several days and only prayed that the conscientious staff would do their detective work well. She was given 3 grams of Q10, Lugol's iodine, 4 times a day to conquer the infection, and urea powder, 5 tsp. a day in water for liver support. Each day I asked if she had survived. In a few days my own illness had improved enough to continue studies. I decided to try glutathione (reduced) for Betty. It seemed to return my own health rather swiftly. She was given $\frac{1}{8}$ tsp., 3 times a day, before meals.

The very next day, she claimed she was "feeling good." I was seeing her myself now; she had arrived in the office in a wheelchair. Meanwhile, her son was undaunted, keeping her spirits high, and her thoughts on success. A new blood test showed three of the liver tests improving now.

But the LDH and alk phos were rising [from emerging dye]. She was losing weight, her son said, and losing ground. In desperation we ordered her tested for 80 toxins. [*The toxin test did not include food or hair dyes at that time.*] From the rising alk phos, I suspected bone or lung metastases, but did not bring up this possibility; there was enough to cope with and this would not change her treatment anyway.

The results of the complete toxin test were: praseodymium, chromium (III), tin, platinum, holmium, terbium, zinc, rhodium, bromine, Positive. The remaining 71 elements were Negative. <u>Only tooth fillings</u> could give such results! How could this be? All amalgam had been removed! Was it left over amalgam? Yet, mercury was missing. Could it be the plastic replacement? Was the dentist not using the customary composite? We asked. Indeed, she had gone to a different dentist, unfamiliar with our dental standards. The cost was less! It was our lowest moment. She was much too ill and weak to sit in any dentist's chair now.

And *Staphylococcus* from improperly cleaned sockets and cavitations had spread to her bones and lungs. She had a constant fever. The pain at her left shoulder blade was relentless. To all appearances she was dying of cancer, yet her blood test of February was not worsening. And a new ultrasound showed further improvement. If the pain was due to a large gallstone stuck in

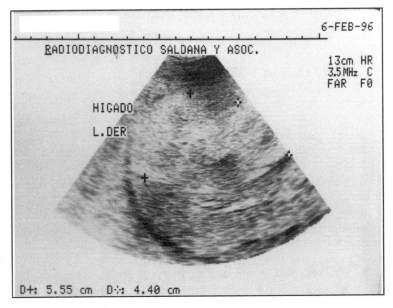

a bile duct, she could do a liver cleanse; there was nothing to lose. Her son prepared it. Indeed she got out a large stone. Her pain level went down, but her general condition stayed the same. She made the mistake of having some high fat food the very next day and was in extreme pain again. We declined

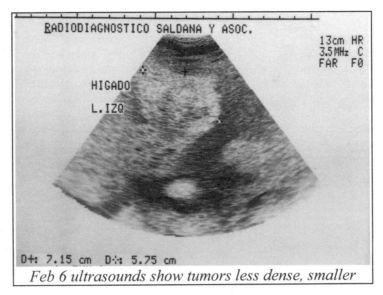

Feb 6 ultrasounds show tumors less dense, smaller

to give morphine or codeine, explaining this would be the kiss of death. Better to do another liver flush right away. It was only four days later. But this time it was successful. She bounced back to her old self. In a day, in spite of bathroom sprints, she felt like exercising. She was definitely improving. Some pain over shoulder blades persisted, but her appetite returned and hope had returned.

On February 19, a new blood test was done. Her BUN and uric acid were extremely high, no doubt due to the urea we were giving by mouth; the creatinine was not elevated showing kidney failure was not responsible.

We stopped her urea supplement. [*With hindsight, we should have merely reduced it.* Besides this, to our utter amazement the GGT, our nemesis, had dropped in half. Her alk phos, our other nemesis, had dropped drastically, too. Calcium and potassium normalized! And one liver enzyme, AST, began to drop as well as the LDH. Was this the turning point? Did the liver cleanses do this? Or the urea? These were the two extraordinary treatments.

A few days later her dental work was complete and now she had a mouthful of plastic.

For eight days she gradually improved, although her left arm was incapacitated with pain again. On February 29 she suddenly lost her walking ability, due to spasms in her left hip. [*Hip pain is always dental!*] We guessed the problem was dental. But she also had picked up vanadium, thallium, mercury, and copper again! She was even full of malonate! We knew not from where. She wanted a cortisone shot for both hip and shoulder. But hot packing and water swishing her mouth was the right answer. She agreed. The next day she <u>walked</u> in, no wheelchair or assistance! It was time for a blood test and ultrasound. Just for good measure, we persuaded her to include a lung X-ray.

March 4 was a red letter day. There on her chest X-ray was a tumor as large as a fist (not shown), not far from the location of her constant pain. This explained the dropping RBC. The tumor was no doubt bleeding in a minute fashion. The platelet count was rising to accommodate this bleed.

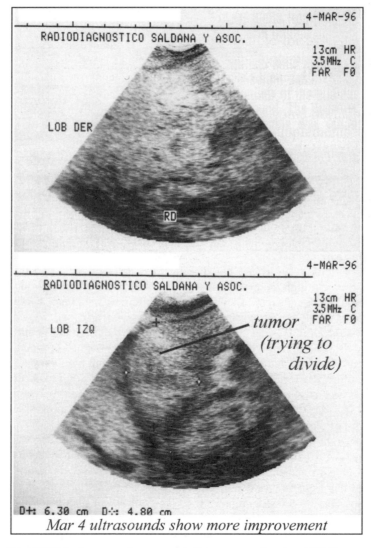

Mar 4 ultrasounds show more improvement

The BUN had returned to normal. To our surprise the AST liver enzyme took another steep drop and the LDH also fell. Now the albumin was worri-

THE TRUE STORY OF...

some, though, because it was only 3.0. We thought it could reflect copper toxicity again, since the iron had stayed very low.

How long had she had this large lung tumor? The beginning of her shoulder pain probably was the beginning of its shrinking and pulling away from the pleura. Then why did the liver cleanse give pain relief? The pain was probably made of two pains; the gallstone and the lung tumor.

We dug into the new tumor problem with determination and panic. Her RBC was sinking. She was hemorrhaging! Unless we could stop this, all would be lost. I brought up the subject of transfusion, so it would not be so

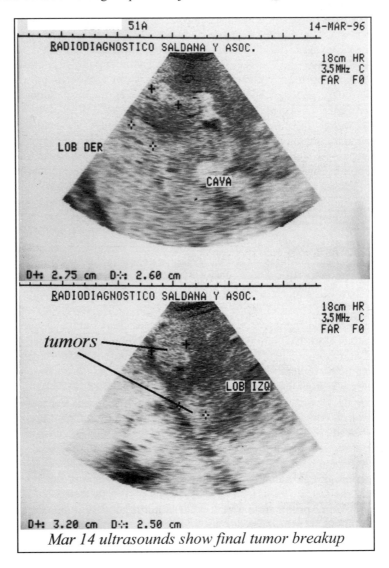

Mar 14 ultrasounds show final tumor breakup

333

scary later. Besides, her son had been spelled by her daughter who had been too busy to read the literature that explained our treatments. She was impatient for her mother to come home. No amount of transfusion can keep up with a hemorrhage. [*We had not yet learned the usefulness of the Chinese herb, Yunnan paiyao. We only knew about the anti-hemorrhaging action of cayenne pepper which we had already used extensively.*]

Besides cayenne capsules, we started her on lung tea. It had two ingredients, comfrey and mullein. She cooked them herself and was to drink 2 cups a day. She was to eat a small clove of garlic daily, raw, with a bit of bread, also for lung improvement.

Her liver tumors now took second priority. The right lobe showed much better texture, the former tumor outlines weakly discernible. The left tumor, 6.3 x 4.8 cm was still trying to divide across the middle.

In four days, she was feeling better. Her shoulder pain was gone, simply gone. The lung tumor must have pulled free—and without hemorrhaging! Extraordinary good fortune! A fresh X-ray showed the lung tumor smaller and with barely discernible borders.

By March 14, she was walking quite well by herself. She could speak of nothing but going home. We begged, in vain, for her son to return for her last few weeks. He understood the vagaries of her situation. She was finally on more solid ground with her recovery. It was premature to stop overseeing developments in her path to health. We ordered a last blood test, ultrasound of liver, and X-ray of lung. The lung tumor was gone…completely gone. The left liver tumor had pulled apart, leaving two small pieces, one 3.2 cm in diameter, the other about 2.5 cm. The right liver tumors were reduced to a few fragments also. The texture was good. But the blood test still had its warning signs. The RBC at 3.18 was lower than ever. An RBC of 3.0 is the cut off point, where we give a transfusion. Was she still bleeding? Platelet count was 431, suggesting she was.

The liver function tests were greatly improved. The liver could make albumin again, raising it to 3.7. The calcium was normal, but the iron level was lower than ever; had her copper water pipes been changed at home? Perhaps being home would get her away from the chronic copper burden she was picking up here. Maybe leaving prematurely would not be all bad.

She was instructed to do a blood test every week until the RBC was on its way up. Otherwise, to get a transfusion without delay. She promised to send follow-up ultrasounds and blood tests. Then they grabbed their X-rays and dashed to the airport. And we chalked up another successful failure. Success in clearing up the cancer and shrinking the tumors. Failure to completely restore her health.

Summary: A glance at first and last blood tests shows her remarkable improvement. But if it is obtained by means of IVs that merely "catch up" with a toxicity problem, temporarily, it is not a good solution. Better ways had to be found, so we searched on.

Betty Fries	12/30	1/9	1/13	1/18	1/22	1/29
RBC	5.3	4.98	5.91	5.55	4.72	4.58
WBC	4.6	3.8	3.8	3.8	4.6	5.2
PLT	220	194	260	219	210	219
glucose	109	122	151	90		155
BUN	19	11	8	11		23
creatinine	1.0	1.0	1.0	1.0		1.0
AST (SGOT)	98	111	119	112		110
ALT (SGPT)	50	60	72	62		56
LDH	278	288	299	274		337
GGT	794	885	870	898		816
T.b.	0.8	0.7	0.6	0.9		0.7
alk phos	156	278	271	298		424
T.p.	7.0	7.4	6.8	7.1		7.6
albumin	4.7	4.9	4.2	4.4		4.5
globulin	2.3	2.5	2.6	2.7		3.1
uric acid	6.4	6.8	4.5	6.3		5.3
Calcium	10.0	10.0	9.0	9.5		9.5
Phosphorus	2.8	2.9	3.3	3.6		3.3
Iron	78	75	60	80		37
Sodium	148	141	136	138		138
Potassium	4.6	4.8	4.6	4.7		4.5
Chloride	98	100	97	105		102
triglycerides	183	81	1 verified	90		139
cholesterol	210	204	70	190		199

Betty Fries	2/6	2/19	3/6	3/13
RBC	4.71	4.19	3.6	3.18
WBC	5.1	9.1	8.8	8.7
PLT	214	211	339	431
glucose	77	102	132	79
BUN	15	48	14	13
creatinine	1.1	1.2	.8	.8
AST (SGOT)	146	120	74	66
ALT (SGPT)	59	133	111	81
LDH	332	293	228	237
GGT	806	333	360	257
T.b.	.8	.8	.5	.7
alk phos	423	280	562	391
T.p.	7.4	6.8	6.1	7.2
albumin	4.7	3.3	3.0	3.7
globulin	2.7	3.5	3.1	3.5
uric acid	6.2	11	3.7	4.2
Calcium	10.1	9.1	9.1	9.6
Phosphorus	3.8	41.1	2.9	3.5
Iron	83	21	22	19
Sodium	141	128	132	133
Potassium	5.4	4.4	4.5	4.9
Chloride	103	93	98	94

triglycerides	89	137	102	84
cholesterol	200	113	126	125

17   Nikki Ashby   Lung/Liver/Bone/Lymphatic Cancer

Nikki Ashby, a thin and wiry woman, always active, came with a dedicated friend to take care of her. It all started five years earlier. She had undergone four surgeries to remove tumor (melanoma) from her eye, but then it had gone to the lung, liver, bone, lymph nodes. There were two marble size tumors at her neck and another small one coming up on her neck on the other side. An ultrasound of the liver (not shown) showed two lesions. We planned to use these little neck tumors as monitors of her progress, but all that would soon change.

She was fairly clear of toxins at her initial test, only freon, asbestos, arsenic and mercury showing up at the "whole body" test. The copper test was negative, but it showed up at her liver and retina (eye). She was positive for aflatoxin and malonic acid. Also shigella and *staphylococcus aureus* bacteria, besides the usual isopropyl alcohol.

Her last surgery was a month ago, the fourth one, and she worried about losing her vision if it grew back again. We reassured her that could be prevented. We focused on the retina, although her major complaint was severe low back pain.

A glance at her blood test shows she also had cobalt or vanadium toxicity, since her RBC was too high.

She was obviously coping with too many bacteria (WBC 10,700). But the LDH and alk phos were only moderately elevated, so there was not a lot of tumor activity.

She had three vicious air toxins at home: freon, asbestos and arsenic and the season was winter time when air toxins are especially high and people mostly indoors. It was good for her to come to Mexico where there is no heating or air conditioning. [*At that time we did not yet know that malonic acid came from food nor that malonate plus cobalt and vanadium could come from plastic dental fillings.*] We encouraged her to start on dental replacement with plastic.

Her IVs were begun at once, three a day, including EDTA, glycyrrhizin (for the liver lesions), vitamin C and magnesium. Soon she was switched off EDTA, after copper tested negative at the retina and liver. Then she was given two glycyrrhizin doses, vitamin C, magnesium, cesium and DMSO. We also gave her silymarin tablets (concentrate of milk thistle).

Her intense low back pain was nearly gone in the first few days. She did everything: Q10 three gm, parasite program, Lugol's, bowel program, freon program and the dental replacement. We were mystified that malonic acid would not disappear; it was always present at the lung. She promised to bring her previous chest X-ray of November.

The second blood test (Jan. 17) shows severe inhibition of urea formation, no relief for the LDH, a considerable worsening of alk phos [*the damaging effect of DAB in colored plastic*], and more bacteria (WBC) probably from dental work.

But improvement occurred in other areas, where glucose was up and calcium was down. Yet the iron had dropped, a sure sign of copper toxicity. We searched immediately; it was present in the liver. She needed to move to a new motel where the water pipes were all plastic, which she promised to do.

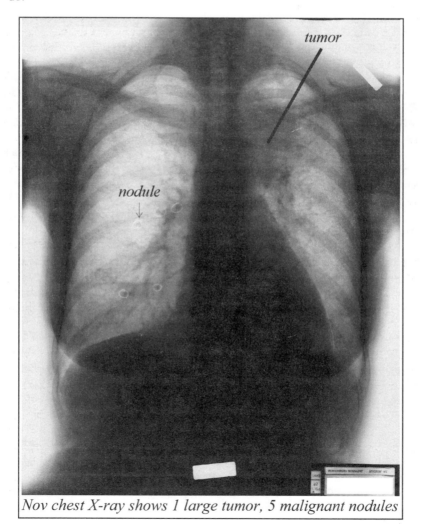

Nov chest X-ray shows 1 large tumor, 5 malignant nodules

The smallish lumps at her neck were now about half-size; the one at her ear was entirely gone. Her low back pain was 50% better. Her muscle spasms all over were gone. Her breathing which had been labored was much improved. She felt she was "out of the woods." Her caregiver needed a rest. She planned to go home for one week against all advice. But this drew out to three weeks and she was much the worse for it. Her home had not been adequately cleaned. When she returned, February 14, she was once again full of toxins: isopropyl alcohol, wood alcohol, benzene, copper, aflatoxin, patulin.

She had brought her previous November chest X-ray; a large tumor was visible! We took our focus off the retina and liver and put it squarely on the lungs.

While at home her LDH and alk phos had gone up steeply, causing the worsening lung problem. It was probably due to the malonic acid derivatives and a slate of carcinogens including dyes placed in her mouth before leaving.

The calcium level was again too high now. But the most startling was the steep drop in iron; she had been using coppered water at home. So it was back to EDTA IVs to pull out copper, then cesium, laetrile, DMSO to shrink the lung tumor, plus vitamin C, calcium, and magnesium. She bounced back with energy and an appetite. Then we added glutathione 250 mg three a day, vitamin A 25000 units, and carrot juice daily for beta carotene [*not suspecting carrots contain malonic acid*].

By February 27, two weeks later, the LDH was coming back down in spite of persistent malonic acid, maleic acid, and maleic anhydride at her lungs. Their sources were a mystery. But alk phos was at a new high. (Note: the blood sample of Feb. 27 was left standing too long before being tested. When this happens, the red cells that have broken during standing have let out their potassium. The potassium level is then too high. Such "hemolyzed blood" often shows a falsely low glucose, too! Such data must, of course, be discounted.)

Suddenly she was very much better. She decided to go home for one week again. The staff agonized over the prospect of another return under emergency circumstances.

But Nikki surprised us this time. She returned three weeks later with this news: Her follow up visit with the ophthalmologist at home who had done her eye surgery had said there was no sign of regrowth. Her cough was gone. Her neck nodules were about the same. We ordered a chest X-ray and scan of liver. She had chills and fever, some shortness of breath, and was full of pains. But all in all, her three week recess seemed to do her good. Still, when she returned on March 19, her LDH had risen further, though the alk phos (lung condition) had dropped a lot.

Now calcium had dropped much too low and iron was critically low. She was full of copper again, as well as isopropyl alcohol (drinking bottled water on the airplane). We quickly gave her "iron booster" (a chlorophyll beverage), an iron shot, vitamin B12, and folic acid, 0.4 mg. [*This small dose*

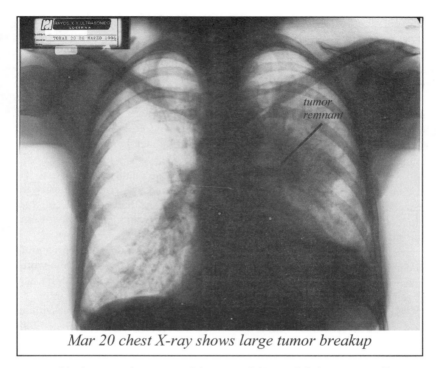

tumor remnant

Mar 20 chest X-ray shows large tumor breakup

was used before our discovery of the great folic acid deficiency in all cancer patients.]

The reward, though, and highlight of her return was her new chest X-ray. The large tumor was broken up. No margins could be seen. It was dispersing. And the enlarged lymph nodes in the right lung were no longer noted by the radiologist. But water accumulation had continued, as it must in the presence of maleic anhydride.

The rest of her story is typical of a cancer patient anywhere in the world today. Pain and pain killers, nausea and anti nausea medicine.

In spite of tumor dissolution, her health did not improve. I was beginning to see that we typically do not die from the malignancy or tumors themselves! We die from the toxicity that <u>caused</u> the tumor growth. Doing away with the tumors, either surgically or by alternative methods, does not do away with the toxicity that generated them.

Notice how her BUN remained very low till June 12, the date of her last blood test. This would keep her toxic with ammonia. Gradually, her liver function worsened, as AST, ALT, GGT values rose. Her body's metabolism could not make energy. [*As soon as pyruvate was made, it was diverted by the hugely increased LDH. The dye causing all this had come out of the tumor but was not being detoxified or eliminated.*] Eventually her LDH was 1293. Alkaline phosphatase, another enzyme rose to 1538. Calcium fluctuated from too high to too low, as the thyroid and parathyroid took turns cop-

339

ing with the burden. The burden of copper, cobalt, vanadium, [*and dyes*] always varying as we chelated them, detoxified them, removed more sources [*but never ever guessed they were put in her mouth willfully, invisibly, in dental plastic and pink dentures; iron fluctuated similarly from the newly implanted copper*].

On March 28 the liver was scanned and no trace of the two tumors was found. Our hopes for her fluctuated with her condition. When she got better, she would go home and come back in worse shape. It took till June 9 before Nikki's family began changing the plumbing at her home. Each time she loaded up with copper and dropped her serum iron.

On May 15 another chest X-ray was done (the quality was poor, so it is not shown). But the large tumor she originally had was gone. To verify this marvelous result, a CT scan was ordered. But she had stopped coughing blood and had enough breath to walk around at a "swap meet" so it was not a priority to her.

By June 1, she slept through the night and was hungry. Her vomiting had stopped and intestinal pain, as well as other pains were gone. She wore a brace for back support and was on B_{12}, glutathione, vitamin C, folic acid, taurine, and sodium alginate mixed with moose elm herb daily.

Summary: ultimately she spent a fortune on her treatment with us, probably $8000.00. Her retina tumor was gone, her neck nodule was gone, her lung tumor was gone, but a glance at her blood test on June 13 shows that her health was worse.

She left for the last time June 12. We feared the worst and dared not inquire. The lesson she taught us was priceless: We can stop the malignancy, dissolve the tumors, but this cannot save a cancer patient from the ongoing toxicity from copper, cobalt, vanadium, malonates, and dyes. We are deeply indebted and grateful. Nikki always kept a smile, even in pain. She led us to discover malonic acid in <u>foods</u> after battling it for such a long time.

Nikki Ashby	1/8	1/17	2/14	2/20	2/27	3/19	3/25	4/1
RBC	5.22	4.99	5.19	4.95	5.0	4.66	4.25	4.42
WBC	10700	12100	12900	9800	9100	13300	12600	15200
PLT	402	440	388	435	481	519	594	565
glucose	78	107	89	66	56	76	74	147
BUN	13	6	10	11	10	9	5	4.0
creatinine	0.8	0.8	0.9	0.8	0.8	0.6	0.7	0.7
AST (SGOT)	21	21	24	21	23	32	96	67
ALT (SGPT)	22	12	16	13	11	23	62	63
LDH	239	237	329	349	255	500	421	472
GGT	18	25	33	32	32	38	42	72
T.b.	0.6	0.3	0.3	0.3	0.3	0.8	0.5	0.4
alk phos	202	328	495	437	521	347	512	792
T.p.	7.1	7.1	8.0	6.8	6.9	7.2	5.3	6.1
albumin	4.5	4.5	4.7	4.0	4.3	4.0	2.8	3.2
globulin	2.6	2.6	3.3	2.8	2.6	3.2	2.5	2.9

uric acid	2.9	4.1	3.2	3.7	3.9	3.3	3.3	3.3
Calcium	9.9	9.3	10.2	9.6	9.1	8.7	8.5	8.6
Phosphorus	3	3.3	3.8	3.8	3.3	3.6	3.1	2.8
Iron	58	45	19	42	39	10	49	17
Sodium	136	139	139	140	138	135	135	137
Potassium	4.7	4.7	4.6	4.6	6.0	4.9	4.7	4.8
Chloride	105	102	99	104	102	103	96	103
triglycerides	80	87	133	95	111	84	88	90
cholesterol	214	195	192	163	178	142	100	137

Nikki Ashby	4/18	4/24	5/8	5/13	5/21	5/27	6/1	9/7	6/12
RBC	4.40	4.47	4.11	4.05	3.67	4.2	4.0	4.53	3.8
WBC	9000	9700	11400	11300	15600	12100	17000	16200	13700
PLT	574	397	540	744	541	694	598	374	581
glucose	72	88	132	72	148	100	61	107	140
BUN	6.0	8.0	8	7.0	6	4.0	6	9	15
creatinine	0.7	0.7	0.6	0.7	0.6	0.6	0.7	0.7	0.6
AST (SGOT)	22	39	55	31	60	51	48	54	81
ALT (SGPT)	25	23	121	48	34	37	26	25	65
LDH	338	626	806	804	1683	620	889	708	1293
GGT	74	64	220	188	230	232	218	263	324
T.b.	0.4	1.3	0.6	0.6	0.5	0.5	1.1	0.9	0.5
alk phos	543	492	1163	901	1490	1289	1041	1132	1538
T.p.	6.2	6.3	5.6	5.8	4.7	5.1	6	6.4	6.2
albumin	3.8	4.1	2.6	2.8	2.4	3.2	3.7	3.7	3.5
globulin	2.4	2.2	3.0	3.0	2.3	1.9	2.3	2.7	2.7
uric acid	4.1	4.4	4.4	4.3	5.1	3.2	3.2	2.0	4.1
Calcium	8.6	9.6	7.8	8.3	7.1	8.9	7.1	8.1	8.9
Phosphorus	3.9	4.8	3.0	4.1	2.6	2.7	3	3.7	4.1
Iron	74	91	28	45	17	107	----	----	84
Sodium	142	141	136	137	136	144	145	146	144
Potassium	5.1	5.4	4.2	5.0	3.1	4.4	5.3	4.6	5.5
Chloride	107	106	101	100	98	107	117	118	112
triglycerides	134	188	81	114	93	46	111	138	141
cholesterol	149	203	130	140	125	93	139	138	143

18   Martha Berland   Breast Cancer

Martha Berland was still a stunning beauty in her new crop of bristle short hair; some white, some black, some gray. Her husband brought her from Israel on this "last chance" venture. She was on morphine, already a sure sign that doctors had abandoned hope. And so had she. She believed she was dying. And whenever he raised hope or spoke optimistically, she fought back.

Yet her blood test results, as is plain to see, were quite good—her body was still functioning well and she had every chance to recover.

Her breast cancer started two and a half years earlier. She had been on chemotherapy for two and a half years! And survived it's toxicity. She had been on tamoxifen, steroids, and radiation—the works! Now the cancer had

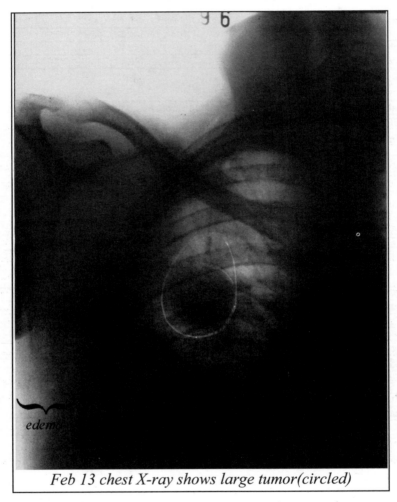

Feb 13 chest X-ray shows large tumor(circled)

spread all over her body in lumps under the skin like small mole hills every-where. She had just had a chest X-ray done (Feb. 13) before leaving home seven days ago; it showed a large tumor in the lung. And "water" had accu-mulated in the lung, the water level was clearly visible (all the dark area be-low the tumor). She had pain in the chest, arm, back and generalized weak-ness. She was wearing a "portacatheter" (indwelling catheter), parts of which can be seen on the X-ray, to make it easy to inject things. It is just a tube that leads to a vein. But, it must be cleaned regularly and doused with heparin to prevent blood clots from forming around it.

342

Only her husband spoke English. We began the task of explaining the program to him, who explained it to her. Most important was getting off morphine, substituting some other painkiller. We tried to explain that it was "morgue-medicine," intended only for the dying and would greatly inhibit her progress. It slowed bowel action, making laxatives necessary and for some unexplained reason, prevented weight gain. She resisted him.

Her initial toxins included fiberglass, arsenic, and chlorine, all of which would be inhaled and "feed" the tumor in the lung. She also had mercury, thallium, and aluminum from dentalware and cosmetics, no doubt. She had patulin and aflatoxin, as well as *Salmonella* and *Staphylococcus aureus*. She still had benzene, xylene, and isopropyl alcohol solvents. But not much malonic acid. Her dentalware was mostly gold—the very "best" gold—some amalgam and some plastic.

Our electronic metabolite test, done with the lung in the circuit showed maleic anhydride Positive at lung (cause of "water" accumulation); t-retinol (a vitamin A member) Positive at lung (good); t-retinoic acid (also a vitamin A member) Negative (meaning insufficient vitamin A); vitamin C Positive at lung (good); tumor necrosis factor (TNF) Negative at lung (bad); NADP and NADPH Negative (insufficient NAD enzymes) at lung; rhodizonic acid Negative (lack of oxidizer activity) at lung; benzoquinone Negative (lack of oxidizer activity) at lung; glutathione, reduced, Negative at lung (bad).

Metabolism in the lung was quite poor. She was given benzoquinone by IM (1 ug) a single shot, and rhodizonic acid, 15 mg four times a day, besides the usual starting program. Her blood test showed there was only a small rate of tumor activity—that is, production of lactic acid (LDH) and alkaline phosphatase, probably due to intensive "tumor killing" clinical treatments at home. Rather, she was dying from toxicities which we must determine and remove.

She was extremely fatigued, due no doubt to lack of oxygen and to ammonia toxicity. Lack of oxygen due to fluid in the lungs. Ammonia toxicity due to not being able to convert it to urea; the BUN was very low.

But, clearly, her chief toxin was copper [*and germanium*]; iron levels were down to 22. And at no time during her stay did we manage to discover the source and remove it. The toxic effects of cobalt and vanadium were noticeable in the elevated globulin and RBC.

All these metals could be part of the gold composition as well as in the amalgam and plastic. She did not want to part with the gold in her mouth. Yet the gold would contain nickel, too, commonly used to harden the gold. Nickel is especially toxic to the lung and is often seen there. We started her on IV therapy, with 3 vials of EDTA, 100 gm vitamin C, magnesium and DMSO.

In two days her energy was up; she was feeling very much better. Yet, in spite of giving her 250 mg glutathione four times a day, we could not detect any reduced glutathione in her lungs. Electronic tests only showed the oxidized useless variety. Selenium, (elemental, toxic!) was in oxidized form, too. But maleic anhydride was already Negative.

With maleic anhydride absent, no more fluid would be accumulating in the lung. Would this be enough to improve lung capacity? Would the lung reabsorb the fluid already escaped? She had already been surgically drained four times before coming here.

In five days her mood had improved so much she agreed to do dental work—but amalgam replacement only. The good and bad effects of this would soon appear. But she was eating well and had appetite. She decided to go off morphine. The pain in her shoulder and in the breast and skin everywhere intensified. She tried coffee enemas for pain relief, but didn't get much.

Two weeks later, on March 4, she was feeling a lot better, but still very fatigued and pain ridden. New tests showed vanadium Positive at lung; mercury Positive at lung; thallium Positive at lung. This showed there was leftover amalgam in her mouth. The source of the vanadium was not guessed. Copper was Negative at lung and liver. Evidently, our chelation-type IVs were keeping up with the steady stream of copper coming from her dentalware. TNF Positive at lung; NADPH, NADH Positive at lung; NADP, NAD Negative at lung. This means there is no oxidized NAD to enable respiration to continue. Notice how parts of metabolism can be over-oxidized while other parts are under-oxidized. The links are missing. Glutathione, reduced and oxidized Positive at lung; cytochrome C Negative at lung (one of the links in the respiration chain). Aflatoxin Negative.

Both glutathiones were now present (finally!). But cytochrome C, necessary to "catch" electrons in the respiratory chain is not high enough to appear positive. This would be an iron problem or a mutation. Iron was much too low.

This much progress invited a new chest X-ray, scheduled for March 5. She arrived, X-ray in hand. The tumor was missing! Simply gone. Could there be a mistake? No. The radiologist's report stated it clearly. He was quite certain. But the water-logged condition (pleural effusion) had not shown much reabsorbtion—she still had difficulty breathing. Yet, there was too much joy in her husband's heart to allow any pessimism. She caught some of his enthusiasm.

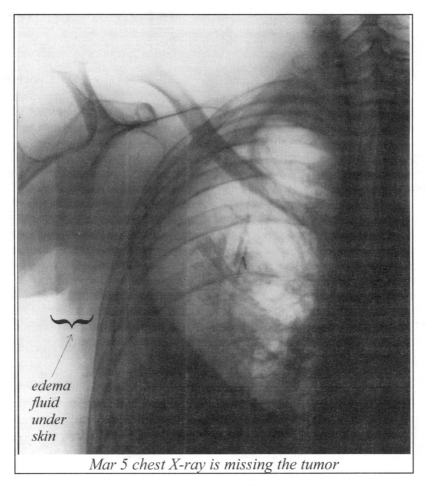

edema
fluid
under
skin

Mar 5 chest X-ray is missing the tumor

The blood test of March 5 shows the effects of amalgam removal (gold was not removed) which probably removed quite a bit of copper and cobalt, too. The RBC is down to normal. But, although there was less copper, there was still <u>some</u> copper [*or germanium*], since iron stayed very low.

On March 9, she had a sudden pain crisis. She wanted her morphine back. She felt entitled to it, since her country gives it liberally. All our pain substitutes were not satisfactory. Her husband tried to cope. After all, she was doing so much better. He must have prevailed.

By March 13, she could go upstairs without help. She only used her oxygen tank for 1 hour a day and that was at my insistence. We searched the complete set of 80 toxic elements trying to find anything besides gold, nickel, and copper to explain why her liver enzymes had been steadily getting worse and LDH had risen, not suspecting dyes or lanthanides.

345

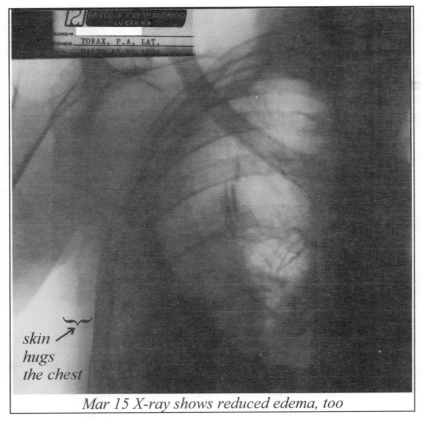

skin
hugs
the chest

Mar 15 X-ray shows reduced edema, too

The Syncrometer found only cerium, europium, niobium, and thulium Positive. The first three were obviously dental alloy or dental plastic. Were they in the gold? Were they in the remaining bits of amalgam, now covered with plastic? Or in the plastic? The thulium came from her brand of vitamin C, which she stopped immediately. The blood test did not show improvement on March 13.

She could not yield the gold in her mouth, nor the plastic. Again, she wanted to go home desperately! She also wanted morphine. None of the doctors agreed to supply morphine. We scheduled the final blood test and chest X-ray.

The tumor was still gone! The water level had receded significantly. The overall reduced edema could be seen along the margin of skin along the X-ray's left side. There is much less distance between rib cage and outer skin than before. Much fluid had been reabsorbed. She was still weak, but coughed less.

Her last blood test, March 18, showed a dramatic drop in LDH, in fact tumor growth had stopped completely. It was not the right time to stop or interrupt the progress she was making. We prevailed upon her to extend her stay by one week at least. But to no avail.

We couldn't guess that she was back on morphine (procured from another hospital) and dreaded nothing more than running out of it. At home it would be plentiful. Her bowels couldn't move because of it, but she could take a laxative. Her appetite was gone because of it, but she could be fed by IV. She didn't aspire to a natural life, a secure life.

She was feeling very well the day before they left. But she was sailing on a magic carpet of morphine, IVs, and supplements. It couldn't last.

On May 9, they called from home by telephone. She was swelling, full of pain, getting worse every day, and bedridden. Clearly going down hill.

Summary: It was not her fault for being addicted. (The medical profession has had 100 years to develop pain killers that are not addictive). It was not his fault for yielding. He thought she had turned the corner and would survive. She didn't care. We respect them both. The tragedy is in the disease and the current professional response to it. We must make every effort to improve this.

Martha Berland	2/21	2/26	3/5	3/9	3/13	3/18
RBC	4.96	5.09	4.33	4.81	4.37	4.09
WBC	7,1	7,2	5,6	3,7	6,1	8,7
PLT	287	299	274	244	254	323
glucose	141	107	111	134	118	120
BUN	7	9	11	9	9	12
creatinine	0.7	0.7	0.7	0.8	0.8	0.8
AST (SGOT)	24	38	45	58	51	37
ALT (SGPT)	16	23	27	32	46	24
LDH	189	177	184	251	247	154
GGT	42	58	47	49	86	67
T.b.	6.8	7.0	6.0	6.6	6.7	7.0
alk phos	76	104	85	65	106	98
T.p.	0.5	0.5	0.5	0.8	0.6	0.7
albumin	3.7	3.9	3.1	3.9	3.5	3.5
globulin	2.9	3.1	2.9	2.7	3.2	3.5
uric acid	2.9	2.8	2.2	2.9	3.6	3.1
Calcium	9.2	9.3	8.2	8.4	8.8	8.8
Phosphorus	2.8	3.1	2.9	2.8	2.7	2.6
Iron	22	30	31	20	28	18
Sodium	135	136	137	129	136	135
Potassium	3.9	3.8	4.2	3.4	4.2	4.0
Chloride	104	99	101	111	100	98
triglycerides	86	95	8 verified	105	93	66
cholesterol	200	218	124	164	182	148

19	Holly Bessant	Cancer of the Spine

Holly Bessant, fifty-five, was a tiny woman whose cancer (multiple myeloma) of the spine began in 1994. As small as her frame was, she could create a general panic for the entire staff. Just the sight of her colorful hat coming along the pathway stopped everybody's conversation. We knew she was coming for a crisis. And when that was past, it would be "living as usual" for her, till her next crisis.

Multiple myeloma is a cancerous condition of the bone marrow. This is where our RBC, WBC, and platelets are made. As the dyes, parasites, metal, and bacteria destroy the bone marrow, it is less and less able to keep up with the demand for blood cells. Holly had malonic acid at the bone marrow. [*At this time we did not know about the risk of getting malonic acid "placed" into your mouth in the form of non-metal restorations of decayed teeth.*]

Holly was on quinidine for her arrhythmia and an antibiotic, preventively, from her heart specialist in the US; in fact her heart was about twice normal size. She had severe lower back pain, too. But she displayed an impish smile as if aware she was panicking us.

From her first blood test we could see that her problem in the bone marrow was mainly due to vanadium (albumin low, globulin high) and malonic acid derivatives (low calcium), not so much copper and cobalt. Notice that the RBC is not elevated, though. The elevation phase is an early one. As the disease progresses, the bone marrow becomes totally incapable and all cell types drop, as we see here.

In fact, her water samples tested Negative to copper; yet she was Positive at her liver and parathyroids. Where was it coming from? We guessed her amalgam alloy. And she began the removal process.

When she arrived she was all done in. She was being seen at several other alternative clinics as well as her oncologist at home in California. She tried to do them all justice, no doubt. And perhaps it was even best, in the long run, somewhat like a rotation diet, thereby avoiding too much toxicity from any one food; in her case, health programs.

We took one look at her calcium level (7.9) and started her on an IV of 3 gm calcium, magnesium, B complex, and DMSO to be given twice daily. We also gave her coenzyme Q10, 3 gm to be taken every third day for 6 doses and ½ gm daily in between to assist her heart. Also, Lugol's for her *Salmonella* and the Bowel Program for *Shigella*.

Testing at her bone marrow showed TNF Negative; glutathione, reduced Negative; glutathione, oxidized (useless) Positive (high levels); glutathione reductase (enzyme that makes reduced glutathione) Negative; patulin Positive. We supplemented her with glutathione.

We found vanadium and freon in her kitchen dust (refrigerator). *Shigella* came from eating unsterilized cheese. She was to be off fruits entirely until her patulin was gone. The IVs must have given her an immediate lift. She disappeared without a word. We also guessed the IV therapy was too expensive for her, but we did anxiously await some kind of communication. She had been, after all, rather close to needing a transfusion, (RBC 3.23) which we give when the RBC can't even be kept up to 3.0.

Six weeks later she reappeared. This time, April 24, we put her right in our emergency room. She was very ill, wracked with pain and gasping for breath. We ordered a chest X-ray, did a blood test, put her on oxygen, and started IVs going. They contained 3 gm calcium, procaine, magnesium, cesium, vitamin B-complex, DMSO, and vitamin C. The calcium was based on her last blood test, much too low. Procaine was for pain relief, magnesium to help the heart, B-complex to help metabolism, DMSO to help the B vitamins penetrate the cells. While taking her IVs she was given Q10, 3 grams, glutathione, and a 2 tsp. dose of black walnut tincture extra strength. We thought this could be her last leg on life's journey.

Copper was now present in her liver and parathyroids, but we could not use EDTA to get it out quickly—it would interfere with the calcium being given. There was malonate at the bone marrow. We had just found that malonic acid could come from foods; we quickly warned her about orange juice, her favorite beverage.

Surprisingly, she walked in quite ably the next day, her X-ray in hand, declining any IV, probably for financial reasons. The X-ray showed a distinct tumor in the lung, side view. There was very little air capacity due to the enlarged heart and "water" effusate taking up lung space. Yet, she was rallying. Especially at the bone marrow on April 24; the WBC (3,800) and platelet count (185) were up significantly.

Best of all, her LDH was down, way down (205), meaning there was less tumor activity in the bone marrow and now, the lung. In fact, the lung must be healing already, since alk phos had not come up at all.

But the iron level was shocking. Was this why her RBC failed to come up? Lack of iron? But she had quite enough earlier. Perhaps her bone marrow was using the iron to make more cells, but the quinidine drug was simply killing them. We quickly gave her an iron <u>shot</u> to be repeated weekly and a liquid supplement, "iron booster," 1 tbs. daily (chlorophyll).

The plan was to repeat the test in four days, since she did not want a transfusion, and yet was poised right at the transfusion level. Perhaps if we switched her from quinidine to a different heart medication, it would save the RBCs and let them come up. She had not seen her specialist.

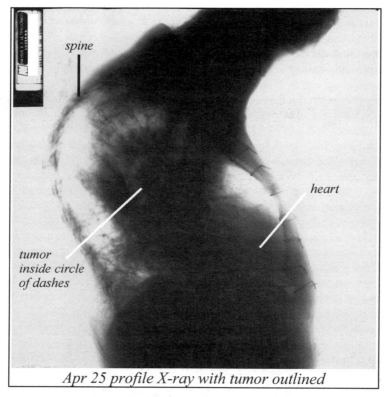

spine

heart

tumor
inside circle
of dashes

Apr 25 profile X-ray with tumor outlined

Five days later, her breathing was much better, she was not fatigued or wracked with pain. In fact, she was walking daily on the beach. She was an enigma to us. We repeated the blood test; it was April 29.

There was no significant change anywhere to be seen. She stayed an extra day to make progress with her dental work. We persuaded Holly to take another IV, containing calcium, magnesium, procaine (for persistent pain between shoulder blades near her lung tumor), B complex, cesium, and vitamin C.

She was also started on niacin 100 mg, three times a day and vitamin E, 400 units one a day (to reduce fragility of RBCs). She was on the kidney herb recipe and Q10, all intended to help the heart.

In a few days, she was breathing better still; she was no longer on pain killers, although she hadn't really started on the niacin or vitamin E. Her lower back pain was gone.

And she vanished.

A week later, she appeared, breathing almost normally. Her pain was much less. Had the tumor finished its antics finally? She had enough energy to take the Syncrometer class. She was here to continue dental work; she declined any treatment. We scheduled a chest X-ray.

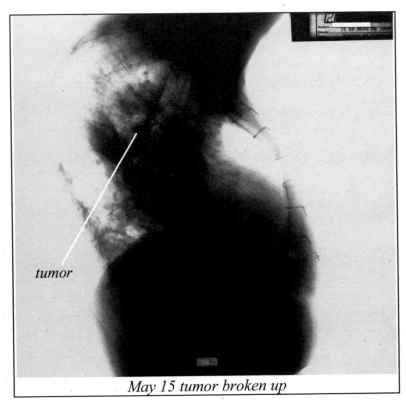

May 15 tumor broken up

Although expecting a small degree of improvement, we were very surprised to see the shrunk tumor (reduced to three small shreds). There was much less edema of the lung. Air capacity was much better; this can only be seen on a front view, not shown.

The former location of the tumor was circled by the radiologist, but there was no clump of dense tissue there now. Only some fluffy fragments. This was probably what had given her so much pain between the shoulder blades and right through the chest. Now it was over. She wanted to leave for home immediately. But I wanted to see her last blood test before okaying her departure.

To our great surprise, a new abnormality was present—a very significant one. Her total protein was suddenly very elevated (11.9), characteristic of her multiple myeloma.

351

What was the cause? Could it be an error? Not likely, since albumin and globulin are measured independently and then added. [*With hindsight, it was probably due to placing vanadium and/or dye polluted dental plastic in her mouth. The very things she had so carefully removed from her environment when she first came. And, of course, the drained tumor.*]

Such a blood test result can be expected to take a lethal course. We persuaded her to stay over the weekend and repeat the test on Monday. The results were even worse (T.p. 12.4). She was coughing a lot—a tell tale sign of heart failure. She was switched to digoxin and off quinidine. She was also given hawthorn berry, taurine, cysteine, and vitamin C by mouth. She refused IVs. We started her on spironolactone, though, for extra diuretic action.

By May 27, the globulin level had dropped. Was it due to our supplements, or switching off quinidine, or neither? Strangely, the phosphorus level was now much too high; this must surely be a lab error. The LDH had climbed, too. Did this represent new tumor activity or new heart stress? Perhaps the quinidine was actually a better choice for her; the RBC was beginning to recover, though, as if responding to the removal of quinidine. Still she refused to go back to her heart specialist.

There was one clue; a rather strong clue. One tooth had been giving her a lot of trouble. It could be spewing forth staphylococcus bacteria; bacteria that would go right to her heart. We switched her antibiotic to a broader-range one and added carnitine and Echinacea to her supplement list. Then sent her back to the dentist for <u>extraction</u>, not repair.

In a week, June 4, there was <u>no vestige</u> of illness left! She sat in the office chair like a well person. The blood test bears this out. In fact, she wanted to go off all medication and "just try it out." No, no, we cried in horror. She left for home, promising to be back in three weeks.

We will never know what happened in these three weeks. But she kept her promise and was back July 1. She related that she had gone into heart failure, while at home, but had gotten out of it spontaneously, while in the hospital. Surely, she had used up her extra leases on life! But she seemed in good health. We found methyl malonate in her lungs, but the *Staphylococcus* was gone (the extracted tooth). She declined IV treatment and left for home. Before she left, she did one more chest X-ray (not shown). The tumor was completely dissolved now; the heart was unchanged.

Summary: The cancer story was a success, although the remainder will never be known. We shall remember seeing her colorful hat approaching and her impish smile.

Holly Bessant	2/29	4/24	4/29	5/6	5/14	5/16	5/27	6/4	7/1
RBC	3.23	3.00	2.94	2.94	3.11	2.96	3.18	3.37	3.01
WBC	2800	3800	4100	3100	3200	3400	5300	3700	4900
PLT	105	185	184	193	209	186	202	243	119

BUN	10	12	12	10	9	9	19	12	15
creatinine	0.7	1.0	0.9	1.1	0.9	0.9	1.0	1.0	0.6
AST (SGOT)	36	27	26	24	34	29	39	36	33
ALT (SGPT)	27	22	22	14	22	7	24	35	43
LDH	346	205	219	211	237	255	395	217	220
GGT		18	26	22	24	24	25	22	13
T.b.	1.0	0.6	0.6	0.6	0.3	0.3	0.9	0.5	0.6
alk phos	58	52	57	57	59	65	60	70	63
T.p.	7.1	7.0	7.1	7.1	11.9	12.4	6.7	6.9	6.6
albumin	3.6	3.7	3.9	3.3	2.9	3.0	3.8	3.3	3.1
globulin	3.5	3.3	3.2	3.8	9.0	9.4	2.9	3.6	3.5
uric acid	3.8	2.7	3.1	3.7	3.7	3.3	0.9	2.6	2.9
Calcium	7.9	8.8	8.2	7.4	8.0	8.5	8.4	8.6	8.1
Phosphorus	3.4	4.0	4.6	3.4	4.2	5.2	16.5	5.0	4.7
Iron	84	14	61	74	69	59	59	100	135
Potassium	4.4	4.6	4.5	4.2	3.7	4.1	6.5	3.5	4.6
triglycerides	94	57	60	66	96	83	112	116	103
cholesterol	198	232	204	187	190	199	239	271	265

20   Felipe Gustafson   Brain Cancer

Felipe Gustafson, age seven, was droopy and glum. He didn't play; he preferred to sit. A letter from his doctor revealed that Felipe was diagnosed with astrocytoma of the brain stem at 1½ months of age. He came from Iceland.

Surgery at that time removed it; it was graded I to II. It had re-grown and required another craniotomy at age three. Now it had re-grown again. They brought two MRIs, the latest one was dated January 30, about a month ago.

The scan of Felipe's brain showed a 5 cm tumor at the brain stem. (The scale at the right of picture represents 5 cm. By holding this scale over the tumor its size can be seen.) The tumor has been circled by the radiologist.

When he arrived, he tested Positive for xylene, as well as isopropyl alcohol. Xylene is a common pollutant solvent that is attracted to the brain. Xylene is always found in brain tumor cases. We did not learn how he was getting xylene. We cautioned that Felipe be off all store bought beverage powders and ready made beverages regardless of whether they came from health food stores, and this included all purchased water. Of course, his home water came through copper pipes and was promoting tumor growth, too. His family at home was instructed to change water pipes to plastic during his stay with us. No shortcuts were to be taken. No distillers or filter was to be installed. Water was not to be transported for drinking purposes. The water used to wash hands, shower and do laundry must not be coppered either. PVC endures temperature extremes very well.

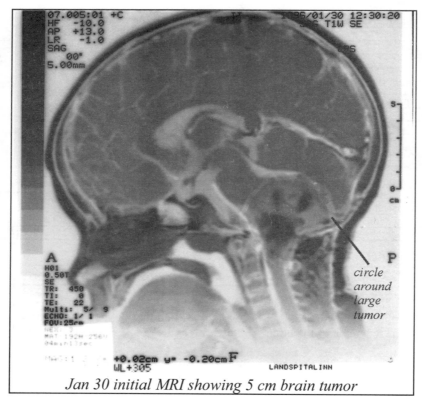

Jan 30 initial MRI showing 5 cm brain tumor

circle
around
large
tumor

He tested positive for copper and vanadium at high levels. Evidently, there was chronic gas leakage from their utilities, spewing out vanadium; they were advised to switch to electric utilities in spite of the cost. He would not soon outgrow this "sensitivity."

He also had patulin and aflatoxin in the cerebrum (brain) as well as salmonella bacteria. This implies a growth of fungus as well as bacteria at the tumor site.

Malonic acid, too, was built up at the cerebrum, implying a tapeworm stage. [*We did not know about the food source at that time.*]

On his first day he was instructed to: (1) go off all items listed on the isopropyl alcohol list in *The Cure For All Cancers*. (2) Take a 2 tsp. dose of black walnut tincture extra strength and 3 capsules of the other herbs, then (3) zap daily. Repeat herbal program once a week. He was to be re-tested for ortho-phospho-tyrosine later that day to verify its absence. (4) Take Lugol's three times a day, 6 drops in water. (5) Go off all fruit for 2 weeks to eliminate patulin fungus growth in brain. (6) Eat only white bakery bread to eliminate aflatoxin; no peanut butter. (7) Take coenzyme Q10, 2 gm to kill tapeworm stages in brain.

Testing showed that glutathione was Negative at his cerebrum. The oxidized form was Positive. So there was no shortage of this major factor. There was simply a shift to the oxidized, useless form. Indeed, the enzyme glutathione reductase, whose job it is to change the oxidized form of the glutathione back to the reduced form, was absent. Absent because it was being inhibited, or not being formed? FAD, representing the flavin enzymes, also essential for metabolism, was missing, too. So vitamin B_2 (riboflavin) was supplemented, 100 mg daily.

At the end of his first office visit, I decided to give Felipe a chance to improve without using IV therapy—but only ten days; if he was not visibly improved, we would begin. His mother agreed. We did no blood tests, either, to spare his over-punctured, over-prodded body this extra trauma. Electronic testing seemed enjoyable to him.

The very next day, aflatoxin and patulin were already Negative at the cerebrum. The big dose of black walnut tincture extra strength kills any fungus that is growing in the intestine, destroying the source from which the brain could be re-seeded. Hopefully, he would not eat it again. But malonic acid was still Positive; tapeworm stages had survived, seemingly.

Another dose of Q10, 2 gm, was given. Also glutathione, 125 mg, three times a day and vitamin C to make up for malonate damage in the brain.

On the second day, March 6, malonate, as well as aflatoxin and patulin were Negative at the cerebrum. *Salmonella* and *Shigella* were now absent, too. Nevertheless, the 2 gm Q10 dose was to be continued daily for 6 more doses.

Tumor necrosis factor, TNF, was now Positive, meaning his body had regained some of its ability to destroy tumors.

Copper was absent; they were housed in a copper-free motel.

Felipe was started on methylene blue, 65 mg, one a day, to assist brain metabolism by shuttling electrons and hydrogen atoms to and from the NADs.

By March 7, Felipe was a changed boy. He smiled. The staff and other patients all smiled back at him. He was sleeping better, eating better and, without help or coaxing, playing. It is a marvelous sight to see a sick child begin to play.

Solvents, malonic acid, copper, and patulin were all Negative at the brain. TNF continued Positive.

On March 8, he continued sleeping and eating well; he was playing, smiling, and running; not sitting much.

On March 11, re-testing showed he was Negative to all previous toxins.

On March 12, he was acting like a normal child, very energetic with loud screams and laughter amidst running and jumping off the garden wall (against the rules). Both oxidized and reduced forms of NAD and glutathione were present at the cerebrum. Malonate and copper were Negative, TNF Positive. His daily series of Q10 could end.

We reduced Lugol's to once a day and glutathione to twice a day. We reconsidered the need for IV therapy with his mother and agreed to keep off it.

On March 13 and 14, all electronic tests came back as they should.

On March 15, behavior assessment with his mother revealed he was holding his head straighter most of the time. His behavior had no hint of abnormality. All test results were appropriate. They went to visit friends (or was it the San Diego Zoo?) for two days.

On March 18, isopropyl alcohol was Negative. This is the toxin most people acquire on a visit away from the Diagnostic Center. His family had taken good care of him. Malonate was Negative, too. We reduced his glutathione to one a day.

On March 20, patulin was Positive at the thyroid, though not at the cerebrum. And copper was present at the brain. This was probably acquired on the recent visit to a copper-plumbed home. We would watch it, before resorting to a chelating IV.

On March 21, patulin was still there but copper was now in the cerebellum, not the cerebrum. Other toxins were absent.

On March 22, copper was still present at the cerebellum. He was still very susceptible to it, attracting it to the brain instead of excreting it. Would the plumbing job be complete before going home? He was allowed to have watermelon and banana as his first fruit now.

During the next week, there was no recurrence of malonic acid or copper. Was he now able to metabolize malonate and excrete copper?

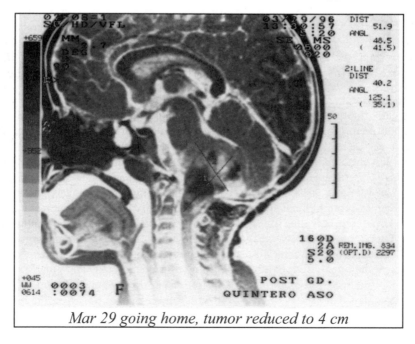

Mar 29 going home, tumor reduced to 4 cm

356

They were given parting instructions for home and scheduled for a final scan. He would take a series of Q10, 2 gm doses for 7 days in a row every 6 weeks. On other days he would stay on glutathione, 250 mg, one a day for one half year. He could go off methylene blue, but stay on vitamin B2, 100 mg a day.

The new scan shows a significant reduction in tumor size from 5 cm to less than 4. (See scale at right for 50 mm.) Good work, Felipe! Good work Felipe's Mom! Now the responsibility passes to his family at home. Did they prepare a safe environment at home?

A telephone call, months later, related that Felipe was entirely well, had not regressed in any way. It sounds hopeful.

Summary: we can't help wondering what made this case so easy. Was it the absence of any metal or unsafe plastic in his teeth? Was it the perfect compliance? Was it luck, so he escaped polluted supplements? Was it absence of IV therapy? Or something else? Till we learn these secrets…good luck, Felipe.

[*Since then his family received the malonate-free food list. They were eager to follow it. We hope to get a follow up scan eventually.*

A telephone call two years later related he was a happily growing child.]

21	Donna Balders	Breast & Lymphatic Cancer

Donna Balders, fifty-eight, came with her right arm wrapped in elastic bandage from the hand to the shoulder. This left the fingers bulging and stiff. Fifteen years earlier she had cancer in her left breast, which was surgically removed. But eleven years after that, the right breast developed a small tumor which she did not have removed until two years later when it was 4 cm across. But recently another tumor had grown, plus an enlarged lymph node in her armpit the size of an egg. It was easy to see, bulging out. This was probably the cause of pressure on her lymphatic vessels, so they couldn't drain the arm fluids well enough—thereby causing the swollen arm. The swelling had recently reached her hand. She also had a prominent goiter, a swelling of the thyroid gland. She was always cheerful, pointing out the smallest improvements.

Her initial toxin test showed: wood alcohol, benzene, copper, cadmium, aluminum, asbestos, mercury, thallium, aflatoxin, malonic acid, *Shigella sonnei, Salmonella enteriditis*, all Positive. CFC's and patulin were Negative at breast, Positive at parathyroid. And isopropyl alcohol was Positive, in spite of going on the cancer program over a year ago. (Cosmetics or a favorite vitamin supplement is many a patient's downfall [*and now we have seen that clostridium bacteria themselves make it*].)

357

Her arm was getting to a critical size and the fluid could get infected; we doubled our efforts to get quick results. The breast felt hard all around it, as if there were a submerged shelf.

The first day she was started on coenzyme Q10, 4 grams per day for 7 days in a row. (This dose gave very good results with everyone; only the expense caused us to reduce its use later on.) She was to be off all dairy foods to prevent picking up harmful bacteria, off grocery store bread and nuts and off most fruit to avoid getting mycotoxins. She was to go off the benzene and isopropyl alcohol lists immediately, do the parasite program regularly and zap daily. She was to start on Lugol's iodine to kill *Salmonella* and the kidney herb recipe to drain water from her body (diuresis).

She had already changed her amalgams to composite; how could she still have mercury and thallium? It could be left in tiny amounts, tattoos; or remnants could be covered over with composite. She still had some gold in her mouth; she did not want to replace it quite yet. She was started on glutathione, and given a drug diuretic, spironolactone, one a day.

An ultrasound of the breast was done to show us the starting situation; there were 3 tumors. Even her IV therapy was started the first day. It included calcium, magnesium, vitamin B-complex, laetrile, DMSO, and vitamin C. Before these supplements, though, 3 doses of EDTA were given to pull the copper and other heavy metals out of her. Her IVs cost her $330.00 per day.

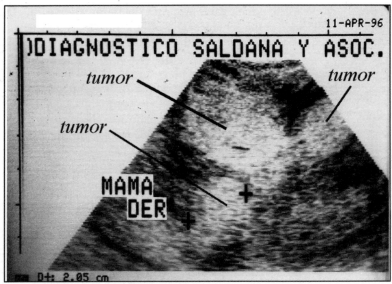

3 roundish tumors (white areas) in right breast (mama der.) and armpit (at right edge of picture).

Apr 11 initial ultrasound of breast

Her blood test results showed only the beginning of toxicity from copper, cobalt, vanadium, and malonic acid and only a small WBC elevation in response to bacterial infection. LDH (226) revealed tumor growth [*due to Sudan Black B*]. Albumin too high and globulin too low revealed cobalt in the liver.

In two days Donna could bend her swollen hand, so we knew the edema had lessened.

Glutathione and TNF were now Positive at the breast, as well as B_{12}. Cesium was added to her IV.

Six days after arrival she could see the veins in her hands and there was no pitting edema. Both the armpit tumor and breast felt much softer.

She was using a magnetic mattress pad to reduce pain.

Meanwhile, she had seen how effective our biology-based methods were and decided to finish her dental work. She got her gold replaced by plastic in her mouth. Her next blood test , April 19, showed her RBC was too high. She now tested Positive for vanadium. We suspected a gas leak at the time; she was to bring a dust sample from home. [*We had begun to wonder if vanadium was coming from her new dentalware. We didn't suspect malonic acid derivatives, yet.*]

Her uric acid had suddenly dropped showing that glutamine levels were much too low [*and clostridium bacteria were revealed*]. She was given a glutamine supplement. But she had gotten rid of copper water pipes, so her iron level rose to 105.

By April 20, the entire breast was soft as it should be. Only a narrow lump at the armpit could still be felt. But she was all broken out in a rash suggesting a benzene exposure. We also searched for bacteria (which can cause rashes) and found plenty, at the lymph nodes. Testing showed *Salmonella, Shigella, Staphylococcus aureus* Positive at lymph nodes, glutathione Negative at lymph nodes, benzene Positive everywhere.

Had she eaten some benzene polluted food? Or simply bacteria-contaminated food? [*Benzene and zearalenone are released from a draining tumor.*] A dose of Q10 (6 gm) came to the rescue.

By April 24, she still had *Salmonella* infection, and she still had no glutathione at the lymph nodes. A new blood test showed her total bilirubin had suddenly risen to 1.1, a serious danger sign. She was immediately requested to stop eating all breads and nuts, since she must be getting aflatoxin again. Aflatoxin was found in potato peels, even after cooking, so she was reminded to peel all potatoes.

The vanadium problem did not go away, in fact a copper problem also loomed (iron dropped to 50). D-malic acid was now found at the lymph nodes. [*This too, could originate in the teeth.*]

The potassium was suddenly too high (5.2) a sign of thyroid malfunction besides the goiter. She was given 1 grain of thyroid a day. All in all, by the blood test, she was in worse shape now than when she arrived. But the tumor

359

was shrinking, because the arm was less swollen and the breast was nearly normal.

On April 29 she began to give herself coffee enemas [*not recommended now, unless filtered for asbestos*], an idea taken from the Gerson program, another alternative cancer therapy available in Mexico.

On May 2 a new blood test showed a lot of improvement. The bilirubin was back to normal. LDH was down, implying less tumor activity. Albumin and globulin were normal. Uric acid was normal. Potassium was back to normal. And iron was back up, implying less copper interference. Her arm was much smaller, less swollen; her fingers could all be used. The breast was soft. Would an ultrasound show the improvement? It did.

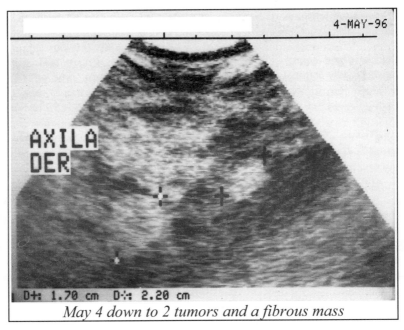

May 4 down to 2 tumors and a fibrous mass

The fibrous texture (white streaking) was still quite evident in the breast, but only two "lumps" were rated as tumors by the radiologist. The largest one had pulled apart and was now considered normal tissue.

She could use her arm and hand normally again. The immediate threat was gone.

Her next blood test, on May 14, showed more improvement. The LDH dropped to 160, normal by our standards, meaning no tumor activity.

Her third ultrasound reflected this. Both lumps were now gone. Only some diffuse fibrosity remained in place of each of the original tumors. The largest one, measured between the plus signs, did not qualify as a tumor to the radiologist. The breast itself was free of everything. She was feeling fine and eager to go home.

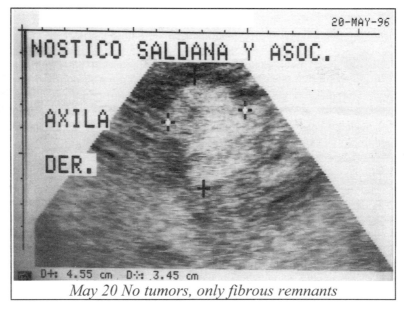

20-MAY-96

NOSTICO SALDANA Y ASOC.

AXILA

DER.

D+: 4.55 cm D·: 3.45 cm

May 20 No tumors, only fibrous remnants

But the May 27 blood test had suddenly worsened. Her LDH was up; RBC and WBC were up.

What was the problem? We didn't know.

By May 31 it had not improved much. Vanadium was Positive again. Albumin was up again, the thyroid was affected again (calcitonin was negative at the thyroid, calcium was too high and potassium too high) and copper had returned from some unknown source, so iron had dropped.

But there was no time left on her schedule. Her mission was accomplished. And more: her goiter was no longer visible no matter how she turned her head. She could swing her arm. She was going home.

Summary: We know now there was more to do. Toxins had inadvertently been placed in her mouth to suck on the same way she had gold and amalgam before. But for the present she savored success. Surely she will come back if she loses her new found health.

Donna Balders	4/10	4/19	4/24	5/2	5/14	5/27	5/31
RBC	4.61	5.06	4.96	4.93	4.91	5.25	4.89
WBC	8,200	6,400	6,300	5,400	5,200	7,200	6,300
PLT	256	231	248	246	233	237	242
glucose	86	115	94	90	93	77	110
BUN	15	15	14	13	12	14	13
creatinine	0.9	0.9	1.0	0.9	0.9	0.9	1.0
AST (SGOT)	23	25	25	27	25	32	35
ALT (SGPT)	35	33	30	37	25	32	35

LDH	226	219	206	178	160	218	199
GGT	14	17	16	16	16	15	17
T.b	0.6	0.7	1.1	0.5	0.5	0.3	0.8
alk phos	55	61	60	63	58	63	53
T.p.	7.1	7.0	7.0	6.9	7.1	7.3	7.3
albumin	5.1	4.9	4.9	4.5	4.4	4.6	4.9
globulin	2.0	2.1	2.1	2.4	2.7	2.7	2.4
uric acid	3.7	2.0	2.5	3.5	3.5	3.4	0.8
Calcium	9.2	9.3	9.8	9.0	9.3	9.6	10.3
Phosphorus	4.2	4.6	4.5	3.4	3.6	3.9	4.6
Iron	54	105	50	87	90	110	55
Sodium	139	133	142	139	138	137	140
Potassium	4.2	4.7	5.2	4.6	4.2	4.5	4.9
Chloride	97	107	99	100	102	104	104
triglycerides	152	123	219	189	207	120	175
cholesterol	259	186	208	182	174	190	173

22 David Forness   Prostate Cancer

David Forness, a middle-age man, was tall and just a bit on the portly side. He had diabetes along with his cancer, a rather unusual coincidence. His cancer was in the prostate, colon and liver, starting about a year ago. In

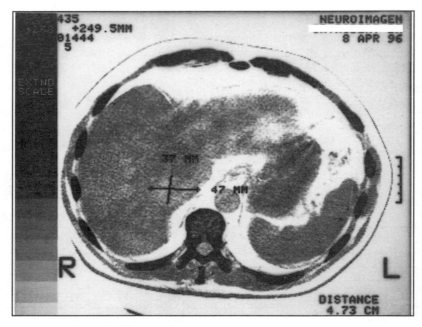

fact, he was just out of the hospital where 18 inches of colon had been removed. But he still didn't have a colostomy. He was just in time. We would focus on the liver, though, to monitor his body's recovery. The colon would recover along with it. His first CT scan showed two fairly large tumors, 3.7 x 4.7 cm and 2.8 x 3.5 cm visible in different frames.

In fact, a closer look at these frames shows the liver was packed with small to medium size masses (light gray spots). He also had tumors in the spleen, a most unusual location. He was not sick at all. He had no symptoms. This was in spite of testing Positive to four solvents, five bacteria, malonic

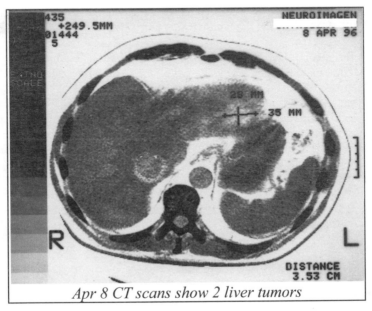

Apr 8 CT scans show 2 liver tumors

acid, aflatoxin, PCB, chlorine, asbestos, CFC, and six heavy metals! His first blood test was equally bad. It showed that toxicity had already affected several of his vital organs including:

- The bone marrow (very low RBC).
- The thyroid gland. Potassium too high from lack of absorption by the body tissues. Diabetes contributes to this.
- The parathyroids. Calcium very low.
- The liver (portion controlling albumin production). Albumin low.
- The spleen (where iron is released to travel to the bone marrow). Iron moderately low.
- The liver (where cholesterol is made). Cholesterol too low.
- Location where triglyceride levels are regulated (much too low).

Things could get worse quite quickly for him. But the LDH and alk phos were not very high, meaning the tumor growth was slow at this time.

An unusual feature was the high blood sugar due to his diabetes. Since this means that sugar has difficulty entering cells, perhaps it also has difficulty entering the tumor cells. Tumor cells need a lot of glucose to grow. The mineral chromium is in short supply in diabetics. Chromium helps sugar enter the cells. Should it be given to help the rest of the body reabsorb the tumors, or withheld to starve the tumor? I planned to do a little of both, watching carefully for abrupt changes.

He was started on the freon program, parasite program, Lugol's, Q10, and glutathione. His IVs began with EDTA, vitamin B-complex, glycyrrhizin, DMSO, laetrile, and vitamin C. The EDTA would pull heavy metals out.

On the second day, the EDTA was exchanged for calcium and magnesium. Methyl malonate could repeatedly be found at the liver and spleen. He was given B_{12}, folic acid and silymarin.

Although some things improved by April 17, some things were worse. The thyroid and parathyroids were better, allowing calcium and T.p. to rise and potassium to fall. Somehow he was getting more copper [*or germanium*] than before; his iron had dropped. His LDH had risen somewhat. In fact, gradually worsening liver function can be seen throughout his stay [*in spite of and possibly due to shrinking tumors!*]. One significant change is the drop

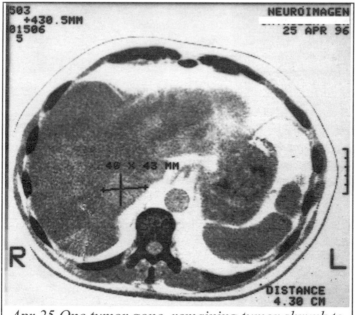

Apr 25 One tumor gone, remaining tumor shrunk to 4.0 x 4.3 cm, smaller masses more diffuse

in blood sugar; more sugar might now be entering tumor cells and causing a burst of activity. Glucose was 190, down from 316, but still needing to fall below 140.

Maybe trace minerals would be of help now. We gave chromium yeast, selenium yeast, molybdenum yeast, germanium yeast, manganese.

By April 24, he was testing negative at last for cobalt and vanadium. Improvements in the blood test can be seen everywhere, except in the liver enzymes and LDH.

The new liver scan already showed one tumor absent on all frames (no longer mentioned by the radiologist) and the larger one beginning to shrink. The liver texture was much better, but there was still a lot of improvement needed.

He was feeling so energized, he enrolled in the two day Syncrometer class and decided to do a liver cleanse. He got out hundreds of gall stones. But the liver function tests continued to worsen (May 6). He had been doing dental work. He completed exchange of dental metal for plastic by May 13.

We doubled his trace mineral intake and added zinc, 30 mg daily. We doubled his B_{12}, folic acid, and vitamin C intake. We added thyroid, taurine, and cysteine. It was no use. Vanadium, malonic acid, and copper continued to appear and they would not be "neutralized" by any of our supplements or IVs. There must be an ongoing source; but where?

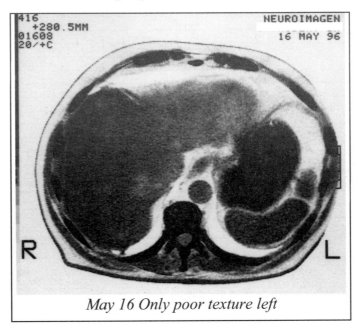

May 16 Only poor texture left

Another scan of the liver was done May 16 showing even further improvement. His last tumor was no longer recognized as such by the radiologist. Only poor texture was noted (light gray areas).

He had gained a lot; his life was not in danger from liver cancer. It was time for him to leave. But his future was not secure.

Summary: This case teaches us an important lesson. Tumors may dissolve and liver texture may improve, yet toxicity is hidden in certain organs. They fight bravely, using every adaptation, but until the source of the toxicity is found, and removed, the battle continues. [*We know now that a plastic tooth can be that source.*]

David Forness	4/2	4/17	4/24	5/6	5/11	5/18	5/25	5/30
RBC	3.48	5.05	4.7	4.75	4.67	4.96	4.83	4.72
WBC	9,4	7,7	8,7	7,6	8,7	8,9	7,0	7,0
PLT	370	261	283	280	250	308	215	212
glucose	316	190	151	273	277	141	235	251
BUN	22	17	21	27	23	23	33	24
creatinine	1.2	1.1	1.5	1.2	1.2	1.2	1.4	1.4
AST (SGOT)	18	27	32	35	38	51	51	45
ALT (SGPT)	29	27	41	47	45	63	71	73
LDH	213	230	257	262	215	292	255	239
GGT	46	46	40	46	47	51	60	64
T.b.	0.5	0.2	0.5	0.3	0.3	0.3	0.3	0.7
alk phos	96	80	76	85	79	78	93	84
T.p.	5.9	6.4	6.5	6.1	6.3	6.6	6.8	6.7
albumin	3.6	3.9	4.1	4.0	3.8	4.2	4.3	4.4
globulin	2.3	2.5	2.4	2.1	2.5	2.4	2.5	2.3
uric acid	4.1	4.1	2.5	4.1	3.7	3.9	4.8	2.3
Calcium	8.4	9.0	9.2	9.0	8.9	9.1	9.2	9.7
Phosphorus	3.0	3.9	4.0	3.2	2.9	2.7	2.8	4.1
Iron	59	29	----	50	52	53	82	45
Sodium	133	137	143	133	131	138	138	135
Potassium	5.1	4.7	4.7	4.6	4.5	4.6	5.1	4.6
Chloride	101	102	99	102	94	101	102	95
triglycerides	72	138	90	106	133	80	108	96
cholesterol	135	120	134	142	135	114	141	126

23 **Todd Wilcox**	**Testicular Cancer**

Todd Wilcox, age forty, had gone to the Gerson clinic immediately after "stopping by" our clinic in March. He had been diagnosed with testicular cancer at home in Canada. He had gotten his right testicle surgically removed first, but it then spread to the lymphatic system. Now it was called "embryonic carcinoma". At that point he headed for Mexico on the advice of a friend. In fact his abdomen was full of tumors with one very large one when he arrived there. After three months at the Gerson clinic he came back

366

to our clinic. An ultrasound now showed that the large tumor was gone, but he was still full of enlarged lymph nodes (not shown).

He had already been on the parasite program plus zapping for three weeks. His ortho-phospho-tyrosine and isopropyl alcohol were Negative. Still testing Positive in his lymph nodes were:

Solvents	Heavy metals	Bacteria	Others
benzene	nickel	*Salmonella enteriditis*	malonic acid
xylene	copper	*Salmonella paratyphi*	formaldehyde
	cadmium	*Shigella flexneri*	CFC's
	cobalt	*Staphylococcus aureus*	asbestos
	thallium		aflatoxin
	mercury		

The malonic acid, copper, freon, cobalt, solvents, and other toxins had used up the glutathione in his abdominal lymph nodes, glutathione tested Negative here. This lowered their immunity to bacteria, which now could colonize there, making growth factors. They also caused the lymph nodes to grow and enlarge. At one time fluke parasites had inhabited them, too, causing malignancy, but this had been stopped. The bacterial invasion could not be so easily stopped. The toxins had to be removed first.

He was encouraged to continue with his Gerson program and diet, except to go off carrot juice because we had just discovered it contained malonic acid. He already was on a potassium supplement, Lugol's iodine, and thyroid tablets! His pulse and body temperature were being monitored at the Gerson clinic as they rose to a point where sweating, nervousness, and insomnia were felt.

After his blood test, he was given our "Day 1" cancer program [*for that time*]. It included:

1. A large dose of coenzyme Q10.
2. The malonate free diet.
3. Lugol's to kill *Salmonella*. We had to wonder why he still carried *Salmonella* after all the iodine he took from the Gerson clinic. Either it wasn't enough or he constantly reinfected.
4. Instructions to get metal out of his dentalware and do the Dental Aftercare program.
5. Instructions to change his refrigerator at home to a new non-freon variety and start on the freon removal program.
6. Instructions to stop using a hair blower.
7. Instructions to change his copper plumbing at home (in Canada) to PVC plastic in spite of the weather there. Water from his local residence had copper, so he was instructed to move.
8. Going off detergent for every purpose.
9. Throwing out his foam mattress and detoxifying his formaldehyde with taurine plus cysteine both for 3 months.

10. Paying special attention to moldy foods to avoid aflatoxin. And taking glutathione (reduced) on an empty stomach in the morning.
11. Of course, he was to continue the maintenance parasite program plus zapping.

He was then given an IV of EDTA, vitamin B complex, and vitamin C, each item being tested for a set of eleven pollutant toxins (copper, cobalt, vanadium, benzene, isopropyl alcohol, wood alcohol, malonic acid, maleic acid, methyl malonate, maleic anhydride, D-malic acid). [*Now we also test for dyes and urethane.*] The IV bag of saline was tested for these also.

After a single IV, Todd was re-tested for copper at the lymph nodes, liver, and parathyroid. He was Negative now and could stop taking this kind of IV.

It was a day of swallowing, drinking, taking supplements, zapping, and IVing; but at the day's end, he felt better instead of being fatigued. He went back to his Gerson residence, but stuck to the malonate-free diet. He took copper-free drinking water with him until he could have his own tested.

Next day, he was free of benzene and xylene, having stopped drinking bottled water. His copper was still Negative, so we gave him our tumor shrinking IV to be done daily. It contained calcium, magnesium, laetrile, cesium chloride, vitamin B complex, vitamin C, and DMSO. Again, all items were tested for the 11 tumor toxins.

His first blood test showed a very low potassium in spite of his Gerson supplement of potassium. He was instructed to double his intake of it. His blood sugar was extremely low, as is common for cancer patients.

His blood urea nitrogen was much too low, also, in spite of taking 26 grams (5 tsp.) a day on his Gerson program.

The supplementary urea was evidently a drop in the bucket and not even noticeable after many weeks. This was understandable, since he had been dousing himself with carrot juice (malonic acid inhibits urea formation). He also took creatine, by mouth. His albumin was too high, no doubt due to cobalt in the liver. Serum iron was quite satisfactory, showing his copper intake had been slight. His LDH and alkaline phosphatase were gratifyingly low [*showing that Sudan Black B and DAB were not the problem*]. His good results so far were a tribute to the Gerson program and Todd's personal determination to comply. He continued his IVs for a week and then did a follow up blood test (May 15). Now his BUN was still lower. Only a strong inhibitor of urea formation could be responsible, such as a stalled urea synthesis cycle in the liver or large quantities of malonic acid. Checking back in his test records, malonate was found to be present each day he had come in for testing. [*But we did not suspect it might be in the very plastic we had recommended for amalgam replacement!*] His calcium had risen too high, along with phosphate: (calcium 10.3, phosphate 4.1) showing that bone was being dissolved. Something toxic was still in his thyroid! This would inhibit calcitonin formation, removing the protection his bones relied on. Testing showed: cobalt Positive at thyroid, vanadium Negative at thyroid, copper

Negative at thyroid, parathyroid hormone Negative at parathyroid, calcitonin Negative at thyroid.

This electronic test supported the toxicity conclusion. But where could the cobalt come from? It was wreaking havoc with his blood test results, which seemed worse than before, in spite of getting his dental work done! [*His neck got stiff and painful, which should have pointed us to his teeth. But "body language" was still too vague for us to interpret at that time.*]

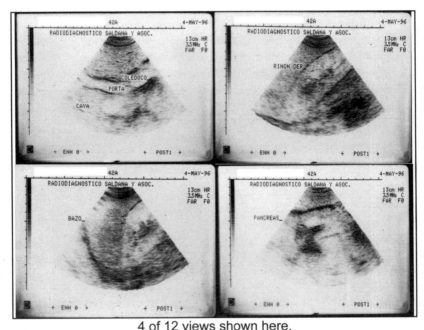

4 of 12 views shown here.
May 4 many views of the abdomen reveal no tumors

His new ultrasound arrived. The abdomen had been searched and viewed from the liver down. Not a tumor or enlarged lymph node could be seen! Was it lack of resolution (power) of the ultrasound? His previous ultrasound (not shown) pictured them quite well. We recommended a CT scan for greater certainty. But the truth was already before us. He had first dissolved his large tumor; then gradually all his remaining tumors.

Was it Gerson's program or our program that did it? Their program was certainly responsible for dissolving his large tumor; why couldn't it simply continue dissolving the rest? Perhaps our program merely helped. He was a happy man again, although a mysterious enemy, cobalt, had not yet been vanquished. And *Staphylococcus* was still present in his lymph nodes; the source of this would have to be dental, so we checked and to our surprise he still had a root canal to be pulled!

369

But joy overcame him. His five month vigil was over. When he came, he had quit his job and decided to stay as long as it might take; after all, his chances for survival at home were nil. We didn't want him to leave with an elevated calcium, though. We prevailed upon him to delay departure.

He delayed 3 days. We tested again.

His calcium had dropped somewhat, along with phosphorus. Evidently, his thyroid was doing better. But we searched the thyroid and parathyroid glands electronically. Cobalt Negative at thyroid, parathyroid; parathyroid hormone Positive at parathyroid; calcitonin Negative at thyroid; malonate Positive at thyroid.

[Although the thyroid had been freed of cobalt temporarily by IVs, it was sure to return since it really derived from his new plastic fillings. The thyroid would continue being poisoned by malonate too and therefore jeopardize production of calcitonin.] The LDH and alkaline phosphatase stayed reassuringly low.

Todd Wilcox	3/18	5/3	5/15	5/18
RBC	4.2	4.49	4.49	4.58
WBC	14,600	6,600	4.0	4.2
PLT	196	220	201	217
Sodium	142	139	146	147
Potassium	4.9	3.4	4.6	4.9
Chloride	105	105	107	109
glucose	88	69	91	91
BUN	7	8	6	6
creatinine	1.0	1.3	1.2	1.2
AST (SGOT)	17	27	20	20
ALT (SGPT)	20	22	17	15
LDH	138	151	112	116
GGT	19	19	18	17
T.b.	0.5	0.5	0.5	0.5
alk phos	52	59	50	47
T.p.	6.9	7.2	7.3	7.0
albumin	4.3	5.0	4.4	4.4
globulin	2.6	2.2	2.9	2.6
uric acid	4.5	4.5	4.0	4.2
Calcium	9.0	9.0	10.3	10.0 (8.5-10.3)
Phosphorus	3.9	2.8	4.1	3.8
Iron	71	70	73	70
triglycerides	181	104	152	129
cholesterol	138	174	143	138

BUN was still too low. His hCG marker (not listed) was under 2. Gerson clinic had been using hCG and AFP as tumor markers for him. Without finding and eliminating his last sources of cobalt and malonate, he nevertheless desired to go home.

As a parting reminder, we gave him several extra supplements to take: vitamin B_{12}, folic acid, vitamin C, taurine. His coenzyme Q10 was reduced to 3 gm once a week. Glutathione was reduced to two a day. And glucuronic acid was added. He still had not pulled his root canal. But he felt he deserved a vacation. Perhaps it will be a lasting one. Perhaps not. Toxins and bacteria are as relentless as any other predator. I believe his intelligence will serve him well again if new tumors pop up.

Summary: Todd was the perfect patient—he blended two alternative treatments, even though this is distasteful to both providers. He caused no friction by taking full responsibility for his choices. He listened to the reasons given for the various treatments without pitting them against each other. He fused them and found success. I have since been asked where the initial scans are. He took them home. Yet having in my possession his final scans that show <u>nothing</u>, is success, no matter <u>what</u> was on the initial ones.

24	Sonja Eckenroth	Lymphatic/Lung Cancer

Sonja Eckenroth, a tall stately woman of about fifty, arrived (with her daughter's help) extremely emaciated, but not in a wheelchair. She originally had lung cancer, diagnosed in 1990. She had the usual treatments, but had a recurrence in 1993. It spread through the lung again, this time to lymph nodes.

In the last two months she had severe shortness of breath, weight loss, insomnia, and pain down her left arm. This arm and fingers would frequently go numb. A lump on her neck was called a thyroid "cyst". Sonja's daughter was determined to get her mother well, hovering over her with the supplements, checking supplies, and asking questions. This was fortunate because Sonja had a do-as-I-please approach and often this meant late afternoon arrival when there was no time left for an IV. We engaged the nurse for overtime work for her.

She had received one series of chemotherapy, but was given only six months to live even if she completed the other two, so she "jumped ship" and headed for Mexico. She had already been on the Kelly program which uses large doses and varieties of digestive enzymes to digest tumors. A glance at her first blood test shows she was still in fair condition.

Her electrolytes were normal. Kidney function was good, although creatinine was much too low, probably due to a shortage of glycine, arginine, and methionine. Two liver enzymes were very good, but the GGT was "out of sight" (254). Her calcium level was extremely low and this would contribute to permeability of her tissues that were already letting fluids seep out and also fan the flames of tumor growth. But her liver could still make enough protein, though barely. If this didn't improve in a few days, we would put albumin in her IV.

Her tumor activity level, judged by LDH, was quite low, though judged by alk phos was extremely high. [*Evidently, she was suffering from DAB, not Sudan Black B dye toxicity.*]

Copper [*or germanium*] toxicity is easily seen in the very low iron level (27), but her nutrition was still adequate, in spite of her emaciation. She should be able to get well, provided no accident happened, like hemorrhage. The platelet count, at 448, looked dangerously like evidence of minute bleeding. The low RBC reinforced this idea, though of course the bleeding might be anywhere, not necessarily in the lung. Our policy has never been to scan from head to toe, although such knowledge would be very welcome. We started her immediately on the Chinese herb, Yunnan paiyao, to help prevent more bleeding. Perhaps it was responsible for the rather good history for the platelet count all the way to October 2.

She had brought her own X-ray showing a large lung tumor and much pleural effusion (water accumulation), but we needed a current one which she did the same day.

The tumor was circled by the radiologist and lies under two of the metal pins left in her from a previous surgery. On the other side, the enlarged lymph nodes (small round masses) were circled, also. The white area represents air; there is rather little of it, due to "water" accumulation (dark area), at the base of both lungs. She had been drained of this fluid twice already. The numerous finger-like dark projections are the bronchioles, much too

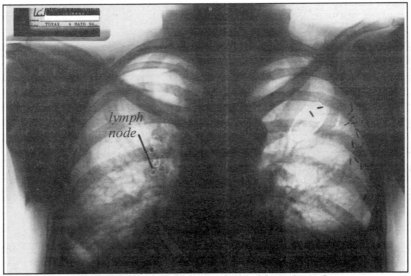

lymph node

Small circles on left are enlarged lymph nodes.
May 4 initial X-ray shows large tumor

prominent due to inflammation and infection. The entire lung looked moth-eaten on close inspection.

On her first day parasites were killed, the freon removal program was started and dental work was scheduled. She had very bad teeth. She had quite a list of toxins built up in her, including freon, asbestos, nickel, and formaldehyde, all of which are lung toxins. Just being away from home would help a lot! The cadmium, copper, aluminum, lead, and mercury would be chelated out with IVs. That left patulin and aflatoxin for her daughter, Sharon, to take on. The ever lurking salmonella and shigella bacteria were present, in addition to malonic acid and, of course, isopropyl alcohol.

As supplements, we started with glutathione, glucuronic acid, coenzyme Q10, Lugol's iodine, and taurine and cysteine, specifically to detoxify formaldehyde.

In five days her chronic diarrhea had stopped and for the first time in two months she could sleep at night.

Vitamins A and B_2 were added to her supplements. And after seeing her blood test results IVs were begun. They contained 3 grams calcium, magnesium, vitamin B-complex, DMSO, and laetrile.

By May 11 all her dental metal was out. She immediately could breathe better. The rattling sound of her breathing was gone.

The blood test, May 13, was in agreement. The calcium level and total protein was up significantly. The big improvement in health could also be seen in the lowered GGT. But the LDH went up [*probably due to azo dye in new dentalware*].

By May 18, she was feeling well enough to walk a mile to a restaurant. Her appetite was very good; she had lost 20 lb. just before coming and needed, desperately, to gain weight.

We could stop putting calcium in her IV now, giving her only B-complex, DMSO, and laetrile. By mouth, we gave chlorophyll "iron booster" syrup, B_{12}, folic acid and vitamin C.

By May 28 her appetite was still good, she was not panting so much after walking. Yet, her LDH went higher and calcium dropped back down, a sign of malonate toxicity [*and dye*]. Both vanadium and cobalt were detected in her parathyroids. Several malonic acid derivatives were again present at her lungs. *Staphylococcus* had already returned, too. We desperately searched for their sources.

In a week, she began to fail quite seriously. She came in a wheel chair and lay huddled on her cot while getting her IV, without talking or moving. We feared the worst. Her family probably did, too. But she found the strength to point out a painful tooth—just the clue we needed. We hustled her to the dentist and were very grateful for her acceptance in her condition. He found an abscess, drained it and cleaned it with Lugol's, but she would not allow extraction. Immediately, she became alert and willing to eat. That was a close call! She had lost weight during this week. To help her gain it back we prepared the lemon-oil beverage recipe for her. She would get one a day. She enjoyed it. She got better again. We were all elated. Even Sharon began to smile. But not for long. The copper and malonic acid continued to plague her. LDH, alk phos, and iron were going up and down unpredictably. Was she eating junk food? (That is, off the malonate-free list.) **Yes**. Was she not taking her supplements? **True**. But I was not convinced these transgressions were entirely responsible. It was something more.

By June 25, she could exercise again. She would feel pain over her heart occasionally, but her arm had long since been pain free and she no longer got numb spells.

But by June 30 her breathing was worse. She had a bad cough. Both malonic acid and maleic anhydride were present at the lung. In the next few days she became very weak again, was in the wheelchair, and vomited with coughing. We took her off thyroid medication–she was on 1½ grains, the lump on her neck was gone. We took her off the lemon-oil beverage. Her uric acid had dropped abnormally low; was this a factor? We did not understand it. She frequently didn't take her glutamine. We searched everywhere for her malonic acid source...and found it...right in the eggnog beverage we made for her to replace the lemon-oil variety. We had not yet learned to detoxify it (a dairy product) with vitamin C. But learned the same day.

It was mid-July. She had stopped vomiting, but couldn't regain strength. She was now on oxygen continuously and seemed to be losing ground. The family was considering giving up and taking her home. But once more she pointed the way. There was a hard spot on her right lower jaw. Was it another abscess? This time a special dental surgeon was called in to make a "house call" due to her frailty. The surgeon reported to us, in surprise, that she had several plastic crowns, and a bridge! We had not been informed of this during her dental work. Could this explain her chronic malonate problem and recurrent acute illness? Under one of the crowns, the surgeon found a black tooth, full of decay. Another abscess was opened and cleaned up, but she refused extraction.

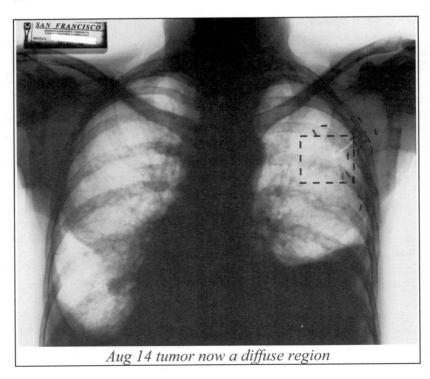

SAN FRANCISCO

Aug 14 tumor now a diffuse region

The next day she was not nauseous, for the first time in a long while. Her breathing was better again. She needed less oxygen. Her *Staphylococcus* disappeared. It was time to check her lungs with an X-ray again and drain if necessary.

The lung tumor was much smaller, in fact, nothing but a diffuse (fluffy) region of remaining inflammation. (Search for the radiologist's white arrow.) Her lungs had twice as much air in them (white space) and the enlarged lymph nodes were gone. Nevertheless, one more liter of fluid was drained from her chest. She could drink better now and was started on "lung tea" (mullein, comfrey) and a clove of garlic daily.

On August 15 she left. Her family was disappointed. Yet she was clearly better according to the X-ray and blood tests. They didn't think so; she was wheel chair bound, had lost more weight, and needed oxygen occasionally. The grapevine whispered she was going home to die.

Summary: Two months later, the family called. I expected the worst. But it was Sonja herself! She wanted something, but I could only sputter back: How was she? She was fine, she said. Had she gained weight? "Oh, yes, 4 lb. already." That was the telling news. She had turned the corner. She was getting well. But she was calling about another tooth! "Yes, do come back. Don't refill it, pull it!" But she refused. In her blithe way, as always, she just refused. Her hard won victories may have been in vain. But she treated us to one more follow up blood test. She had improved in many ways and had a better chance to get well than in the beginning.

Sonja Eckenroth	5/1	5/13	5/28	6/3	6/11	6/18	6/25	7/2	8/5	8/14	10/2
RBC	4.07	4.34	4.55	4.37	4.07	4.04	4.38	3.96	3.99	4.04	4.24
WBC	4,1	9,6	8,9	8,7	7,4	8,6	7,8	8,3	9,3	9,0	6,2
PLT	448	500	368	418	458	414	473	393	415	377	306
BUN	11	11	14	26	14	18	10	14	10	15	8.0
creatinine	0.6	0.7	0.7	0.8	0.9	0.8	0.7	0.6	0.8	0.8	0.6
AST (SGOT)	31	35	45	55	56	64	56	71	54	50	37
ALT (SGPT)	27	27	13	18	25	22	23	22	19	18	13
LDH	161	228	279	327	252	336	277	335	256	246	203
GGT	254	126	82	79	77	79	85	65	134	118	144
T.b.	0.2	0.6	0.6	0.6	0.7	0.8	0.5	0.5	0.8	0.4	0.4
alk phos	498	484	452	451	517	595	464	614	514	510	563
T.p.	5.3	6.6	6.7	6.9	6.7	6.8	6.9	6.6	7.1	7.0	6.9
albumin	2.9	3.9	4.0	3.9	3.9	3.9	4.2	3.8	4.0	4.0	4.1
globulin	2.4	2.7	2.7	3.0	2.8	2.9	2.7	2.8	3.1	3.0	2.8
uric acid	4.0	5.2	2.7	2.0	2.0	1.9	0.9	1.0	1.6	1.0	3.0
Calcium	7.4	9.5	8.9	8.6	8.6	8.7	8.6	7.8	8.6	8.9	8.1
Phosphorus	2.4	4.1	4.4	5.0	4.6	5.8	5.0	5.0	5.2	4.8	4.4
Iron	27	30	31	39	22	33	56	40	69	30	58
Sodium	134	134	133	138	138	136	135	136	135	139	128
Potassium	4.3	4.3	3.7	4.1	4.4	4.4	4.4	4.8	4.7	4.4	4.5
Chloride	102	94	95	99	96	103	97	100	99	102	92

| triglycerides | 136 | 179 | 157 | 199 | 142 | 158 | 125 | 180 | 175 | 104 | 105 |
| cholesterol | 170 | 230 | 191 | 173 | 141 | 169 | 143 | 137 | 160 | 169 | 191 |

25   Robert Marcoux   Hodgkins Disease

Robert Marcoux, in his early forties, came from French Canada with a friend. He had been diagnosed in 1990 with Hodgkin's disease. In spite of regular clinical treatment at home, the lymph nodes of his abdomen were getting bigger again. He was now having night sweats. [*This is caused by* Mycobacterium avium, *brought in by* Ascaris.] He was losing weight. His appetite was poor. He was extremely fatigued. There was constant pain and pressure in the groin area.

His last CT scan was done in February, so we immediately ordered a new one. This one, done May 7, showed a large tumor in the abdomen between the kidneys, measuring 6.7 x 4.5 cm, about the size of a potato. The scan also showed considerable ascites (water seepage and accumulation) around the kidneys. The radiologist noted that the liver texture was quite poor, on the verge of developing tumors there.

They were nervous and frightened, unable to comprehend a word of Spanish. Yet they had to stay in a Mexican motel, because, although an environmentally safe one had just been opened, it was already full. They could only stay for three weeks, giving us a rather impossible task. We reasoned

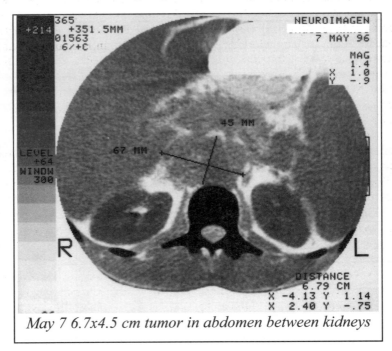

May 7 6.7x4.5 cm tumor in abdomen between kidneys

that it was long enough to learn the essential change in his lifestyle and environment to save his life if he was diligent. And we hoped they might extend their stay if they got good results.

On his first day, May 6, he was given the parasite killing herbs and co-enzyme Q10, 3 gm, to be repeated every fourth day. [*At that time we were still not certain of the great importance of glutathione; we only gave him one 500 mg capsule a day.*]

His initial toxin test showed he had two salmonella and one shigella varieties invading his body tissues. He had benzene, wood alcohol, isopropyl, and xylene solvents. He had fiberglass, aluminum, nickel, arsenic, copper, chlorine, and mercury. And he was full of aflatoxin, the fungal toxin that can raise the total bilirubin and cause a lethal jaundice. He was taken off grocery store bread immediately. Malonic acid was Positive, too.

Next day the blood test results arrived. The extremely poor liver function was apparent in the GGT (574). [*And somewhere (in the WBCs) the carcinogenic dye DAB had accumulated so much it raised the alk phos to a wildly high 701. Was he using hair dyes?*]

The copper [*or germanium*] toxicity was easy to discover; serum iron was only 24; yet his RBC count was adequate. The calcium level was much too low—conducive to seeping of body fluids. The total protein was rather low, probably causing the ascites we could see around the tumor and kidneys, although maleic anhydride was probably the real culprit.

Time was most important to them, so we started IV therapy to speed up the tumor shrinkage. After 2 doses of EDTA to pull out copper we administered by IV 3 gm calcium, magnesium, 25 gm vitamin C, 2 vials laetrile, DMSO, 3 gm cesium chloride, and 1 ampoule vitamin B complex. But the next day he was Positive for copper again. He was moved to a motel without copper water pipes. Here rotenone pesticide was often used. He was to request NO pesticide treatment while there. Rotenone is another very strong metabolic inhibitor. We planned to watch and test him for it. More EDTA chelation was used.

In one week, all his dental work was done; we omitted to record in his file what was done, however. We can only guess that amalgam was taken out and composite put back in. The blood test showed some improvement (GGT 539), but the alk phos went higher [*dyes are used in dental plastic*] and the iron level lower.

Somehow, he continued getting copper, in spite of moving to the "copper-free" motel. [*It was no doubt in his new dental plastic.*] Would we be able to keep ahead of it with our IVs that pulled it out in order to let the tumor shrink? Calcium had risen, probably from intensive IV therapy.

Nevertheless, tumor activity was stronger than before, in some respect, since the alk phos was up. The LDH drop, though, was a hopeful sign.

We increased his glutathione to 500 mg, eight a day to help the liver detoxify everything. He was started on silymarin for the liver also. In spite of having no appetite, he was asked to drink a cream-shake every day as well as lemon oil drink accompanied by digestive enzymes (our own formulation), three with each meal.

By the end of the second week, May 18, he was still frequently Positive to copper; he had to switch motel rooms again. Rotenone was now showing up in his liver besides malonic acid at his lymph nodes. Nevertheless, his appetite had picked up and he was now out walking on the beach. He was started on taurine and cysteine to detoxify the rotenone. And he was given caster oil packs to place in the groin area every night, both to ease pain and provide immune stimulation.

Seven days later, May 25, his fatigue was gone, he was sleeping better. The pain in his groin was better. Yet there was cobalt at his kidney. He was still on EDTA and tumor shrinking IVs daily. It was two days before departure time. What had been accomplished?

A final blood test showed more improvements. Alk phos came down substantially. His cholesterol and triglycerides were improved. Iron was the highest it had been, but still much too low, a testimony to ongoing copper [or germanium] toxicity. This would of course, not go away if it was in his new plastic teeth. Our chelations may have kept pace with this toxicity, but away from the clinic— what was in store for him?

Calcium had come up a little, but was still too low, evidence for continued malonate toxicity. Could it be from

Robert Marcoux	5/6	5/13	5/18	5/27
RBC	4.75	4.36	4.04	4.42
WBC	6,900	5,900	6,800	6,300
PLT	201	162	158	191
glucose	96	152	136	82
BUN	14	12	10	17
creatinine	0.9	0.9	0.7	1.0
AST (SGOT)	25	25	25	25
ALT (SGPT)	32	30	32	35
LDH	147	118	152	134
GGT	574	539	492	517
T.b.	0.7	0.5	0.5	1.0
alk phos	701	729	677	621
T.p.	6.0	5.6	5.0	6.2
albumin	3.9	3.6	3.4	4.0
globulin	2.1	2.0	1.6	2.2
uric acid	4.4	3.4	2.7	2.1
Calcium	8.3	8.6	7.8	8.6
Phosphorus	3.1	3.0	2.5	4.3
Iron	24	16	13	39
Sodium	138	134	136	134
Potassium	4.0	4.2	3.8	4.0
Chloride	103	95	101	100
triglycerides	71	80	60	95
cholesterol	178	164	141	193

the new dentalware? Uric acid was now unmasked and much too low. [*We did not understand Clostridium infections at that time.*] We started him on glutamine to raise it and thereby allow nucleic acids to be made again. The RBC was good. But the GGT liver enzyme was still dangerously high.

Although the blood test showed some improvement from the time of arrival three weeks earlier, his best news was tucked under his arm as he brought in his new ultrasounds. The large abdominal tumor had shrunk to 4.1 cm x 3.05 cm, about two-thirds of the original size. Its contour was now rough; it was beginning to fragment judging by density change. The ultrasound of the liver showed a smooth, even texture as it should be.

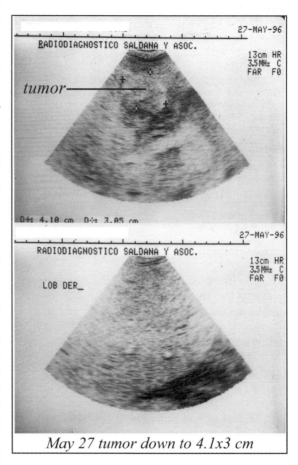

May 27 tumor down to 4.1x3 cm

Summary: They departed with all our best wishes. And with the admonition to do a scan or ultrasound once a month till it was all gone and a blood test that included serum iron. Little could we perceive that obtaining these elementary data records would not be easy even in a country like Canada with a "well developed" medical policy. We heard no more.

---

26   Remi Parker   Kidney Cancer

Remi Parker, a very pleasant, grandfatherly person, came with more than a degree of despair. He was my age and certainly too young to succumb to cancer. He had only one kidney, on the right side. The left kidney had been surgically removed for liposarcoma. But after that, a new tumor grew in the empty location where the kidney had been (called the renal fossa). This was removed in a second surgery. It was the size of a bowling ball. And now it was growing again. It was already over an inch long. It was a despairing situation.

Besides this, he had already lost his spleen and one end of the pancreas to previous surgeries for cancer.

He had started the parasite program eleven days ago, but still had isopropyl alcohol built up in him. His initial toxin test, done at the "whole body" showed:

Bacteria and Solvents	Metals	Other Toxins
Staphylococcus aureus Positive	aluminum Positive	PCB Positive
Salmonella typhimurium Positive	nickel Positive	CFCs Positive
Salmonella enteriditis Negative	copper Positive	fiberglass Positive
Salmonella paratyphi Negative	cobalt Negative,	patulin Positive
Shigella dysenteriae Negative	Positive at kidney	aflatoxin Negative
Shigella sonnei Negative	cadmium Positive	arsenic Negative
Shigella flexneri Negative	mercury Positive	asbestos Negative
	lead Negative	chlorine Negative
isopropyl alcohol Positive	thallium Negative	formaldehyde Negative
wood alcohol Positive		malonic acid Negative
benzene Negative		
xylene Negative		
toluene Negative		

His first blood test showed the effects of some of these toxins. RBC was elevated due to cobalt. Calcium was too low, due to malonic acid and other toxins appearing in the parathyroid glands. Iron was too high; cause not known. A generous level of triglycerides and enough cholesterol would certainly help him succeed.

The slightly elevated BUN and creatinine showed that his one remaining kidney was working hard, perhaps too hard. The rest of his test results were exceptionally good. There was no LDH or alk phos elevation.

But there was no time to gloat over his good health; there was a tumor to shrink, and he had come many miles to do this. We decided to proceed without IVs at first. He was started on:

- the parasite program and zapping
- going off the isopropyl alcohol list in the book, *The Cure For All Cancers*
- going on the malonate-free diet
- the freon removal program
- changing his glasses frames to plastic
- stopping use of detergent for anything
- staying off apples in any form (to eliminate patulin)
- use of coenzyme Q10 (to kill tapeworm stages)
- glutathione, taurine, cysteine, vitamin B_{12}, folic acid

- changing his plumbing at home to PVC from copper. He was advised to move into a mobile home with plastic water pipes temporarily while his plumbing got changed.

All supplements had to be procured from us to be sure they had been tested and were free of the common tumor-causing pollutants.

Two days later, May 22, he was feeling better, his malignancy was stopped (ortho-phospho-tyrosine Negative), but copper was still present.

An ultrasound of the lower abdomen, done this day, showed the tumor was 3.8 x 2.75 cm.

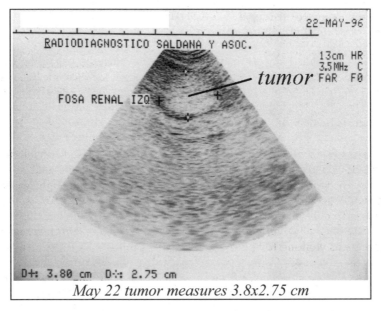

May 22 tumor measures 3.8x2.75 cm

On June 5, he was still Positive for freon, fiberglass, and copper.

On June 26 although copper and fiberglass were now Negative, he still tested Positive for *Staphylococcus* at the kidney location. This originates in a dental infection, reaching out to his tumor. A blood test was scheduled. He had not yet started on the freon removal program. He had just begun dental cleanup, but hadn't been using white iodine to brush; he was quickly started on it.

It is easy to see, he still had either cobalt or vanadium toxicity; his RBC was still too high.

His WBC was higher, probably from ongoing dental work which releases bacteria into the whole body while wounds are open. This was a good immune response, though! His LDH, although indicating no malignancy before, was now even lower (good).

The albumin had gone higher—too high. The calcium level had come up and was now normal. Albumin and calcium are linked by your body so that the more calcium there is, the more albumin there is. In case the calcium should go too high, the albumin is present to sponge it up and take it out of action in the bloodstream.

Although calcium had come up significantly, it was still low, a parathyroid problem. Testing at the parathyroid showed copper and vanadium Negative there, but glutathione, biotin, and glutamine were also Negative. With glutathione Negative, this tipped us off that a heavy metal was still present or a malonate. Cobalt was Positive. How can a tiny gland do it's work with an interfering metal there?

What was the source of his cobalt? It is not written in his file. We probably searched his supplements, body products and other things. [*But never suspected his new plastic teeth.*]

His next visit was a week later, July 3. An ultrasound of the kidney tumor was scheduled since it had been six weeks since he began the cancer program.

Then, a strange event followed. The radiologist, not being able to see anything at the left kidney site (remember it had been surgically removed) thought the patient must be mistaken so he took the ultrasound of the right kidney instead. When the patient returned, the missing ultrasound of the left side was seen as an error so the patient was sent back to the radiologist. But the radiologist explained to the patient there was "nothing to take," since the kidney was gone, so why spend the money? This made sense to the patient who returned a second time without the negative. It seemed unfair to send him a third time just to get the missing tumor namely, <u>nothing</u> on record. Remi and his family were pleased and convinced, although only the radiologist's <u>word</u> could ascertain that the tumor in the left kidney fossa was gone.

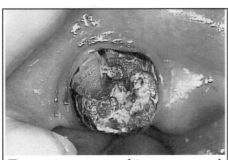

Tumor gone, was this rotten tooth the culprit?

On July 17, his blood test still showed abnormalities. RBC was too high (cobalt Positive); WBC was too high (bacteria); glucose was too low; creatinine was too high (kidney insufficiency); T.p. was too high (cobalt) calcium was too high (thyroid problem); and potassium was too low.

By now we had begun to suspect dental plastic as the mysterious source of cobalt. He was advised to have it all reviewed, tested by the staff with scrapings or chipping of the plastic; and some of it replaced, again!

But Remi was much too happy with his vanishing tumor to take this advice seriously. There was nothing to do away with. His health was good. He was done. And deserved it richly. Except, for one tiny detail...how did he know his tumor was gone? He had no picture of its absence.

But he did have a picture of a very rotten tooth the dentist had pulled for him earlier. Could this have been the real culprit that tipped the scales in favor of tumor growth? Even the dentist was appalled and made this print for him.

He left for home without testing his "bad" dental plastic or replacing it. He promised to send an ultrasound from home in August. But we heard nothing.

Remi Parker	5/20	6/26	7/17
RBC	4.91	4.89	4.96
WBC	8,200	11,200	10,100
PLT	324	315	310
glucose	91	81	73
BUN	24	20	19
creatinine	1.3	1.2	1.5
AST (SGOT)	15	22	22
ALT (SGPT)	22	36	33
LDH	149	120	136
GGT	12	87	26
T.b.	0.8	0.7	0.7
alk phos	89	87	80
T.p.	6.9	7.0	8.0
albumin	4.9	5.1	5.0
globulin	2.0	1.9	3.0
uric acid	6.0	5.0	5.8
Calcium	8.5	9.1	10.0
Phosphorus	3.8	4.0	3.4
Iron	144	102	115
Sodium	140	142	137
Potassium	4.5	4.5	4.0
Chloride	100	102	109
triglycerides	214	251	170
cholesterol	171	182	204

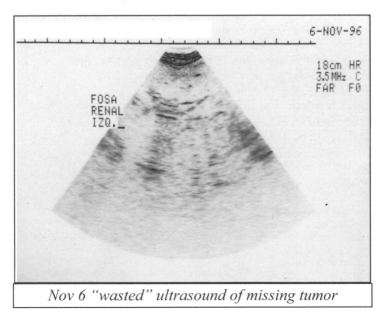

Nov 6 "wasted" ultrasound of missing tumor

383

Summary: Suddenly, on November 6, he popped into the office for a follow-up. He was persuaded to return to the radiologist. This time to request an ultrasound of the location of the space where the left kidney had once been. Nothing else. He soon returned, ultrasound in hand. It was as the radiologist had said—just plain nothing. No tumor in sight anywhere. Nothing to take, just a waste of money! And a good, hearty laugh was had by all to cheer Remi and his wife.

27	Danielle Andersen	Brain Cancer

Danielle Andersen came with her husband, Karl, from Canada for brain cancer. It started as non-Hodgkin's lymphoma, but a year ago there were several brain lesions found by scanning.

One was removed surgically and was diagnosed as diffuse large cell non-Hodgkin's lymphoma, intermediate grade. She then got ten radiation treatments to the head, which brought two of the remaining lesions down to 1.5 cm and 0.5 cm at the thalamus and internal capsule respectively.

That was as much progress as could be made. And she was fine until recently. She began going to sleep for half hour periods during the day, her balance was bad, and her eyes weren't focusing so she couldn't read anymore. Something must be growing.

We reviewed her scan on May 8; we could see what looked like a disorganized tangle in the thalamus filling the depression that hangs down and mushrooming above it. It was about 2 cm in size. Unfortunately, this negative was not printed for my collection. One look at her blood test shows she was still quite well. If the tumor could be shrunk in a permanent way, she would not need to recover from anything. Only one liver enzyme, the GGT, was too high, in fact extremely high. Could this be due to the dilantin she was on to prevent seizures? This drug is ordinarily rather harmless.

Her alkaline phosphatase was slightly high, but not extreme [*showing DAB dye toxicity*], and the total protein was rather low due to the low globulin. The calcium level was too low, showing that the metabolic problem involved the parathyroid gland. Iron showed some depression (it should be about 100), but not enough to interfere with red blood cell formation. Although her blood fats (triglycerides) were much too low, cholesterol level was excellent.

Her toxin test showed:

Bacteria and Solvents	Metals	Other toxins
Staphylococcus aureus Positive	aluminum Positive	malonic acid Positive
Salmonella Positive	copper Positive	aflatoxin Positive
	lead Positive	patulin Positive
isopropyl alcohol Positive	thallium Positive	CFCs Positive
	mercury Positive	chlorine Positive
	nickel Positive	

In addition to the usual Lugol's, Q10, freon program, parasite program, and glutathione, she was given methylene blue, 65 mg (three times a day). She was reminded that her urine would look blue...not to worry about "turning into a blueberry".

Her IVs were started the day she arrived and contained 3 vials EDTA, to pull heavy metal out of her brain, vitamin B-complex, laetrile, and vitamin C. The next day, though, May 4, she was still testing Positive for copper at the brain and liver; it was found polluting the dilantin pills she was taking. A Mexican brand of dilantin was chosen that tested free of toxins. Another course of EDTA was given.

Two days after that, May 6, she had to be assisted to walk straight. She was losing ground. Copper was still Positive. They had already moved twice to different rooms in their motel, each time bringing the tap water in to test for copper. Meanwhile, time was flitting away. An emergency loomed.

On May 9, six days after her arrival, she was still Positive for copper in the cerebrum, in spite of chelating it out with EDTA. She was advised to move to our environmentally safe motel. It would mean sitting in a long line of border traffic each day, but at least the copper problem would disappear. On May 11, copper was Negative. She could read again, her eyes and her balance were much better. She was in the middle of dental work. And malonic acid was testing Negative in her brain.

By May 15, she was much less dizzy and walking better. Glutathione was testing Positive, now, at her cerebrum. But TNF was still Negative. Patulin must still be present at the brain. She was taken off all fruit in her diet till this would be gone. On May 18, she was so much better, she was talking conversationally with anybody. She had no dizziness at all.

Her blood test, done May 16, showed the typical drop in uric acid as it becomes unmasked by folic acid and other supplements. [*Later we found the true cause of a low uric acid to be clostridia bacteria. This results in almost no purines (nucleic acids) being formed or used (catabolized) and hence a low uric acid.*]

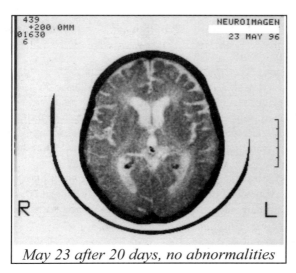

May 23 after 20 days, no abnormalities

By May 22, she no longer dragged her foot even slightly. She said she felt great and was walking a lot without help. A follow up CT scan of the brain was scheduled. The next day, our tests showed maleic acid Positive at her liver [*we did not know, then, that maleic acid is used in some dental materials*], but the brain stayed free of it.

To everyone's surprise, there was no trace of any tumor on her CT scan. Had we missed seeing it because no contrast was used? It was repeated, with contrast. [We would never do this now. The contrast medium brings in all the lanthanide elements, causing serious immune lowering.] Nothing abnormal could be seen anywhere! This shows how very easy it really is to shrink a deadly tumor. If only we understood them enough to do it reliably and quantitatively. Until we know which part of her treatment program was responsible, we do not understand it and cannot abbreviate it in any way.

Did her next blood test, May 25, reflect the improvement? Certainly her iron level had become normal (about 100), indicating the absence of competing heavy metal, specifically copper [*and germanium*]. She would now be able to make more red blood cells and improve her immunity so deadly bacteria could no longer live in her brain lesion. And in turn, this would stop production of bacteria-derived growth factors.

But there were also bad things happening. The BUN and creatinine were even lower, calcium had dropped again, and her blood fats had dropped, too [*new dyes from plastic teeth*].

They were getting ready to leave as a happy couple again feeling, as we all did, that their mission had been accomplished. They were scheduled for an MRI at home in a month; this would give them the extra certainty they needed.

Her last blood test left us quite uneasy on May 31. Her RBC and WBC were still much too low; there had to be a toxin remaining in her bone marrow. Her blood sugar (glucose) was much too low, as were BUN and creatinine. Something was severely curtailing her ability to make these; after all, no cancer patient's kidneys simply get better and better. Liver enzymes and LDH were quite poor.

And total protein had fallen. But at least the calcium and iron levels were improved. Going home would get them away from auto exhaust and public food if these were involved. It was Bon Voyage to Danielle and Karl with just one caution: to hurry back if anything went wrong. Soon we heard that a confirming MRI had been done at home. It was sent for my examination.

A month later we got a Fax telling us Danielle

Danielle Andersen	5/3	5/16	5/25	5/31
RBC	4.14	3.96	3.51	3.70
WBC	4,600	3,600	3,200	3,100
PLT	238	275	244	211
glucose	91	87	85	62
BUN	14	10	7.0	6.0
creatinine	0.8	0.7	0.6	0.7
AST (SGOT)	29	50	32	40
ALT (SGPT)	29	63	46	52
LDH	163	181	183	222
GGT	325	355	318	316
T.b.	0.7	0.6	0.4	0.7
alk phos	106	145	128	128
T.p.	6.3	6.2	6.2	5.9
albumin	4.5	4.3	4.2	4.2
globulin	1.8	1.9	2.0	1.7
uric acid	3.7	1.8	1.7	2.1
Calcium	8.7	9.1	8.5	9.0
Phosphorus	4.4	3.8	2.7	3.3
Iron	60	85	116	131
Sodium	139	143	143	143
Potassium	4.2	4.0	3.5	3.5
Chloride	99	106	108	108
triglycerides	63	114	58	66
cholesterol	257	252	242	249

was fine, not gaining but not losing weight. Her functioning was even better than it was here. But a marble-like lymph node had popped out at the left side of her neck near the collar bone. [*This is invariably dental in causation.*] It wasn't growing. By then we had learned of the toxins in plastic dental ware. And we knew that Danielle's mouth was full of it! There was only one thing to do. Get it out. Hurry back and get it out! But she didn't hurry.

By September there was a second marble. Would they never get back?

But the MRI, done on July 26, had shown her oncologist at home there was no abnormality in the brain. So what was the hurry? They had been coasting on the good news. How could the new plastic dentalware be suspect? It didn't sound reasonable to them.

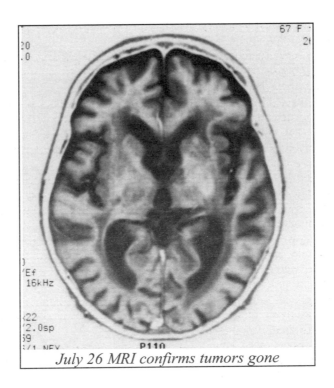

July 26 MRI confirms tumors gone

The Return

They arrived again on September 24. Home had been good to Danielle these four months. She had gained 2 lb. and then could gain no more.

Her toxin test showed she was getting toluene on a daily basis; this would certainly go to her brain. She was losing her balance again. She was not drinking commercial beverages, so toluene was suspected in the prescription pills and capsules she was taking. She was to stop everything for a day till the culprit source could be found. She was happy for the reprieve. Mexican brands were tested and substituted.

Her malonic acid level was high. Now we knew it could come from plain food, as well as dental plastic. We gave Karl the malonate-free food list; his determination was greater than ever.

She was Positive for *Staphylococcus aureus* at the lymph nodes; we knew the problem would be dental since the lymph nodes at the neck drain the mouth fluids. She also had *E. coli* and aflatoxin. But gone were all the other toxins she had originally come with. No freon. No aluminum. No nickel. No copper! No chlorine. No lead. No mercury. No thallium. And no patulin. She and Karl had done an exemplary job of keeping a "clean" environment at home.

But my curiosity was piqued. Could there be a tumor growth—even just one—that did not contain copper: free, metallic copper? This was interesting for its own sake; it would be a "first".

We searched specifically in the lymph nodes next and there we found: xylene, malonic acid, aflatoxin, cobalt, vanadium, salmonella, and copper. Copper was not seen at "whole body" testing, above. The level of her exposure was certainly very low. But the lymph nodes were picking up that small amount and "bio-accumulating" it. [*Dental plastic is a source.*]

Her two neck lumps had been biopsied at home and pronounced melanomas by her doctors. But, with her huge improvement quite visible, they had decided to "wait and see" for a month. One was 1 inch (2.5 cm) in diameter, the other about $^3/_8$ inch (1 cm). The first thing to do was test the upper denture she had received at her first visit. It was Positive for copper, cobalt, vanadium, the malonates, and urethane! She had been getting copper from her polluted dentures. It was replaced immediately (in a few days) with an identical denture, free of the toxins.

She had *Staphylococcus*, *E. coli*, and three varieties of salmonella in her brain again. Plus maleic anhydride which would give her the symptoms of edema again, also due to polluted plastic in her mouth.

Her blood test showed significant improvements almost everywhere. Only alk phos had gone up. And iron had dropped. The blood fat level had stayed much too low (triglycerides 63).

She was started on potassium gluconate powder to raise her potassium level, and on creatine powder. She would put castor oil hot packs on her neck over the lymph nodes to help them shrink.

A new X-ray of her teeth showed a root tip had been left in from previous dental work. All the remaining plastic in each of her lower molars and premolars was scheduled for removal.

She immediately had better balance after this, but it was not perfect. And *E. coli* continued to test Positive at the brain.

By September 30, her iron had come up significantly, but copper and malonic acid were still testing Positive at the lymph nodes. She had not yet changed her metal glasses frames to plastic. She did this at once. This could be the last mysterious copper source.

On October 1, she was still Positive for copper and malonate at the lymph nodes. They had not returned to the copper-free motel! They planned to move into it the same day. But this would not explain the malonates—all four malonic derivatives were present in her lymph nodes. Yet they were meticulously following the malonate-free diet. All supplements had been tested and re-tested. She had been taking Q-10 on schedule to kill tapeworm stages. There was only one conclusion: there must be left over toxic plastic in her mouth. [*We had not learned to test for urethane and bisphenol-A at the teeth to specifically implicate plastic there.*]

But there was nothing plastic in her mouth. There were only eight teeth present, across the front on the lower side and these were pristine, untouched, never-filled teeth!

She was started on olive leaf tea to help shrink lymph nodes. They were already noticeably smaller.

On October 3, the lymph nodes were down to ¾" (2 cm) and ⅛" (½ cm) in diameter. But she had accidentally fallen down the previous night, and we were all concerned that it could have been due to a seizure. She had taken herself off dilantin, although she had been on two a day when she arrived. Could it have been due to rotenone used liberally in all motels except the safe one? She did test Positive for rotenone, from the previous motel. She was given taurine, and GABA. Unfortunately, the GABA was not provided immediately and she was without for another 2 days.

She soon had another "seizure". [*They are caused by* Ascaris *escaping from a draining tumor.*] This time they went to an emergency facility in the U.S. where she was hospitalized. It now required 3 tablets of dilantin a day to get her blood level up high enough. While in the hospital, a new blood test was done for her (October 6). Although the ranges are not strictly comparable and serum iron was missing, the results are informative. The good trends were continuing, the LDH had dropped almost to normal and liver enzymes were getting better.

On October 8, she returned, in a wheelchair now, due to the injury from her fall. But her appetite was good. It was just her general grogginess that disturbed us. If it was indeed seizure activity, then she was still getting maleic anhydride to her seizure center causing edema there. (We did not suspect *Ascaris*.) This would derive from maleic acid, namely dental plastic.

On October 9, she tested Positive for cobalt at the liver, vanadium at the bone marrow, and copper at the liver. This trio implicates plastic or metal. We went to work. Each of her remaining eight lower "pristine untouched" front teeth was rubbed with an emery board. The end of the emery board with the rubbing was cut off and dropped in a baggie for testing (water added first). The last tooth on the lower right side was Positive for cobalt, copper, and vanadium. But this tooth appeared pristine. It had never been tampered with! Nor had any of the other seven in the row. We sampled the tooth again, compared it with the saliva test; there was no mistaking the Positive results for the familiar trio. We recommended extraction of that perfect-appearing tooth. The dentist rebelled. He had examined these teeth several times. He could not in good conscience extract a "perfect" tooth. We discussed the risk and possible benefit for Danielle, namely death versus a gap in her teeth.

On October 12 the tooth came out. It was brought in for my inspection. It had a <u>huge</u> plastic filling on the back side! The dentist visited later. He explained that plastic can easily escape detection by X-ray, as well as by the dentist's eye even with the help of dental dye. Although three individual X-rays had been done to search for it, plus numerous dental visual inspections, it had escaped detection. No sooner was the dentist's drill applied than its true soft nature was revealed. *(Now we would easily find it with a digital X-ray.)*

By October 14, she was alert, active, and completely normal appearing. She was put on dexamethasone instead of dilantin. The smaller of the two enlarged lymph nodes was completely gone. The larger lump was no longer visible (but parts could still be felt below the skin). Now was the time to stay and finish the task for Danielle, so she could be secure at home.

But it was "home again" after a last blood test. The calcium was again too low, the blood sugar was too low, and Bun and creatinine were too low (in spite of taking creatine by mouth).

Danielle Andersen	9/24	9/30	10/5	10/6	10/14
RBC	3.92	4.07	4.04	3.5	3.79
WBC	4,8	3,3	4,4	4,9	3,7
PLT	317	284	278	246	293
glucose	161	88	75	113	71
BUN	13	10	10.5	10	11
creatinine	0.7	0.6	0.7	0.7	0.6
AST (SGOT)	33	38	35	26	26
ALT (SGPT)	50	47	41	46	31
LDH	182	180	232	166	189
GGT	174	196	173	167	133
T.b.	0.5	0.5	0.2	0.3	0.3
alk phos	151	158	168	151	168
T.p.	6.3	6.3	6.4	6.3	6.3
albumin	4.2	4.3	4.5	3.2	4.1
globulin	2.1	2.0	1.9	3.1	2.2
uric acid	3.0	2.9	2.9	2.6	2.7
Calcium	9.1	9.2	9.2	9.4	8.8
Phosphorus	3.2	2.9	3.1	3.5	3.5
Iron	46	77	65		57
Sodium	139	141	134	193	142
Potassium	3.7	3.9	3.5	3.5	4.2
Chloride	106	104	101	107	104
triglycerides	63	59	43		49
cholesterol	212	241	271	226	251

Iron was still too low as were triglycerides. And the anemia and leukopenia (low WBC) were quite apparent. Possibly, not enough time (two days) had passed to reflect the dental improvement (latest extraction). [*Nor had we yet found the pollutants in the* capsules *that held her supplements before they left.*] Nor could we be sure she did not have yet another plastic filling! They left before all this could be checked.

Summary: People as beautiful as Karl and Danielle deserve every chance. Of course, people of all sorts deserve such a chance, too.

The toxicity of dental plastic is unknown, its relevance to tumor growth is unknown. Dentists can't be expected to know. The general pollution of human food products with a dozen tumor-growers is unknown. Manufacturers can't be expected to know this. Who then, is responsible?

28	Herve Curo	Lung/Liver/Brain Cancer

Herve Curo lived just a few hours' drive from the clinic and did not choose to be either an in-patient or out-patient. He wanted to come and go as he pleased; especially, since his doom had been sealed. It lay on his lap in the form of scans and summaries; lung cancer, liver cancer, possibly now the brain, as well as skin.

His January 2 chest X-ray showed a large tumor, the size of a pear lying vertically in the right lung. He was put on chemotherapy, but it made him sick. Besides, it would cost him $800.00 for 20 pills. And it would all be hopeless anyway. So he had put himself on the parasite program and zapper on Jan. 6. He also had considerable "infiltrate" meaning fluid accumulation in the lung tissue.

When he arrived on June 14, he had the appearance of a tired old man, rather corpulent and quick with the lip. He was losing his balance, needed someone to help him get about, and had some pain around the lung area, but he still made quips about all this. His arms became numb for periods of time and his legs felt tired. His knees were quite painful, but he could still walk.

His initial toxin test showed: asbestos, arsenic, copper, chlorine, cobalt, formaldehyde, lead, mercury, thallium all Positive. He also had systemic *E. coli* and staphylococcus bacteria and, of course, malonic acid. He was given

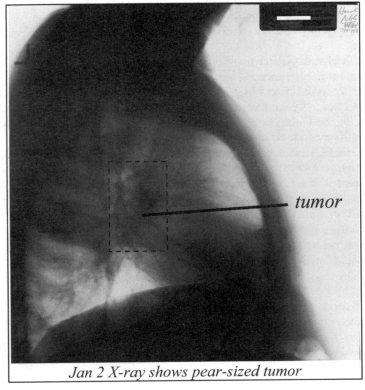

tumor

Jan 2 X-ray shows pear-sized tumor

the parasite killing herbs on the spot and zapped. He was advised how to do his dental cleanup and sterilize dairy foods. He was given the malonate-free food list and told to change his copper plumbing, which was also giving him lead. He was sent out to change his glasses frames to plastic. [*We did not yet know that plastic frames could shed vanadium and dye and also needed careful washing before they are first worn.*]

He was scheduled for a fresh X-ray of the lungs and CT scan of brain and liver that afternoon. He was given the kidney herbs and all his supplements. No other supplements or drugs were to be taken due to risk of pollution. He obtained Lugol's, glutamine, coenzyme Q10, B_{12}, folic acid, vitamin C, taurine, cysteine, methionine, and glycine.

His IV of EDTA was formulated and ready to pull his heavy metals out. Then Herve disappeared. He was nowhere to be found. He had paid his bill and simply walked away without even making a follow-up appointment. He had left his new scans on the desk (not shown). The liver showed numerous small tumors, the lung had its very large tumor. He had even done a bone scan which showed numerous lesions in the skull. What were his chances, we wondered. "Entirely nil" said the pathologist and two assistant physicians. Two weeks to two months was the forecast. We called him at home just to make sure he had understood we wanted him to come in for IV therapy <u>every day</u> and to monitor his progress by <u>daily</u> testing. He had understood.

Twelve days later he returned. We gasped. No faltering gait and stooping. He said his numbness was gone. We reviewed his earlier blood test with him. We asked if he was diabetic, since the glucose level was 350! He suggested not to "give it any mind," since <u>he</u> wasn't. He wasn't feeling bad; in fact, he was feeling better and didn't want any "medicine". He brought a new chest X-ray done June 21, a week after his initial visit.

His LDH showed absence of tumor growth (152)—possibly due to chemotherapy he had been given previously. The lung tumor, though, was implicated in the high alkaline phosphatase (317). [*Research results from the Syncrometer indicate the dye DAB causes a particular mutation that elevates the enzyme alkaline phosphatase. (This enzyme controls calcium deposition in bone.) If alk phos is high you know immediately bones or lungs are involved, and you can expect to find lesions and tumors. Current clinical theory holds that high alk phos is a <u>result</u> of cancer; I see the opposite. But at this time I was still using alk phos as a tumor indicator.*]

The albumin was too high and globulin too low, evidence for cobalt in the liver. Uric acid was much too low, showing there was not enough glutamine to manufacture purines which metabolize into uric acid. (Other explanations come later.) Phosphate was too high, showing that his bones were being dissolved at a fast rate, by the high alk phos. But there at the end of the report were his cholesterol and triglycerides! Especially his triglycerides were nicely elevated! This would give him a fighting chance. Maybe he could survive. Maybe his diabetic status would even <u>help</u>. Dying cancer patients have extremely low glucose and triglyceride levels. Their tumorous tissues consume it so fast. Perhaps a diabetics' tissues cannot consume it fast. Maybe this puts a brake on the tumor activity. And perhaps this speculation was completely wrong. We would see.

We formulated his IV to readiness again. But Herve was nowhere to be seen. He disappeared again! He had done another blood test, picked up fresh supplies of supplements, had been tested for copper and malonic acid and left! (Both were Positive.) We hadn't even reviewed his X-ray! He had gotten it done at home and just kept it tucked under his arm. What could we do about Herve? It seemed he wanted less of life than we did for him. But at least he came in sporadically and we would have a chance to see if it was possible to improve <u>without</u> IV intensive care.

This time he returned in a week, July 3. His knee pain was gone now besides his earlier numbness. He had looked at his new X-ray and was eagerly shoving it at us. It was almost embarrassing to see the improvement. The tumor remains were barely distinguishable in the lung. Was it still tumor? We would have to wait for the radiologist's report. We warned him about coughing up blood. If this should happen, he should come in at once; we would give him a Chinese herb to prevent hemorrhage—as much as possible! We explained that as lung tumors shrink they may pull away from tissue, causing pain and bleeding, not to be alarmed. It was plain to see that we were the alarmed party, not him.

He had not yet started his dental cleanup. They were working on the plumbing at home that afternoon. He did another blood test and disappeared again. We had told him about his blood test improvements, in the hope this would improve his concern for himself. His kidney function was no longer blocked by malonic acid; BUN was up strikingly.

His lungs were improving; there was less tumor activity, alk phos was down. Uric acid was up (he was eating no malonate foods and taking glutamine supplement). His thyroid was better; calcium was down and less phosphate was coming from his bones. Potassium was up. A week later, July 10, he came again. All the symptoms he had come in with were gone, he said. He did a new blood test, got supplies, and left.

Two weeks later, July 24, we reviewed it with him. His glucose had dropped 100 points (glucose 250). His diabetic condition was much better. Kidney function was better (creatinine lower). His LDH was keeping low. His lung tumor must be shrinking (alk phos 260). His albumin was a little lower and globulin a little higher—a better liver. Uric acid was higher; phosphate lower.

Did he have his own kind of magic? Or was his "stubbornness" paying off in avoiding possible IV pollution and plastic dentalware pollution? We had not even reviewed his June 21 chest X-ray with our own radiologist yet. The clinic radiologist was away on temporary leave, so we viewed it in August. What a surprise. The letter with summary stated there was "no tumor or pleural effusion or pulmonary edema or hyperinflation. In fact, he had a negative chest."

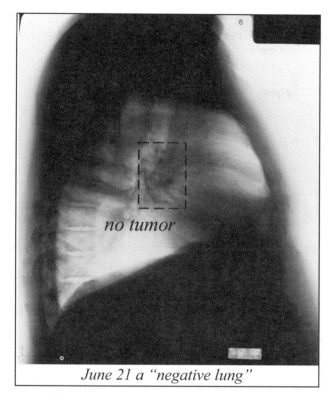

no tumor

June 21 a "negative lung"

His August 2 blood test showed further improvement in the alk phos. He now got his dentalware changed to plastic.

A month later, September 11, his blood test was decidedly worse. It would be a harbinger of things to come. We must somehow trap him long enough to sample each of his new dental fillings and test them for copper, cobalt, vanadium, and the malonate compounds. He had changed his glasses frames quite early, <u>did</u> get his copper plumbing changed, and said he was "doing everything." His WBC showed that bacteria were on the rise; glucose (208) continued to drop showing improved diabetes; ALT showed a liver toxin was up; [*LDH showed tumor activation by Sudan Black B dye;*] GGT showed more liver toxicity; alk phos implied that lung tumor remnants were shrinking.

But trapping Herve was no small challenge <u>especially</u> now that life was being handed back to him.

Summary: We saw him again a few months later; he was still his devil-may-care self. It is tempting to think his negligence somehow benefited him. We hope so. As for ourselves; we would rather choose diligence. Yet, there are lessons to be learned from even the most contrary approach.

Herve Curo	6/14	6/26	7/10	8/2	9/11
RBC	3.87	3.73	4.13	4.52	4.61
WBC	7700	6900	10900	10600	11900
PLT	348	167	318	271	266
glucose	350	374	250	263	208
BUN	9.0	19 (5-26)	19 (7-21)	19 (7-21)	19 (7-21)
creatinine	1.2	1.3	1.0	1.1	1.0
AST (SGOT)	19	23	29	23	52
ALT (SGPT)	35	42	45	39	118
LDH	152	161	147	153	244
GGT	66	63	51	46	242
T.b.	0.9	0.8	0.4	0.5	0.5
alk phos	317	269	260	196	170
T.p.	6.6	6.7	6.7	6.4	6.6
albumin	4.7	4.7	4.5	4.6	4.2
globulin	1.9 (2.5)	2.0	2.2	1.8	2.4
uric acid	1.3	2.1	3.4 (3.5-8.5)	3.7	3.4
Calcium	9.7	9.1	9.1	9.1	9.2
Phosphorus	5.5	5.1	4.1	4.2	4.4
Iron	127	116	72	61	61
Sodium	140	141	137	136	135
Potassium	3.4	4.6	4.7	4.3	4.3
Chloride	96	103	102	100	103
triglycerides	313	378	230	271	207
cholesterol	232	221	232	255	186

29   Jess Ingerson   Breast Cancer

Jess Ingerson, age thirty-one, came for one month, all by herself, from Sweden. Friends had prevailed upon her to come to us rather than lose one and soon both breasts to a mastectomy at her young age. But family was very much against it. Throughout her stay she vacillated between optimism and pessimism, not sure whether to go with the opinion of friends or family.

Her family had insisted on four courses of chemotherapy, which brought the breast tumor down from 5½ cm to half that size. But did not completely destroy it. It did destroy the small nodule in the arm pit. In spite of these improvements, they still wanted to do a mastectomy. No professional person would want to see a young life snuffed out, so whatever dismemberment could guarantee safety for her was gladly recommended. We would do no less, if there were no other way to give her hope for life.

But she wanted to attend to her teeth before coming to Mexico. A relative, being a dentist, gave her eight beautiful, shiny porcelain teeth right across the front of her mouth to replace amalgams; he felt he knew best for her. This would prove her undoing, because she was afraid of his wrath if these teeth were touched. Besides, she was in love with these teeth, as any

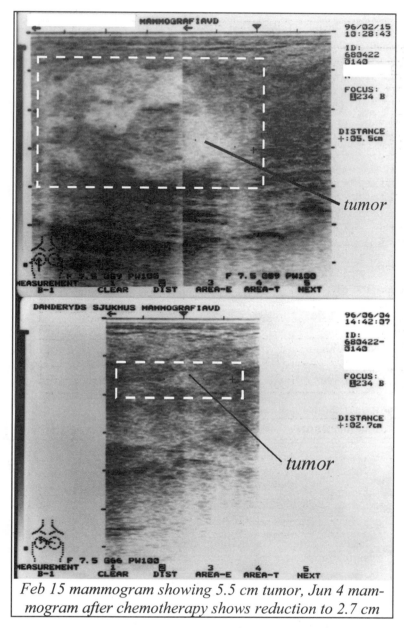

Feb 15 mammogram showing 5.5 cm tumor, Jun 4 mammogram after chemotherapy shows reduction to 2.7 cm

young woman might be after a lifetime of bad dental health and a defensive smile.

So with our hands tied by "untouchable teeth", we decided to do our best with the tumor she brought. Perhaps she would learn the issues herself and then be personally able to control her destiny. It was not to be. At least not in this visit. Although the tumor disappeared, it would surely return under the strong influence of heavy metals and malonates seeping from her porcelains. One couldn't help but wonder what she had been eating to give her eight rotten front teeth in the first place. But this was past history and comes now Jess with mammograms in hand.

The Feb. 15 mammogram shows the tumor as it had been (football shaped white area between the two + signs) at 5.5 cm. By June 4 the tumor was reduced, but still covered a narrow oblong area of 2.7 cm in length. She arrived three days later. Our initial tests showed ortho-phospho-tyrosine Positive at lymph nodes, Negative at breast. Evidently all parasites had been killed at the breast location, perhaps even by the chemotherapy. But they survived at the lymph nodes. Malonic acid Positive at breast; benzene Positive; isopropyl Positive (she would get off shampoo and bottled water immediately); *E. coli* Positive; CFC Positive (she should change her refrigerator at home); fiberglass Positive; aluminum Positive (probably her porcelain teeth); arsenic Positive; copper Positive (she would go to our safest Mexican motel immediately); formaldehyde Positive; cobalt Positive (she would stop using detergent, but was it hiding in her porcelain?); mercury and thallium Positive (leftover amalgam, now permanently hidden under the porcelain); aflatoxin Positive (she would read the section on moldy food in the *Cure For All Cancers* book).

We had no time to lose; thirty days is a very short time to disintegrate a tumor of this size; perhaps it can't be done at all with leftover amalgam and fresh aluminum plus malonic acid placed in the mouth to be sucked on day and night.

We started her the very first day on:
- the freon removal program
- 2 tsp. black walnut tincture extra strength parasite program with zapping
- vitamin B_{12} and folic acid
- vitamin C
- cysteine, taurine, glutathione
- coenzyme Q10
- thyroid 1½ grain in the morning
- wearing no regular bra, the athletic variety that does not lift would be okay.

Because of the handicap in dealing with her porcelain teeth, and the urgency of saving her from mastectomy in thirty days, the decision was made to use IV therapy daily. Cost was not her main issue. Time was. Success was. Perhaps, too, if she saw the tumor shrink she would gain confidence in the underlying theory and come to her own conclusion that the porcelain must go. They hide clostridium bacteria, hide bits of amalgam, and seep carcinogenic materials. Her IV was formulated after her blood test was read, June 8.

It was rather poor for a young woman, who should be at the peak of her health.

Both RBC and WBC were probably lowered due to the chemotherapy and would soon rise. The two liver enzymes, AST and ALT were higher than a healthy person should have. [*But the LDH showed almost no dye toxicity yet.*] Uric acid was too low, showing a lack of glutamine [*we were not yet aware that it also implied Clostridium invasion*]. She was given a glutamine supplement. Both calcium and phosphate were very slightly elevated, showing an upcoming problem in the thyroid.

Her iron level, 55, was acceptable, but suggested copper toxicity, which, indeed, it was. Potassium was much too low. She was given potassium gluconate powder equivalent to 1 gm potassium/day and told to use sodium-potassium salt to help keep it up.

Her first IV contained 2 doses of EDTA to pull out copper, plus vitamin B-complex and vitamin C. After these, she was tested for copper again, at liver and parathyroids. She was now Negative, so the IV was changed to: laetrile, DMSO, B complex, calcium, magnesium, vitamin C. She would get this daily except Sunday. Since her mammogram was perfectly fresh, we did not schedule a new ultrasound.

By the fifth day, she was feeling much better and sleeping better. She was now testing Positive for glutathione, TNF, and methionine at the breast. But there was still no glycine. (This is an amino acid that should always be

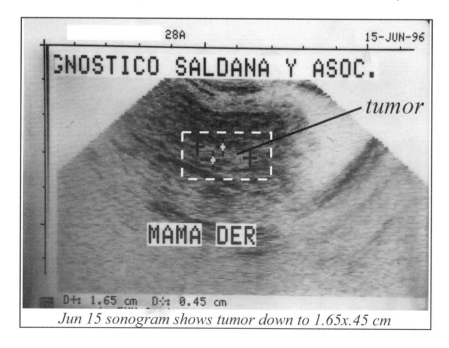

Jun 15 sonogram shows tumor down to 1.65x.45 cm

present.) We added glycine to her supplement list. She also continued to test Positive for mercury and thallium.

Her second blood test showed improved liver enzymes, AST, and ALT, but albumin was too high and LDH had gone up slightly, too. Iron had dropped further. The usual culprits were at work: malonic acid, cobalt, and perhaps hidden copper and vanadium. Mercury and thallium were Positive at breast and lymph node every day, in spite of removing every scrap from her environment (paper goods).

A sonogram of the breast eight days after her arrival, nevertheless, showed great improvement. Only a small bit of the tumor remained. It was measured to be 1.65 x 0.45 cm, a far cry from 2 x 2.7 cm when she arrived. The system was working. Unfortunately, she concluded that this proved it would not be necessary to disturb her porcelain teeth and was more adamant than ever!

Her IVs continued. Her mercury and thallium toxicity continued. We added thioctic acid to her supplement list. In spite of all this, her next blood test, June 18, did not show improvement. BUN—that is, her ability to make urea—was lower than ever, and her calcium and potassium were very low, also.

Her next ultrasound done on June 24 showed no tumors in the breast at all! Two radiologists agreed on this. But she was not at all happy. She was sure it was a mistake. Her family, too, by telephone persuaded her it was all a big mistake; that Mexican ultrasounds were forgeries, rigged somehow, and she should come home at once. And have a mastectomy.

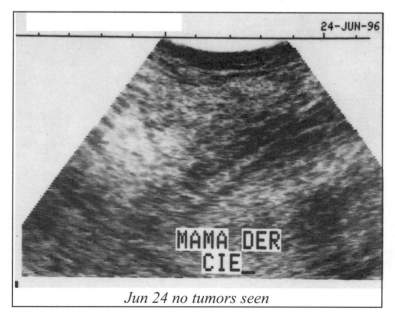

Jun 24 no tumors seen

400

Indeed, there might be a remnant, too small for ultrasound to detect, remaining. We, too, harbored these misgivings. And a CT scan would have been better. But she had money to save and ultrasounds are much, much cheaper. She could do the CT scan at home with fresh resources. The radiologist here could see no tumors. It suggested disappearance.

Several more blood tests showed some ups and downs. Malonic acid continued to be Positive, while uric acid bottomed out at 0.6, and calcium and potassium stayed low. The parathyroids had been targeted possibly due to their nearness to the tooth restorations.

We prevailed on her to stay a little longer; she was still getting sensations in the breast. *Staphylococcus aureus* was still in her lymph nodes. She consented to a panoramic X-ray of her mouth to search for cavitations. Several were easy to spot. The dentist cleaned them.

We took her off IVs on July 3 to see if the tumor would reappear. Her thirty days were up, but her personal intuition prevailed. She extended her stay for two weeks. She could now enjoy her days without being hooked up to an IV bag. Six days later, July 9, her blood test showed significant improvements: LDH down and potassium up. But it was still poor by our standards.

We decided to do a complete heavy metal test. It turned up zirconium Positive; aluminum Positive; aluminum silicate Positive; D-malic acid Positive at both breast and lymph node. The battle was not won. The implication was porcelain. She called her family for permission to change the porcelain

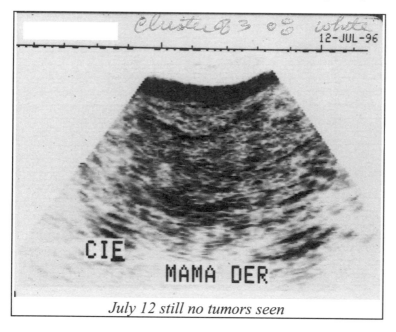

July 12 still no tumors seen

teeth to plastic. It was not given despite copious tears and explanations. One family member was a dentist and one an MD and her body had to be sacrificed for them. Surely, these blind forces of submission, that tie us with irrational might, are no different than live-spouse burials and other human sacrifices we have learned about in history books. She had the power to escape, to make her own decision, but she didn't try. [*That's how I felt at the time. Ironically we now know the plastic might have been worse.*]

One more blood test was done, and another ultrasound. Again, no tumors could be seen. The blood test improved further, but it was not very different than when she arrived.

The accomplishment was only the shrinkage of her tumor.

Summary: We had done our part. And we wished her well. She smiled, but all I could see was the porcelain—it would stalk her like a predator. Perhaps she would understand its true nature eventually. These teeth should all have been extracted.

Jess Ingerson	6/8	6/13	6/18	6/26	7/4	7/9	7/16
RBC	4.09	4.08	3.8	3.91	3.69	3.96	4.16
WBC	2300	4600	4900	3700	5000	4400	4600
PLT	275	274	208	140	227	253	194
glucose	129	78	102	93	107	90	89
BUN	10	10	9.0	12	9	11	10
creatinine	.9	1.0	.8	.9	.9	.9	.9
AST (SGOT)	31	23	26	32	33	31	28
ALT (SGPT)	39	26	23	53	53	41	31
LDH	162	176	179	252	210	192	164
GGT	17	12	15	22	21	17	18
T.b.	.7	.7	.4	.6	.5	.5	.5
alk phos	41	45	51	51	53	50	57
T.p.	6.5	7.0	6.7	6.7	6.9	6.9	7.2
albumin	4.7	5.2	4.7	4.8	4.5	4.9	4.9
globulin	1.8	1.8	2.0	1.9	2.4	2.0	2.3
uric acid	2.5	1.4	2.2	.6	3.3	1.3	3.0
Calcium	9.7	9.1	8.6	8.5	8.5	8.7	9.4
Phosphorus	4.1	5.1	3.8	3.6	3.8	4.8	3.8
Iron	55	45	57	103	86	37	84
Sodium	135	141	142	141	142	139	140
Potassium	3.7	3.7	3.6	3.6	3.9	4.0	3.7
Chloride	108	104	105	99	106	100	104
triglycerides	54	95	17	59	53	47	161
cholesterol	155	172	104	124	140	148	146

30	Tracy Guerin	Ovarian & Lung Cancer

Tracy Guerin, fifty-four, started her bout with cancer five years ago. It was ovarian cancer then; but now it was in the lung. She had already been drained of the fluid accumulation three times. It was accumulating faster now, and she arrived huffing and puffing, and somewhat hoarse. In spite of this, she was making plans to leave for another country where she held a post of international importance. If a good attitude plays a role, it had its benefits here. Her cheery smile belied all the facts in the matter.

Her toxic metals included aluminum, nickel, copper, cadmium, cobalt, mercury, and thallium. She was also full of freon, fiberglass, formaldehyde, three vicious air toxins. She agreed to clean these up at once. She had both patulin and aflatoxin build-up and agreed to stop eating apples, dried fruit, grocery bread, and nuts. She took off her jewelry and cosmetics.

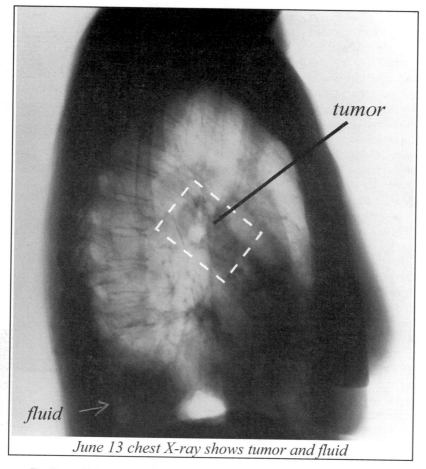

tumor

fluid

June 13 chest X-ray shows tumor and fluid

By June 1996, we already knew what causes pleural effusions—maleic anhydride. We could observe maleic anhydride being formed from maleic acid by the body if vitamin C was present. And maleic anhydride could be further detoxified to D-malic acid, again, if vitamin C was present. [*But we didn't know that maleic acid was a direct component of certain dental plastics and that it would diffuse out forever if you were the unlucky recipient. Nor did we know that acrylic plastic is detoxified to malonic acid by the body, which then could be turned into maleic acid.*] At least one source could be removed, the food source. She began at once to eat only malonate-free food.

It was June 12; she had to leave in six weeks. The task was impossible. Her chest X-ray showed a pear shaped mass, pronounced lymphatic nodules, and fluid at the base that obliterated the lung margin. This news did not discourage her. She agreed to change her plumbing, get her dental problems corrected, and start right now with an IV containing 3 doses of EDTA to pull the heavy metals out of her body. She started the parasite program and coenzyme Q10, and glutathione. She started taking Lugol's and using white iodine for brushing teeth.

Her blood test did not reveal her critical condition. She was still in good health. And she would be able to recover if her lung problem was corrected. It was only that, a problem. Not broken down health. [*Her LDH and alk phos were both very slightly elevated to show there was some toxicity from dyes, but not much.*]

The alk phos spoke for the lungs. The total protein was also very slightly elevated; the globulin just a bit too high. Iron was too low due to copper, and potassium was too low, also. Perhaps she would be saved by her normal triglycerides and cholesterol. We were grateful for these. She got off to a slow start by not getting into the copper-free housing immediately. Three days later she still had some copper at the thyroid and parathyroid glands. So EDTA had to be applied again. After this the IVs would consist of laetrile, DMSO, vitamin C, and cesium.

In spite of perfect adherence to the malonate-free diet, it was still present at the parathyroids. This would account for the drop in calcium to 8.8 at the next blood test, done June 21. Copper and vanadium, too, persisted at the parathyroids. We wondered if the vanadium and malonate had been newly placed in her mouth. She was in the middle of amalgam replacement. The LDH went up instead of down. Yet, the alk phos, reflecting the lung condition, went down. Would this show up on the next lung X-ray? The effect of vanadium would also explain the RBC rise. The rise in serum iron could only mean there was less copper toxicity due to amalgam removal. The uric acid dropped as it became unmasked. We supplemented glutamine.

By June 26 (two weeks later), Tracy was feeling very much better. She was no longer huffing and puffing; her voice sounded strong; her personality sparkled. Should we dare repeat the chest X-ray? It was only thirteen days from the first discouraging one. Only if she promised not to be discouraged. She did. We needed her continued optimism and compliance if we should do an early follow-up. The new X-ray showed almost double her former air capacity—twice as much white area on the print. Her lungs were filled with air again; no wonder she could walk briskly.

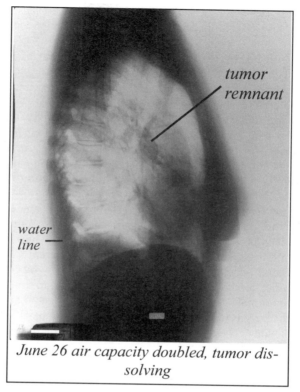

tumor remnant

water line

June 26 air capacity doubled, tumor dissolving

The water-logging of her lungs had stopped, the base of the lung was now fully expanded where water had accumulated before (see arrow drawn by radiologist on earlier X-ray).

The large tumor had lost its top half; it was evidently pulling apart and dissolving. Other tumors were just vaguely visible. The water line was much lower. She had her lungs and her life back. But she did not chafe and beg to leave. We appreciated her wisdom.

By June 28, a blood test showed her iron level up to normal, and other improvements. But by July 4, the gains were eroding. What had transpired in that time? It had been about ten days since her amalgam had been removed and plastic installed. We could attribute the gain to amalgam removal, should we blame the plastic for the deterioration?

She changed her glasses frames to plastic and abruptly lost her breast pain. The pain was actually <u>under</u> the left breast, no doubt where the large lung tumor had its remains. We stopped her IVs—no longer necessary. We started her on Lung Tea, mullein and comfrey, cooked together to make a strong tea. Plus garlic, one raw clove daily; no need to chew, just bite and swallow.

By July 12, a new chest X-ray (not shown) still showed a remnant of tumor, it was now spindle shaped. And a region of infection was still apparent.

She was still Positive for nickel. She did a liver cleanse, but it did not get rid of nickel. We gave her thioctic acid, but it did nothing. Finally, she found it herself. She pulled out a personal air purifier with a shiny metal case that you hang around your neck; it blows "purified" air at you. Hers blew nickel. She stopped using it. The nickel disappeared in two days. But she still had pain in the lung near the breast bone in the morning when awakening. When she arrived in the morning totally fasted, a saliva sample was still Positive for malonic acid derivatives. Where could it be coming from except her own body? That is, what had been placed in her own body. We began to suspect the new dental work. But her stay was near its end.

She had received three crowns (against directions), one bridge, eight fillings, and two porcelain fillings (against directions). With a bacterial problem like hers, it was ill advised to invite them into a new hiding place under a crown. She was game for removal of one crown only. We explained it was not a moral issue, as she carefully brushed the tiny bit of plastic that was covering her tooth stub. Then we rubbed it with an emery board. It tested Positive for maleic acid. This would seep out and get to her lungs. The body would detoxify it to maleic anhydride and then not be able to detoxify it further in the lung. The anhydride would cause effusion of liquid from the lung again.

Her mouth had to be redone! But she would hear none of it. Her mouth looked beautiful again, her tumor was gone (last X-ray not shown), her lungs worked, and her departure date was just days away. She felt she could risk it. I didn't. But we wished her Bon Voyage. And we had learned a mighty lesson: that malonic acid could come not only from tapeworm stages and food, but from a totally unrelated, inanimate source—plastic. And it was a precious discovery made by electronic testing of dental plastic directly. Would we now be able to clear up the mystery-source of malonates that had plagued us for so long?

Tracy Guerin	6/12	6/21	6/28	7/4	7/9	7/16	7/23	8/2
RBC	4.55	4.91	4.47	4.74	4.74	4.99	4.75	4.75
WBC	5300	7000	7800	6900	5400	6300	6100	5900
PLT	325	254	213	236	251	422	291	277
BUN	16	22	10	12	113	11	14	11
creatinine	1.0	1.0	1.2	1.0	.9	.9	.7	.8
AST (SGOT)	29	26	23	26	27	22	22	21
ALT (SGPT)	35	29	23	24	20	19	21	24
LDH	181	195	194	215	205	202	203	198
GGT	64	43	30	25	19	18	15	13
T.b.	0.9	0.6	0.8	0.9	0.7	0.5	0.6	0.5
alk phos	104	85	73	85	82	89	85	75

T.p.	7.8	7.0	6.8	7.5	7.3	7.5	7.1	6.7
albumin	4.6	4.7	4.5	4.4	4.5	4.6	4.8	4.4
globulin	3.2	2.3	2.3	3.1	2.8	2.9	2.3	2.3
uric acid	3.2	2.5	2.6	4.2	4.7	5	4.2	4.2
Calcium	9.2	8.8	8.8	9.3	9.3	9.5	9.1	9.1
Phosphorus	4.2	3.3	4	4.0	3.2	3.4	3.2	3.5
Iron	38	54	102	61	55	58	47	37
Potassium	3.9	4.0	4.0	4.6	4.2	4.3	4.2	4.1
triglycerides	148	152	141	246	125	112	117	67
cholesterol	186	165	167	154	153	146	174	152

31   Wendy Skoglund   Brain & Liver Cancer

Wendy Skoglund came from Finland with cancer of the brain and liver. There were nine hemangioma-like cysts in the liver, which were the cause of her anxiety. She felt the brain tumor was not bothering her, although she had some facial paralysis. She also had numbness in her left fingers.

Our testing, though, showed there was malignancy (ortho-phospho-tyrosine) in the brain, not in the liver. Therefore, we focused our attention on the brain. Chronic headache and tremors added weight to this decision.

An MRI done a year earlier showed a single tumor at the posterior oc-cipital on the right side. The radiologist's inner circle marks the boundary. The full skull view showed the bones bulging out in little billows from the

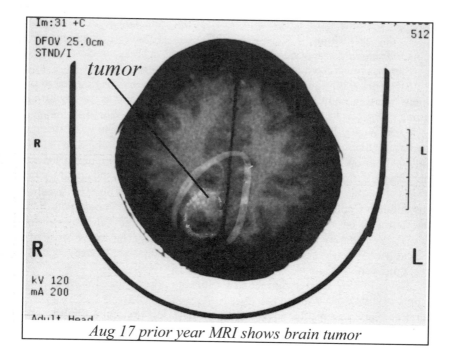

Aug 17 prior year MRI shows brain tumor

407

internal pressure (not shown).

Her initial toxin test done at the liver showed:

Solvents and Pathogens	Metals	Other toxins
isopropyl Positive	cobalt Positive	malonic acid Positive
wood alcohol Positive	copper Positive	patulin Positive
	arsenic Positive	CFC Positive
Salmonella typhimurium Positive	mercury Positive	chlorine Positive
Staphylococcus aureus Positive at		aflatoxin Positive
cerebrum and liver		

She was immediately taken to a Mexican "copper-free" motel nearby. Actually it was only copper-free in dry weather. If it rained and a main water pipe broke, water would be brought in by tankers; this always contained copper and all clinic patients did a hasty exodus to other quarters. Her metal glasses frames needed to be changed to plastic, too, to eliminate copper.

A mouthful of gold and plastic would also have to be cleaned up. She had some implants that our dentist did not want to remove. But with dental bacteria in the brain, no metal whatsoever could remain. It would cost a small fortune. In fact, they had already cost her a small fortune. Wendy was a forward looking person, though, ever practical; she scheduled it all for removal regardless of obstacles. She was only fifty-six.

On her first day, she was started on the following: 1. The parasite killing program plus zapping. This would eliminate the malignancy. Then began our race to shrink the tumor before her return airline ticket date. 2. Glutathione. 3. Lugol's iodine until *Salmonella* was absent from her brain. Then only once a day, at bedtime. 4. Coenzyme Q10. This would kill tapeworm remnants [*our method at that time*].

She was given the malonate-free food list to observe.

Since her symptoms were gradually worsening, there was no need to get a new "starting point" MRI of the brain. It was unlikely that the tumor had shrunk in light of her worsening symptoms. Would we be able to shrink it?

Then Wendy had to make an important decision. Did she want IV therapy or not? She had come a long way to stop this life threatening disease. We could put her on IV therapy including laetrile, DMSO, cesium, our "tried and true" tumor shrinkers. This would cost $330.00 per day. Or she could try our new IV-free therapy consisting of large doses of supplements. Her question was pointed: Could I guarantee tumor shrinkage with IVs? I could not, in the time frame of her stay. Would IVs be faster than no IVs? This was still unknown. We had only recently begun our no-IV therapy. Her long history of a natural life-style (except for dentistry) won the debate. She chose to go IV-free, unless she got worse.

Never had we hustled more than for this brain tumor, one of our first attempts to shrink one without IVs.

Her blood test results arrived the next day, July 31. Only the uric acid was too low. Everything else was nearly perfect. It would not be necessary to do repeated blood tests. We supplemented her with glutamine. [*We did not yet understand <u>the</u> most critical significance of a low uric acid level– Clostridium bacteria!*]

Potassium was somewhat low. She was given potassium gluconate powder to take. Triglycerides were too low. She should eat high fat food, such as avocados, butter, and cream.

Wendy was a perfect example of a patient

Aug 12 inner white spot with square is tumor remnant

given a dismal "terminal" prognosis by her regular doctor, although the blood test shows a truly healthy person. Only the <u>location</u> of the tumor makes it life threatening.

For the first eight days she continued to test Positive for copper and malonic acid. She was still in the process of dental work. She was given EDTA powder by mouth to remove it meanwhile. The dentist had found four cavitations, besides, at her four wisdom teeth. Finally, no metal or urethane (plastic) could be detected in her brain or anywhere. Her teeth were "empty", not extracted (all fillings out, nothing replaced). But she thrived on her "empty mouth" status. Her left hand numbness disappeared. Her heel pain disappeared. The tension left her head. Energy was up. And she just felt better all over. She was getting impatient to have her dentalware put back! We explained the hazard of using anything new till full healing was complete. All foreign things seek out a trauma site—morbitropism.

We were now becoming impatient to see if her tumor was shrinking. After two weeks she did a CT brain scan. The tumor was about half its earlier size of a year ago. It was now 1.9 x 1.9 cm. It had been

Wendy Skoglund	7/31
RBC	4.49
WBC	6,400
PLT	322
glucose	145
BUN	9 (5-26)
creatinine	0.9
AST (SGOT)	28
ALT (SGPT)	22
LDH	159
GGT	9
T.b.	0.8
alk phos	69
T.p.	7
albumin	4.7
globulin	2.3
uric acid	2.6 (2.5-6.1)
Calcium	9.0
Phosphorus	4.1
Iron	80
Sodium	140
Potassium	3.9
Chloride	106
triglycerides	72
cholesterol	232

2 x 6 cm. A liver scan was done, too (not shown), revealing the nine heman-giomas—not tumors. [*Hemangiomas may be due to oxidation products of vitamin C.*]

A few days later, her finger numbness returned. And also the right heel pain. We searched for toxins; it was mercury. Her foods and products were tested for mercury and thallium. Only paper towels tested Positive. She stopped using them.

We supplemented her with taurine, cysteine, thioctic acid. Nothing helped. She continued to test Positive for mercury. She had not yet parted with all her dental gold. Could it be that?

We raised her thioctic. Yet she was Positive. We searched her for the full list of heavy metals. She was Positive for nickel, too. Then it was obvi-ous. This could only come from gold because nickel is used as a hardener for it. The curse of Midas was in her mouth. There was probably amalgam under the gold. But she only had one day left. She ran to get the gold out! In her haste and anxiety over unfilled teeth, she accepted unsafe plastic dental ma-terial for restorations. She boarded her plane. She felt good. Her symptoms were gone again. She had achieved what she came for. And we had achieved our first brain tumor shrinkage without IVs. But she will be back.

Summary: Time and financial constraints shaped Wendy's life as much as ours. What was the final outcome? Could healthful living keep up with toxin release from her mouth? Would she suspect the truth in time? We wish her well.

32	Suzanne Codding	? Cancer

Suzanne Codding was a beautiful twenty month-old girl, but there was quite a lump on the right side of her neck. It might have started with strep throat for which she had been given Augmentin and Amoxicillin (antibiotics). After the strep throat, the lump appeared and grew rapidly. It was surgically removed and clinically tested for everything: malignancy, fungus, and bacteria. Everything was Negative, except possibly a kind of bird tuberculosis. It was only six weeks since the surgery and the lump had already returned; in fact, it was 1½ x 1½ inches in size. Another surgery was being scheduled. The parents were alarmed.

Taking the tuberculosis hint, I searched for resonance with my three *My-cobacterium* slides. I also tested for *Mycoplasma*. The baby's saliva sample was used instead of the baby's hand for testing. *Mycobacterium phlei* was Positive. No others.

The same saliva sample was used to do the initial toxin test. Ortho-phospho-tyrosine was Positive, indicating a malignancy, despite the earlier clinical tests. Additionally, all of these were Positive:

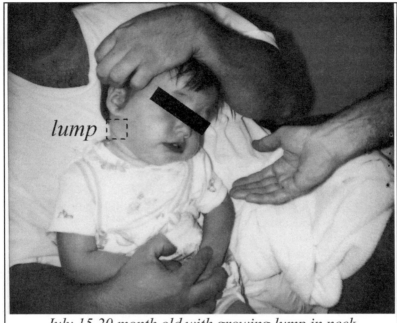

July 15 20 month old with growing lump in neck

Bacteria and Solvents	Metals	Other Toxins
Salmonella dysenteriae	copper (water pipes)	aflatoxin
Salmonella paratyphi	cobalt	CFC
	mercury (diapers)	malonic acid
isopropyl alcohol		

Mycobacterium phlei is considered an innocuous soil bacterium. But I frequently find it present in brain diseases. It is <u>always</u> present in schizophrenia. Usually, family members and their dog have it also. It can be found in the dental area, possibly under tooth fillings or in tooth infections. Of course, Suzanne had neither.

Suzanne's parents both tested Positive to *Mycobacterium phlei*, although there was no family dog. However, relatives had dogs and they would visit occasionally. Perhaps she had been licked on the face: The parents were advised not to let the child near a dog.

She was immediately given the herbal parasite treatment and zapped. Twenty minutes later she was re-tested for ortho-phospho-tyrosine. She was still Positive. Two and three-quarter hours later she was Negative. They could go home for one week. The parents were instructed to treat themselves the same way immediately. The baby's diet was made safe from reinfection. The water pipes were to be changed to plastic. The refrigerator was to be changed. No commercial diapers, or any personal products made of paper

411

were to be used on her. No detergent was to be used. And no crackers, cookies, grocery bread, or cold cereals; only white bakery bread, to eliminate aflatoxin. No malonate-containing food.

The next week, both parents and Suzanne were Negative for *Mycobacterium phlei*. Isopropyl alcohol and malonic acid were Negative. But copper and aflatoxin were still Positive. They were advised to hurry with the changes. They had done everything else, including daily zapping and once-a-week parasite herbs, scaled down to her age.

On July 29, another week later, the lump was very much smaller and softer. But she was still Positive for copper and malonic acid although they had finished the plumbing job. They had been visiting relatives with her and her milk had been boiled, but no vitamin C had been added (this allows malonic acid to persist). They were all still Negative for *Mycobacterium phlei*.

On August 5, the lump was down to $1/2$ x $1/8$ inch, a mere sliver. It was a joyful visit. The tumor was not growing. It was still soft and receding She had picked up some aflatoxin while visiting relatives, but the parents promised to be more watchful. She was started on glutathione once a day. They were all still free of *Mycobacterium phlei*.

August 12 was their last visit, nothing could be seen or felt at the site of the former tumor. I scheduled a CT scan of the neck region, to be done without contrast, but let them choose whether to do it. After all, it was only for the record, not for Suzanne's benefit. Seeing and feeling was reliable enough for her safety.

Summary: Did it come back? Or did it stay away? We won't know unless the parents inform us. The parents did an exemplary job, and we wish them well.

33	Adam Larsen	Lung & Liver Cancer

Adam Larsen had 16 small to medium nodules on the <u>outside</u> of his lungs and liver. They were not calcified, meaning they were active in some way. But were they merely plaque? Some of them looked rectangular, not round. Or were they metastasized from the prostate, a most unusual kind of metastasis? His prostate had a very malignant (stage 4) little tumor in it although his PSA was only 10.0 (over 4 is considered cancerous). If the sixteen nodules were benign, then surgery to remove the prostate seemed wise to one of his doctors. And urgent. But if the 16 nodules were malignant, then he was in a late stage of disease, with very little hope and prostate surgery useless. It would be pretty hard to biopsy one of them, though. Two or three weeks passed in indecision. He started the parasite program at home, corrected his life style to shut out isopropyl alcohol and zapped a lot. He had decided against surgery, and therefore, biopsy, since this couldn't save him anyway, he believed.

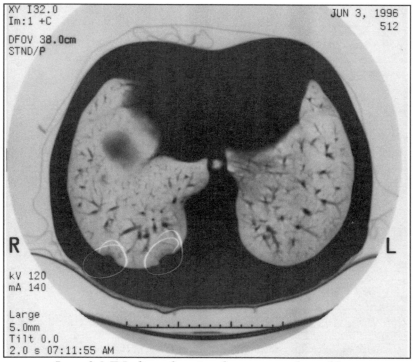

June 3 MRI slice showing lumps on edge of lung

When he arrived two months later in August, he already tested Negative for isopropyl alcohol and malignancy. He had successfully stopped his cancer, but the task was now to shrink his tumors. One look at his CT scan of the liver showed small <u>internal</u> tumors ("marbles") as well. He was Positive for patulin, lead, and CFC. He had a *Staphylococcus* infection spreading from his jaw although he wore full dentures. He had gotten his PSA down to 8 by himself. And a fresh scan of the prostate showed no tumor at all—only enlargement. He was doing well on his own.

He was started by removing both dentures until they could be tested for malonate and the usual carcinogens. This meant he would blend his food and simply drink it until he had teeth again. He did not mind a bit. We reassured him that these liver tumors were small by comparison with the usual liver tumors we see. The nodules on the surface of liver and lungs certainly were perplexing; we would just wait and see what happened to them after getting rid of the internal liver tumors. And the prostate, too, ought to shrink along with the liver tumors.

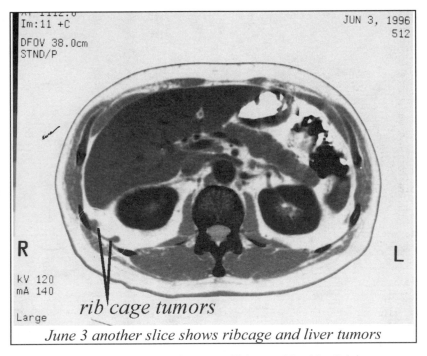

Im:11 +C
JUN 3, 1996
512
DFOV 38.0cm
STND/P

R

L

kV 120
mA 140

Large

rib cage tumors

June 3 another slice shows ribcage and liver tumors

His blood test showed that he was still in good health. Calcium was too low; implying a toxin in the parathyroids and alk phos was slightly high implying tumor activity in his lungs [*dye toxicity*].

His potassium was borderline low. Other values were quite good. He was still a healthy man, age sixty-one. The high WBC was explained by the bacteria in his jaw and prostate.

He was given the usual supplements to detoxify malonic acid: B_{12} (4 mg), folic acid (25 mg twice daily), and vitamin C. He was also given glutamine and glucuronic acid. The glucuronate would help his liver detoxify harmful chemicals. And he was given potassium gluconate to raise his potassium levels. All this besides doing the parasite program, Lugol's, and other programs.

His metal glasses frames were scheduled for change to plastic. He was still very Positive for copper at the parathyroid gland even without wearing his dentures. He and his wife were staying at an unapproved motel with copper water pipes. They agreed to move immediately.

The following day he was Negative for copper and malonates. Having dentures made the task easy. Simply remove them and make new ones— malonate free.

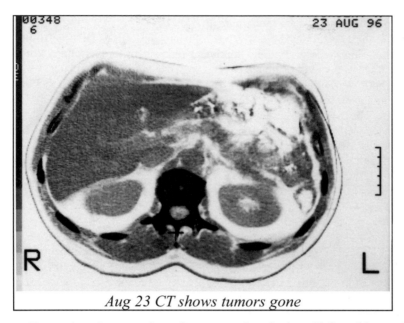

Aug 23 CT shows tumors gone

He continued to stay free of copper and malonic acid from his supplements and diet. He simply threw away his supplements, except the list given which had been tested. And he never veered off the malonate-free food list.

By the seventh day, he definitely felt better, although he had no real complaints to begin with. Another blood test showed small improvements: LDH down; calcium up; iron up from 57, due to copper [*and germanium*] removal. He was given chromium-yeast capsules containing 500 mcg chromium, two a day, experimentally, to raise blood sugar.

On the tenth day he tested Positive for methyl malonate and had picked up benzene, too, no doubt from eating unsafe food. He detoxified it immediately and was Negative the next day. A new CT of the liver was scheduled, without contrast, to minimize this burden

Adam Larsen	8/12	8/19
RBC	4.58	4.63
WBC	10,200	10,100
PLT	160	149
glucose	83	76
BUN	12	14
creatinine	.8	.9
AST (SGOT)	31	29
ALT (SGPT)	30	26
LDH	154	147
GGT	14	17
T.b.	0.4	0.4
alk phos	113	125
T.p.	6.7	7.0
albumin	4.6	4.5
globulin	2.1	2.5
uric acid	3.9	3.3 (3.5-8.5)
Calcium	8.6	9.0
Phosphorus	2.9	3.5
Iron	57	76
Sodium	137	138
Potassium	4.0	4.4
Chloride	104	102
triglycerides	66	105
cholesterol	184	180

for his liver [*and to avoid lanthanides*].

On the twelfth day he fairly bounced into the office, CT scan in hand. Two radiologists could find no "marbles", plaques, or tumors of any kind on the surface of his liver or rib cage. The lung scan could wait till later.

There were no small "marbles" inside his liver, either, although fibrous remnants were visible to me. These were considered to be "bad texture," not tumors, now. He had tested Negative to copper, isopropyl alcohol, and staphylococcus bacteria in the prostate and had probably been free of them for ten full days in a row. He had two new dentures that tested free of malonates and metals and he was eager to eat his food again, instead of drinking it.

It was time for him to leave to practice his new life style. He promised to return in two months for follow-up. As soon as he got home he did a new PSA test. It was down to 5.8.

Summary: Adam was a perfect patient and deserved his good results. Or did luck play a role when no dental problems presented themselves that couldn't be corrected in one minute—just by removing his dentures? They were out of his mouth for twelve days. Or was it the extra-large dose of folic acid? Of course, he had already dissolved the grade 4 malignancy in his prostate by himself before he arrived. We wish him well.

34 **Lorene Ralls**	**Fibrocystic Disease**

Lorene Ralls, forty-one, had a family history of breast cancer. Her doctor told her not to worry, but she worried more and more as new family members got the disease. Finally, her massage therapist found three lumps and she knew the inevitable was beginning to happen. Both breasts had pain and stinging sensations. She didn't know why. Besides, she was generally fatigued and in poor health. She wanted to do something about her lumpy breasts before she, too, had cancer.

She had started herself on the parasite program three months ago, so there was no ortho-phospho-tyrosine and, therefore, no malignancy anywhere when she arrived. But she had not eliminated isopropyl alcohol so she was at great risk for getting cancer or getting it back if she had it earlier. By using unsterilized dairy products daily, she was picking up the fluke parasite stages. They would multiply in the presence of isopropyl alcohol.

She immediately stopped drinking purchased water or beverages and taking untested supplements. She also had benzene and toluene built up in her. These would be gone, too, by stopping the beverage habit. She was zapping daily.

She had two systemic bacteria, *E. coli* and *Staphylococcus aureus*. The staphylococcus bacteria would be under a metal or plastic tooth or in a cavitation. Both would find a breeding place in her breast lump to make it grow.

Her other toxins were: CFCs, nickel, copper, cobalt, mercury, thallium, aluminum, arsenic, and formaldehyde.

She had no patulin or aflatoxin build up. We scheduled a blood test and ultrasound of breast. Then started her on the current cancer program. The reasoning was that if she could shrink these tumors she could prevent getting cancer in them, and be spared the family fate.

Her program consisted of: starting freon removal, changing water pipes to plastic, doing the parasite program, taking coenzyme Q10, taking glutathione, taking Lugol's iodine, once a day for prevention of *Salmonella* invasion, replacing metal in teeth with plastic, sticking to the malonate-free diet, and stopping all supplements unless she could test them for copper, cobalt, vanadium, and the M-family (ours were already tested).

Of course, she would change her refrigerator to a non-freon variety. She was very interested in cause and effect relationships, so she planned to learn the technique of testing in order to protect herself from breast cancer in the future.

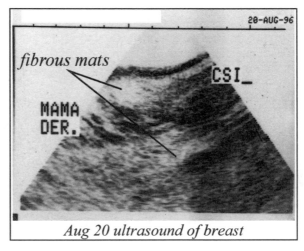

Aug 20 ultrasound of breast

The hardness in her breasts was quite easy to feel. The ultrasound showed fibrous masses throughout both breasts, the right side being more extensively involved. They should all go away, leaving the breast soft. She was eager to start.

Two days later, we reviewed the blood test with her. The early stages of cobalt and malonate toxicity are clearly present: globulin is too low and calcium is too low also. The damage from copper and vanadium is not yet visible.

The RBC, WBC, and platelet count are perfectly normal showing that the toxins have not yet reached the bone marrow where these cells are made. Blood sugar (glucose) is extremely low, showing she was using it up much too fast without getting the energy benefit from it. This is characteristic of tumor disease. Triglycerides, another fuel, are also low. This would explain her general fatigue. The BUN is still unaffected. The LDH is still normal, below 160, showing the absence of dye buildup and aggressive tumor activity. Alk phos, which also reflects dye buildup and tumor activity, is low, too. Total protein, which is the sum of albumin and globulin, is completely normal, but the globulin is a little too low. This is caused by cobalt in the liver. It agrees with the finding of cobalt in the initial toxin test. Calcium should be 9.1 to 9.6. Low levels are caused by toxins, such as malonate in the parathyroids, one of its earliest toxic actions; perhaps it simply chelates out our valuable calcium. Potassium is too low. Perhaps this is due to vanadium. Vanadium is known to displace potassium, but the evidence is not yet clear. It could also be low due to insufficient potassium pump action by the tissues and a subsequent loss through the kidneys to keep the ratio between inside and outside of tissues correctly balanced. The thyroid, too, plays a role in potassium usage. For the present, we must be content to supplement potassium, since this is known to stimulate respiratory metabolism and could help the tumor tissue to normalize.

She was given the following supplements:
1. Vitamin D to raise the phosphate level to 3.
2. Potassium gluconate powder.
3. Vitamin B_{12}.
4. Folic acid, 1 mg, 25 a day. It would be easier to take a single 25 mg tablet, but that is not available. It takes 25 mg to team up with vitamin B_{12} to begin to detoxify all the malonic acid and its derivatives in the body. Even this amount cannot keep up with detoxifying malonic acid if it is eaten as food or constantly being sucked on in the mouth (dental plastic). The cancer patient has a huge deficit of these two nutrients. Chemotherapeutic agents frequently are "antifolate" compounds, intended to kill cancer cells. Our approach is not one of killing tumor cells; it is one of removing the factors that stimulate these cells to abnormal growth rates and repairing their metabolism so they begin to make their normal metabolites again (differentiation).
5. Vitamin C.
6. Biotin 1 mg once a day to repair the body's ability to utilize malonic acid in fat metabolism (this is hypothetical).

Lorene did her best to get rid of cobalt from her life style, at one point even finding a trace in a blue T-shirt and blue jeans (detergent residue). She carried her own dishes and glasses to avoid detergent washed ones. She cooked only at home. To no avail. The situation got worse instead of better.

She was testing Positive for <u>more</u>, not less, malonic acid derivatives although she had stopped eating any. And now she was showing copper again, although her water had been copper-free for four days already and the body level should have been going down.

We had become suspicious of dental work, since this seemed to be the only big event occurring. We decided to chip a bit off an old plastic tooth she had had for several years. It tested Positive for titanium and lead! And titanium and lead had been found in the breast!

The race was on to find other toxins in the dental plastic that were traveling to the breast. Here they would use up her precious glutathione. We began testing the dental materials presently being put into her mouth.

The new plastic had malonic and maleic acids, besides copper, cobalt, and vanadium! But not much had been put in yet! It was stopped–put on hold–till all plastic ingredients could be tested.

Meanwhile, the breasts had gotten much softer. The only hardness left was one area near the top of the right breast. The left side was already clear.

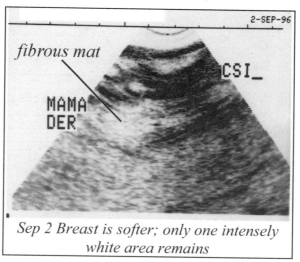

Sep 2 Breast is softer; only one intensely white area remains

An ultrasound and blood test were scheduled. Her frustration with stalled tooth filling and the frequent interruptions for testing and removal, all faded as she produced the negatives. Almost all the fibrous mat underlying the right breast was gone. A small area still persisted at the top. This matched her interpretation by palpation (feeling it). It was all worthwhile. She was escaping the family curse—on the women's side, and doing it in two weeks! The curse had existed for decades.

But the blood test showed a different side to the story. All was not well. The blood test is a tough-minded teacher.

The WBC was up showing some infection, probably from the dentist's hands. It can be avoided by swishing with Lugol's solution or 1% chlorine bleach (see Recipes) right in the dentist's office before, during, and after the procedure. The blood sugar was not yet up, so metabolism was not yet normal. She could make less BUN (urea) than before. Most significant was the big rise in LDH [new dyes put into teeth]. I suspected correctly that it was caused by new toxins put into her teeth. But the albumin and globulin levels were corrected; implying removal of cobalt. Uric acid was not yet up in spite of giving glutamine. And calcium, too, had not risen a bit; more evidence of malonate being put in her mouth to suck on continually. In spite of taking vitamin D, the phosphorus dropped instead of rising—toxins were reaching the parathyroids.

But iron had dropped a large amount. Only copper [*or germanium*] could do this. These must have gone into her mouth with the dentalware. Potassium did not come up in spite of considerable supplementation. But triglycerides did rise, always a good sign. She was going through less fuel in some ways.

The low calcium pointed to the parathyroids. Indeed, we found the copper there. Would Lorene stay and search for its source? Would she pursue her problems till LDH and calcium were correct? Not this time. She accepted the joy the ultrasound brought, but not the thundercloud on the horizon. The breast was normalizing at a very fast rate.

Summary: And we again learned that important lesson: the tumorous situation is distinct and different from the toxic situation revealed by the blood test. The tumor cannot be equated with the underlying toxicity. In fact, the tumor is not the lethal entity, unless of course it obstructs something or becomes infected or hemorrhages. The underlying toxicity is the life threatening part of tumor disease. The changes, subtle at first, brought about by copper, cobalt, vanadium, malonate [*and germanium and azo dyes*] are the real killers. Per-

Lorene Ralls	8/21	9/2
RBC	4.56	4.53
WBC	5,900	8,000
PLT	242	283
glucose	69	72
BUN	13	9
creatinine	1.0	0.9
AST (SGOT)	19	19
ALT (SGPT)	13	17
LDH	156	200
GGT	14	13
T.b.	0.8	0.4
alk phos	46	61
T.p.	6.7	6.4
albumin	4.8	4.4
globulin	1.9	2.0
uric acid	3.1	3.1
Calcium	8.6	8.6
Phosphorus	2.6	2.3
Iron	124	63
Sodium	140	136
Potassium	3.9	3.9
Chloride	101	103
triglycerides	89	114
cholesterol	254	217

haps she will return when the good news has been savored sufficiently. Or perhaps she can make the final changes herself; she may learn where the problem resides, what to do about it, and get it done all by herself.

35	Kristie Barnes	Ovarian & Liver Cancer

Kristie Barnes had surgery a year ago for tumors, possibly ovarian, pressing against the colon. They were the size of lemons, but gave her no symptoms. Since the surgery she had continued to bleed from the rectum. She had refused chemotherapy and radiation, since she never had symptoms. But now a CT scan had been done and to everyone's surprise the <u>liver</u> was full of tumors. Some rather large, most rather small.

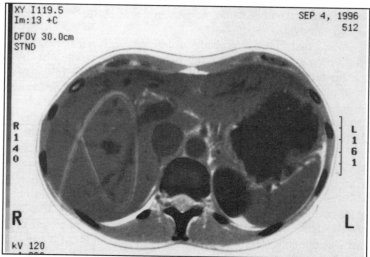

The radiologist circled several tumors (dark blotches).
Sep 4 CT revealed a liver full of tumors

She had been zapping for a time before she arrived, so the largest tumor looked a bit cyst-like, rather than malignant. But she still had isopropyl alcohol in her system.

Her initial toxin test showed freon at the colon; cobalt at the colon; and lead, thallium, arsenic, and copper at the bone marrow. *Salmonella* was Positive as well as malonic acid. But ortho-phospho-tyrosine was already Negative, giving her a nice head start to clear these liver tumors. The tumor marker, Ca 125 was still elevated (61), representing the remaining tumors. They should be easy to mop up.

She was in good physical health, otherwise, except for an intense tinnitus, which was her most troublesome symptom. I thought we could reduce this considerably, as well. She had brought a recent blood test (Aug. 27) with her. The main feature was an elevated total protein. The globulin was too high. Calcium and phosphate were also too high. And her body was definitely anemic (RBC 3.98).

The high albumin and globulin were due, no doubt, to the presence of both cobalt and vanadium in the liver. And the source of these must be her dentalware [*and Ascaris*], since all her supplements had been tested for these metals. She used no detergent or washing soda, no cosmetics or medications. So we did our new "tooth test" for her when she was in the fasted state in the morning (and after killing all tapeworm stages first). We tested for malonic acid and/or its derivatives in the saliva. She was Positive. Therefore, she must have plastic tooth restorations seeping malonates. Perhaps these restorations even covered bits of amalgam (thallium)!

She could not recover without removing these metals; the liver was not able to control albumin and globulin production due to them. She was scheduled for plastic removal.

Besides the usual first day procedures and supplements, she was given potassium gluconate powder to raise her potassium. She would also be off malonate containing food. In spite of this and killing all tapeworm stages and removing all plastic from her teeth, she <u>still</u> tested Positive for malonate in the fasted state. Bits remained and had to be searched for.

She had arrived on September 9, and her new blood test showed that her anemia was worsening (RBC dropping); hemorrhaging from the rectum was our greatest fear. Could we stop it in time? We didn't even know the cause. A CT scan of the bowel (not shown), taken after her last surgery showed a much disturbed, improperly positioned bowel. Perhaps it just wasn't healing. The bowel was also very dilated. But the cause for bleeding could not be seen. She was started on the Chinese herb, Yunnan paiyao, to stop bleeding.

It was her eighth day, September 17, and the bleeding had lessened. But one change was dramatic. Her tinnitus was down by about 50%! It happened after a dental visit. She had been back to the dentist a number of times to remove small bits of leftover metal and plastic. Although we had carefully selected safe composite ingredients for her, the completed job would often not be safe. Only one tooth at a time was being worked on so we could identify the cause of any new problem more easily. After each visit she was retested in the fasted state and often found Positive for malonates and metals. It seemed never ending. Sometimes unsafe plastic would be put back in, although we had tested the ingredients. This was not the dentist's fault [nobody knew that acrylic plastic is turned into malonic acid by the body]. At first, we tested only the kit components (dental supplies for composites come in kits), not realizing that every tiny dab of sealer, every bit of adhesive or liner the dentist supplied personally, could carry the fateful carcinogens and be sealed into the tooth permanently. And they <u>would</u> seep. In contrast to the anesthetic which would dissipate.

Her September 21 blood test probably reflects this as the total protein is again too high (8.2).

The drop in calcium probably resulted from some malonated restorations. But uric acid was normal now and her RBC was finally coming up, a basic sign of improved health. Obviously she could make enough blood to replace the small amount she was still losing.

On October 2, ten days later, she was done with all her dental work, but was she really free of all metal and malonic acid in <u>each</u> and <u>every</u> tooth? A single tooth could change her prognosis from very good to very bad. She was feeling very well.

The ultrasound was scheduled. No traces of tumors in the liver could be found. Was it too good to be true? Even the large cyst was gone. Had it been missed somehow? The texture of the liver was exceptionally good; this was obviously a healthy liver now. If there were remnant bits of tumor, they would be just that...remnant bits. The ultrasound showed many views of the liver taken from different angles. They were all uniformly good. One is shown.

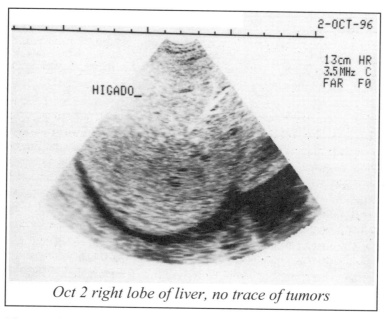

Oct 2 right lobe of liver, no trace of tumors

The new blood test, done Oct. 2, was not yet perfect. But the total protein was no longer too high. The iron level was perfect. And bone was no longer dissolving. Maybe her dental cleanup was perfect. She will do a CT liver scan in a month and another blood test including Ca 125.

Kristie Barnes	US Lab 8/27	Arrival Date 9/9	9/21	10/2
RBC	3.98	3.82	4.21	3.91
WBC	5.3	6	5.1	5.7
PLT	226	237	220	219
BUN	15 (7-22)	18 (5-26)	15	13
creatinine	0.7	0.8	0.8	0.7
AST (SGOT)	15	17	17	20
ALT (SGPT)	7	9	15	18
LDH	147	142	154	145
T.b.	0.9	1.0	0.5	0.5
alk phos	56 (37-107)	62 (39-117)	71	64

T.p.	8.2	7.5	8.2	6.8
albumin	4.4	4.4	4.8	4.2
globulin	3.8	3.1	3.4	2.6
uric acid	3.1 (2.4-5.1)	1.9 (2.5-6.1)	3.5	2.9
Calcium	9.8	9.5	8.8	8.9
Phosphorus	4.4	3.9	3.7	3.5
Iron		113	85	96
Potassium	4.0	3.8	4.2	3.7
triglycerides	175	156		87
cholesterol	130	159		194
Ca 125	61 (<35)			

Summary: Kristie did very little more than clean-up her dentalware, kill parasites, and stop eating malonate-foods. It was all her liver needed to dissolve and digest all the tumors and function well again.

---

36 Denny Hemstead	**Liver Cancer**

If cancer has its personality type, it is sweetness and lack of guile, not festering anger or self-hate as is sometimes portrayed. Denny Hemstead was pure sweetness even in the greatest stress of his life. He offered his much awaited turn to a new patient once, after being "in line" for hours, and when I inquired about his missed appointment, he guilelessly said there was a <u>sick</u> woman in line behind him and she needed to see the doctor before dark. Denny had been given one month to one year by his doctor at home, for a metastasizing adenocarcinoma with an unknown primary source. There was no tumor anywhere, but his whole body was full of cancer cells. His abdomen was distended and tight as a drum. He had recently had a peritoneal paracentesis done at the Cleveland clinic; this means "water" had been removed from his abdomen by needle due to its abnormal accumulation there. Before he was discharged from Cleveland clinic, "palliative care" was discussed. This means taking care of pain and comforts only, no treatments of any kind to be pursued. He was discharged on coumadin and lasix, a blood thinner and diuretic.

But these simple treatments were no match for his condition. He arrived toxic with isopropyl alcohol, wood alcohol, freon, nickel, copper, cadmium, cobalt, mercury, and aflatoxin. He was septic with *E. coli* and staphylococcus bacteria.

He had brought his chest X-ray with him. His lungs were pushed upward by his abdomen (see vertical arrow on X-ray), which was full of "water" again. In fact, his entire chest was water logged. The heart was enlarged, as the pathologist pointed out with the long arrow drawn from it's point, right across it to the other end.

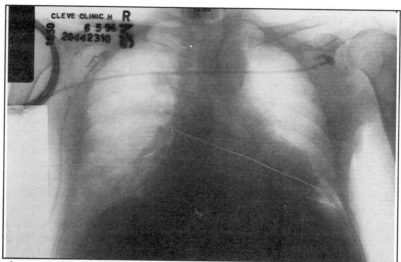

Lungs hazy with "water" and heart enlarged. (Extra markings are scratches on negative.)
Jun 5 X-ray three months ago

He related that he had been on my parasite program about three weeks and also on an Essiac program for three months. He had been zapping for about one month. He asked in bewilderment why these treatments hadn't worked since he had done them very conscientiously. It was quite painful for me to point out to him, "Denny, your mouth is full of carcinogenic metal and plastic; you are sucking on it day and night. It goes to your bone marrow, thyroid, parathyroid, liver, spleen; it fills up your body so your glands can't function. You don't have a tumor anywhere–your doctors have already searched. But you are toxic with those things that cause tumors. Cancer patients die from these things, not from tumors!"

He gave the correct response to this explanation, saying "I am dying, then, not from my cancer?" I agreed, "You are sent home to die from those things that cause tumors, not the tumors themselves. And we know what these things are. It is not difficult to get rid of them. But you need to hurry." He danced out of his chair with eagerness to hurry. But first he was informed about his blood test results (Sept. 30).

The RBC was much too high, due to either cobalt or vanadium toxicity. In his case it was cobalt; it was very high in his bone marrow where red blood cells are made. The source would most certainly be his metal and plastic teeth. First priority was to get all metal and plastic out of his mouth; first the metal, then the plastic. We would not use IVs unless he didn't make good progress.

Globulin was too high, for the same reason, causing the total protein (albumin plus globulin) to be too high. Potassium was too high due to toxins in the thyroid; this gland is very close to the mouth with its toxic drainage; any toxins can have this effect. His liver enzymes were too high; I suspected lead from his copper pipes or some medicine. But he had every chance to recover, if he acted swiftly.

Besides the usual start-up instructions in the cancer program, he was given a thyroid tablet, 1½ grains, taken upon rising, daily. He was also given glucuronic acid, and niacin. This would replace the coumadin (readers are reminded not to try this on themselves at home) and we could check his blood clotting times whenever a blood test was done to verify this. He was instructed to change his metal glasses frames to plastic.

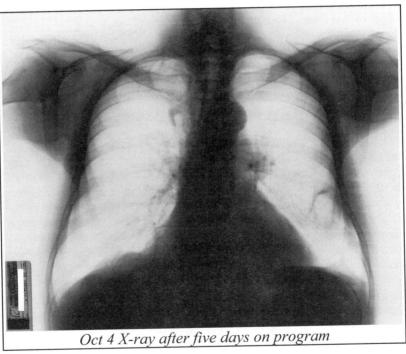

Oct 4 X-ray after five days on program

Five days later, October 4, he had his first chest X-ray from us. But it was too late! His lungs had already improved. We did not catch the first day presentation. Nobody could have anticipated such a speedy improvement.

The heart was much smaller, water level much lower; there was much more air in his lungs. A little "fuzziness" still remained to the outlines of ribs—showing a general "dampness" of his lungs. The ribs were still spread far apart, persisting evidence of his recent emphysema. He was breathing well now, in spite of his abdominal distention. He was not coughing. He was halfway through his dental clean-up. We were removing metal first.

By October 11, all metal was out of his mouth, at least we thought so. His abdominal distention was now much less and he was in less pain. Yet his blood test did not show the drop in RBC to be expected when all toxic cobalt and vanadium are gone! Had a bit of metal been overlooked?

Using an emery board, each remaining tooth was rubbed, followed by testing for copper, cobalt, vanadium, and the M-family. Three teeth still had cobalt! One had vanadium! And one had maleic acid! This single tooth would be the source of maleic anhydride which was causing the liquid escape (ascites) into the abdomen. Evidently the tooth scraping was a more sensitive detection means than simply searching for these toxins in the bone marrow or lungs, as we had been doing.

Denny was sent back to the dentist for a repeat metal cleaning. Maybe this time it would all come out. There was very little change in his blood test results. On October 17, his saliva was still Positive for copper, too, although he was staying at the environmentally safe motel. We repeated his tooth fillings. He must still have metals and maleic acid somewhere in them!

The painful truth had to be accepted. His <u>plastic</u> fillings contained the copper, cobalt and vanadium or were covering up remnants of metal. There was only one option: to remove all his plastic fillings, too. His abdominal ascites and pain would not leave permanently without it.

Removing plastic was even more difficult than removing metal because remnants are much harder to see.

By October 29, all four quadrants of his mouth had been reworked, removing every bit of synthetic restoration ever placed. Meanwhile, his waist size had increased by two inches and he was most uncomfortable. His ankles were still swollen. They should have slenderized in spite of being off diuretic. We searched at his kidneys for the explanation.

Malonic acid Positive at kidney. Methyl malonate Positive at kidney (this is known for its kidney toxicity). Maleic anhydride Positive at kidney (known to cause seepage and edema). Cobalt and vanadium Positive at bone marrow.

There was only one conclusion possible: there was <u>still</u> plastic in his teeth even after all the dental searching. It could not be found or removed by a dentist. (We had sent him to three, including one who used a microscope attachment for precision viewing. It just couldn't be done.) [Now we use digital X-rays.]

The blood test of November 4 reflected it for the sixth time: the red blood cell count stayed much too high and globulin stayed too high. Iron stayed low and triglycerides were too low.

The only solution was to extract the teeth that had had the plastic fillings. He wanted to do this at home, in Canada, where the comforts of wife and familiar surroundings would lessen his stress.

His abdomen was still hard, although the pain was gone. Delaying even a few weeks could tip the scales for him to (1) further ascites (2) hospitalization (3) a massive drug regimen (4) morphine (5) morgue. And delay might be unavoidable at home.

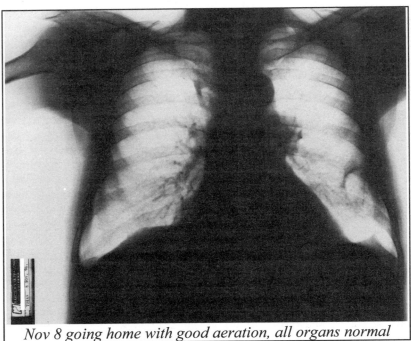

Nov 8 going home with good aeration, all organs normal

But he missed home cooking. With his painful jaws (he had extracted three teeth before leaving) and "open" unfilled teeth, we had cautioned him against chewing too much. I worried that he might be eating less and losing weight, so I asked him what he was actually eating. He replied he did not know. How could he not know? Were his eyes closed while eating? He explained that he ordered his food to be blended—the entire dinner, together—so he never knew what was passing his lips at any one moment. He enjoyed giving precise answers. I was relieved. Perhaps with this personality trait he could be trusted to finish his dental task at home. We scheduled his final chest X-ray.

It was even better than before, with very good aeration, stretching the full length of both lungs. Gone was all "fuzziness". The heart was normal in size, giving greater credibility to the previous X-ray. Heart and lung disease were, in fact, absent. Even the emphysema was improved. No enlarged lymph nodes could be seen. He left us behind, wiser and sadder. Wiser about plastic dental materials. Sadder to know the truth: pollution is everywhere, with the tumor-promoting group of toxins. Our determination strengthened to find "clean" dental plastic to replace metal. But, until then, extractions would be the only way to salvage a critically ill patient.

Denny Hemstead	9/30	10/7	10/15	10/21	10/28	11/4
RBC	6.04	5.59	5.56	5.52	5.58	5.55
WBC	8,2	6,1	6,3	7,4	6,0	8,7
PLT	201	171	360	242	197	242
glucose	99	104	215	96	94	126
BUN	22	13	10	14	16	11
creatinine	1.2	0.8	0.8	0.8	0.9	1.0
AST (SGOT)	62	33	41	39	45	43
ALT (SGPT)	92	44	54	38	42	37
LDH	162	157	172	188	169	177
GGT	65	68	80	76	75	60
T.b.	0.9	0.6	0.6	0.5	0.5	0.2
alk phos	96	109	119	114	112	89
T.p.	7.7	6.8	7.2	7.1	7.2	7.6
albumin	4.6	4.2	4.0	4.2	4.3	4.2
globulin	3.1	2.6	3.2	2.9	2.9	3.4
uric acid	5.2	4.0	5.0	5.0	4.9	3.0
Calcium	9.5	9.0	9.1	9.0	8.8	9.1
Phosphorus	4.6	3.2	3.2	3.4	3.2	3.6
Iron	63	34	78	38	39	45
Sodium	140	142	139	142	140	140
Potassium	5.1	4.7	5.0	5.4	4.6	4.7
Chloride	102	105	103	106	106	105
triglycerides	126	47	81	86	54	50
cholesterol	158	129	146	154	142	193

37	Anabelle Orenza	Breast Tumor

Anabelle Orenza, sixty-five, did not come for a cancer problem. She called her aching bones, arms, legs, shoulder "environmental illness." She was allergic to almost everything she ate, touched, or used. She tested Positive for malonic acid, isopropyl alcohol, *Staphylococcus aureus*, copper, cobalt, mercury and aflatoxin, and of course, benzene when she arrived.

With environmental illness, the first step is to stop using all cosmetics, skin treatments, and other body products whether purchased at pharmacies, health food stores, or by mail order. They are all polluted with antiseptic solvents and petroleum products (petroleum derived products all contain ultratrace amounts of benzene); even small amounts of these solvents are too much for the liver to detoxify. She had already done all this.

A second major source of toxicity in environmental illness is copper water pipes, which usually bring lead with them. She was advised to move to a new home or change the copper pipes to PVC.

The third and possibly most important source of toxicity could be her own teeth.

Anabelle tested Positive to malonic acid and methyl malonate the morning of her "dental test." This test was done by us in the fasted state in the morning, on a saliva sample. Only artificial teeth could be a source of malonates in this setting (not food or tapeworm stages).

Two days later she had all plastic fillings drilled out, leaving holes. But due to confusion (and the dentist's persuasion), she had two holes refilled by another plastic at the same office.

Another dental test was arranged to evaluate the new plastic fillings. Malonic acid was Positive again. To be absolutely certain it was coming from the new fillings, we chipped them for testing; after all, they could be easily repaired. They contained copper and malonates, but we felt she might be able to tolerate this small amount—after all, she was not a cancer patient. To test this assumption, the bone marrow along with liver, parathyroids, and thymus were tested for malonates and copper for seven days in a row to see if they would accumulate there. Only on one day did the thymus test Positive for malonic acid and D-malic acid. So we thought her two new plastic fillings were safe enough for her—besides, she did not want to lose them. A final X-ray (full mouth series), of her teeth was scheduled. It revealed several amalgam tattoos! The next day these were removed by the dentist. She left for home, with reduced symptoms, although taking no supplements on a regular basis due to allergies.

She was using cosmetics made with recipes from *The Cure For All Cancers*, looked well, and now had more energy. She left with several open teeth which she would keep clean with 35% peroxide brushing, and promised to return in a month.

During her three week stay her blood test had shown a very significant improvement. Her WBC, which frequently dropped below 3,000 she said, had come up to 3,600 by September 23. This would strengthen her immunity. The RBC dropped from too high to a perfect value.

But all was not well. She returned from Canada two months later. This time she had very high levels of isopropyl alcohol again, as well as benzene, copper, formaldehyde, and urethane (plastic component known to cause cancer). Recently, she had felt a lump in her left breast and, in fact, had not felt well for all the time she was away.

Tests showed copper and vanadium at the breast and cobalt in her WBCs. The liver had D-malic acid and she was Positive for aflatoxin and patulin, too. How could a lump come up so quickly?

Ortho-phospho-tyrosine was Negative, so the lump was not malignant. But certainly it was growing. An ultrasound of the breast was scheduled as well as a new blood test. By now we could interpret the low uric acid correctly. It implied high bacterial levels, something that would only happen if glutathione levels were much too low. The glutathione was busy mopping up new toxins. In fact, it had already been revealed the day she left for home two months ago, after two new plastic fillings were put in.

She kept her gain in the WBC, and calcium was finally rising, showing that toxins had left the parathyroids.

The metabolic effects of bacteria and their ammonia could easily be seen in the breast. We were beginning to suspect clostridium bacteria as the true culprit at this time. All the <u>purine</u> nucleic acid bases (adenine, guanosine, xanthosine, and inosine) tested Negative at the breast!

Something was even preventing the <u>pyrimidine</u> bases (uridine, cytidine, and thymidine) from being made. The tumor was growing (DNA Positive) while important enzymes were not being made (RNA negative).

Transferrin was Negative, as was xanthine oxidase, the enzyme that helps prepare iron for transport. I already knew that without xanthine or xanthosine, no xanthine oxidase would be present.

The ultrasound of breast did not show any masses identifiable as such, although it could be felt by hand. She needed a CT scan.

She started immediately on the cancer program, including glutathione, Lugol's, glutamic acid (instead of glutamine, to help reduce ammonia levels), arginine, ornithine, vitamin B_{12}, folic acid, etc. [*our Day 1 program at that time*]. Plus the usual zapping, parasite killing, and stopping wearing a regular bra. The plastic fillings were quickly removed from her teeth. She was told to eat sardines to help supply nucleic acid bases.

Two days later, on Nov. 22, all four nucleic acid bases (plus two precur-

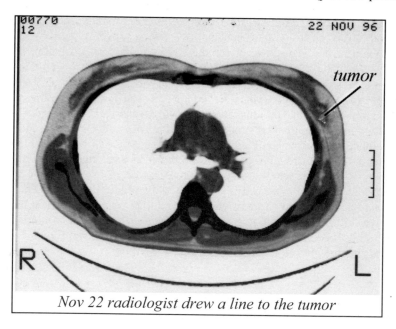

Nov 22 radiologist drew a line to the tumor

431

sor bases) were Positive once more at the breast. Xanthine oxidase was also Positive there, as well as transferrin; she was now transporting iron again the way she should, from storage sites in the liver to the work stations in the bone marrow where RBCs are made. Eight common food bacteria were now Negative at the breast. Healing and tumor shrinking could begin.

She had a CT of breast done. It showed the mass she was feeling, although it already felt smaller to her.

Three days later, Nov. 25, a new blood test was done. To her surprise and joy her WBC was higher than it had been for the last five years. Uric acid was starting to come up, reflecting on conquest over bacteria. (Note that her initial uric acid level on September 3 was masked.)

But calcium and phosphorus had fallen back down. The cause was not known. Perhaps just a trace of plastic was left in her mouth, or another amalgam tattoo—too small to show up in electronic testing, but not too small to affect the parathyroid glands. We decided to send Anabelle to a dentist who could do air abrasion of teeth to remove even the smallest particle of leftover metal or plastic (provided he could see it; this would be challenging).

A number of amino acids were also searched for in the breast, to see if they were all present, so healing could occur. Lysine, aspartic acid, glycine were Positive, but glutamic acid, arginine, glutamine, and ornithine were Negative. Was supplementation with glutamic acid, arginine, and ornithine not working? Experience had taught Anabelle to be very, very cautious in trying any new supplements in her hyperallergic state. So she had eaten sardines, but not taken the supplements. Fortunately a few days later arginine, ornithine, and glutamine were Positive even without the supplements.

Now, too, clostridium and lactobacillus bacteria tested Negative at the breast! Had they been responsible for the RNA-to-DNA switch before the recovery? Anabelle's case helped us to see the connection between *Clostridium* and DNA presence.

Then Anabelle was gone again. Perhaps she had a side-trip planned. Perhaps there were other pressing matters. Two weeks went by before she returned with her bright cheery smile that lifted all of us. We quickly scheduled a blood test and new CT scan of the breast. Meanwhile, a complete search for DNA in her body organs uncovered it at the lungs and thyroid gland! Obviously, there was still a serious problem.

Cobalt and urethane were still Positive! Only plastic could explain it. But she had gotten a final air abrasion cleaning of her teeth. The dentist had superlative skill. Was he leaving small plastic fillings in her teeth? Or was it an impossible task? The pain in her breast <u>had</u> disappeared right after this visit. And she thought she felt a lot better afterward, too.

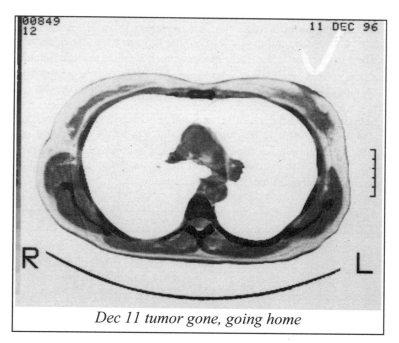

Dec 11 tumor gone, going home

We were mystified. The blood test showed she had kept her gains in RBC and WBC counts. And the uric acid level was, indeed, a lot better, implying much less ammonia from bacteria. Calcium had come up, showing toxins were now out of the parathyroids. But it went too high, 9.8, showing they were still in the thyroid.

Were the cobalt and urethane going to her thyroid? We had to find the source or leave her in great jeopardy. It was her going-home day. We

Anabelle Orenza	9/3	9/23	11/20	11/25	12/11
RBC	4.83	4.49	4.37	4.44	4.71
WBC	3,300	3,6	3,600	4,600	4,600
PLT·	244	183	191	215	206
glucose	87	61	100	111	99
BUN	17	13	13	10	15
creatinine	0.9	0.9	0.9	1.3	1.3
AST (SGOT)	23	20	21	21	25
ALT (SGPT)	14	15	11	11	14
LDH	146	122	117	128	130
GGT	15	15	10	8.0	19
T.b.	0.6	0.8	0.6	0.6	0.8
alk phos	54	45	33	66	54
T.p.	6.9	6.6	6.6	6.9	7.2
albumin	4.4	4.4	4.1	4.5	4.7
globulin	2.5	2.2	2.5	2.4	2.5
uric acid	3.5	1.7	1.4	1.8	2.7
Calcium	8.8	8.4	9.2	.8.8	9.8
Phosphorus	2.5	3.0	3.3	2.6	3.3
Iron	96	69	100	48	80
Sodium	138	140	141	140	140
Potassium	4.2	3.5	3.9	3.5	4.2
Chloride	101	105	106	102	103
triglycerides	78	88	49	79	66
cholesterol	180	193	166	202	249

also needed to review her new scan.

The breast showed no tumor; the radiologist did not even consider it a significant fibrous remnant. He merely made a check mark to indicate which breast had been involved. That was a pleasure. The breast tumor was gone. She could no longer feel it, either, although I think the scan shows remains of fibrous tissue.

Summary: We were all elated. But not with a sense of security for her. That plastic must come out. In the meantime, she was to take 10 drops of HCl (5%) once a day to help kill food bacteria in her stomach. And digestive enzymes with vinegar water at mealtime for the same purpose. This could even help her environmental illness…what remained of it.

38	Sarah Armbruster	Breast & Bone Cancer

Sarah Armbruster, a young mother of thirty-six, was not prepared for her diagnosis with breast and bone cancer, not with young children to raise by herself and a job to keep. Actually it was her second bout of breast cancer. Her first bout was five years earlier. She had a lumpectomy plus six weeks of radiation at the left breast at that time.

Now there was a new lump in the same breast and pain at her right shoulder. The bone scan (not shown) she brought with her showed hot spots all over her skeleton, though she was not in generalized pain, yet. She could easily feel the spot on her right fifth rib, though.

Her anxiety was intense, almost palpable, and to top it off, we told her she had to quit smoking—that very minute! Not one more cigarette. Nothing hidden away anywhere. We could cure her cancer (by this time our success rate was over 90% because we had learned the hazards of plastic dental restorations), but only with her full cooperation. She agreed to TRY—not to QUIT.

Her initial toxin test results were Negative for:

Bacteria	Metals	Solvents	Other toxins
E. coli	aluminum	isopropyl alcohol	formaldehyde
Staphylococcus aureus	cobalt	xylene	CFC's
Salmonella typhimurium	lead	benzene	fiberglass
Salmonella dysenteriae	thallium	toluene	PCBs
Salmonella paratyphi	cadmium		asbestos
Shigella flexneri	nickel		arsenic
Shigella sonnei	vanadium		chlorine
But	Positive	For:	
Shigella dysenteriae	mercury	wood alcohol	aflatoxin
Salmonella enteriditis	copper		malonic acid

These tests were "whole body" tests. They do not detect items unless the quantity is quite large. In this way, only the most abundant toxins are seen.

434

Cobalt and vanadium were not abundant. They need not be abundant to be killers at the bone marrow, spleen, or liver.

The surprise was that she had already eliminated isopropyl alcohol, all on her own, before coming. She must have some hidden determination. This meant that all her tumors and lesions were already reduced to nonmalignant status. But they certainly would grow and spread since the bacteria inside them would continue making growth factors [and DNA] and spread to new locations.

She also had done an exceptionally good job of cleaning her home. But copper water pipes were still there. That would be top priority upon her return home. There was also the mercury in her mouth and the ever present aflatoxin and malonic acid.

She made the intelligent decision to stay as long as it took to clear her cancer. On her first day she was started on the malonate-free diet, glutathione, Q10, and Lugol's iodine. Of course, she would continue the parasite program plus zapping. She would stop wearing a regular bra since it limits circulation under the breast. We would not need IVs.

By day two she had gotten rid of aflatoxin and wood alcohol. She was still Positive for copper. She had not gone to our copper-free, environmentally safe motel; there were no vacancies. Her motel water had copper.

Her blood test results arrived. They did not show a depressed serum iron. In fact, the iron was too high. Is this also due to copper? The answer awaits further research.

But the blockage of creatinine and blood urea is easy to see; they are too low. I suspect malonate [*and azo dyes*] as part of the cause but simple lack of amino acids and urea synthesis enzymes are also possible causes.

She was supplemented with urea powder, 2 tsp. a day (10 gm, which is about half of a regular dose) stirred into water, and creatine powder, 1 tsp. a day (about 5 gm). Urea is not merely a waste product, it has important functions besides.

Her potassium was low so we supplemented her with potassium gluconate powder. Her LDH, alk phos, calcium,

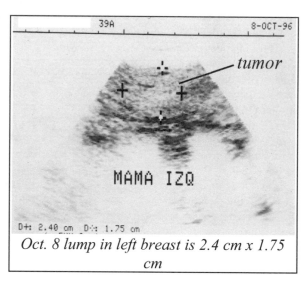

39A   8-OCT-96

— *tumor*

MAMA IZQ

D+: 2.40 cm   D·: 1.75 cm

Oct. 8 lump in left breast is 2.4 cm x 1.75 cm

435

and total protein were entirely normal. And liver enzymes were very good. The good blood test results contradicted the appearance of an ill person with disseminated bone cancer.

Her new ultrasound of the breast showed the breast lump clearly; it was 2.4 x 1.75 cm.

We began her dental cleanup immediately. She had a very "bad" mouth. There were metal fillings everywhere, four root canals, and four caps. It was obvious that all her teeth should be extracted. Bad dental health may have caused her early development of cancer, at age thirty-four. Fortunately, she did not rebel.

By day 4, she was in withdrawal (from smoking), she had headaches. We were happy to have this evidence of quitting smoking, not just cutting down. Each day she was being tested for all the cancer-related toxins at the breast and bone: copper, cobalt, vanadium, five malonates, solvents, urethane, aflatoxin, and patulin. She was testing Negative to all, including copper.

By October 14, her blood sugar was still too low. Uric acid was too low. Phosphorus was too low. She was started on vitamin D. She was also started on thyroid, 1½ grains a day.

By October 19, her new dentures arrived. We tested them for copper, cobalt, vanadium, and five malonates. They were Negative. But we still couldn't risk her wearing them. What if the dental lab was aware that soaking them in vitamin C water overnight would guarantee that they tested Negative—for a day—and would pass our test deceptively! She was instructed to wait for our duplicate testing of them a few days later. She did not rebel. She blended her meals and drank them.

It was October 24. Her eyes shone; she looked animated. She said she felt "very much better." She seemed to be entirely well. She could not feel her rib and shoulder pain anymore.

But bone lesions take time to heal. In spite of healing, the bone density would be less at those spots. Only after half a year would it be worthwhile to repeat the bone scan.

On October 28, a second ultrasound of the breast was done. There was no trace of the tumor. (Actually, six ultrasound views were

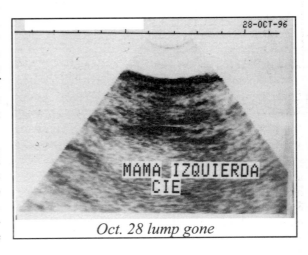

Oct. 28 lump gone

done; only one is shown here.)

The breast wasn't even fibrous anymore. It was soft and normal. Her new blood test continued to be satisfactory, although the serum iron was still too high. All her supplements were reduced or stopped. She could go home. We wanted her to send a picture of her two girls. And of course, follow up with blood tests and ultrasounds, and a bone scan in six months. But, most of all, change her water pipes and stick to a smoke-free life.

Summary: A follow up done a few months later found her well, no evidence of any cancer. She had no pains. There was no DNA found "Positive" in any tissues. And her blood test (not shown) showed improvement.

Sarah Armbruster	10/7	10/14	10/22	10/28
RBC	4.42	4.24	4.38	4.04
WBC	7,800	7,000	11,100	7,600
PLT	248	214	259	271
glucose	79	62	97	82
BUN	8 (7-21)	17	11	15
creatinine	0.8	0.8	0.8	0.8
AST (SGOT)	16	18	21	17
ALT (SGPT)	10	15	15	18
LDH	153	152	160	155
GGT	13	14	13	13
T.b.	0.4	0.4	0.8	0.4
alk phos	64	63	66	59
T.p.	7.2	7.0	7.3	6.9
albumin	4.8	4.7	4.5	4.7
globulin	2.4	2.3	2.8	2.2
uric acid	3.1	2.9	1.9 (2.5-6.8)	3.7
Calcium	9.0	9.2	9.8	8.8
Phosphorus	3.0	2.9	2.7	3.3
Iron	158	187	175	202
Sodium	138	139	139	138
Potassium	3.8	4.1	4.3	4.3
Chloride	103	103	103	106
triglycerides	105	73	82	73
cholesterol	159	172	185	186

39   Bernard Johnson   Lymphatic Cancer

Bernard Johnson, fifty-seven, was given a terminal prognosis at home and had the chest X-ray to prove it. Lymphatic cancer was easily visible in his right lung (dark areas with protrusions into the lung along the inner edge and a bit on the left side, too). The heart was quite enlarged; his doctors at home talked about congestive heart failure. The cancer had spread to three enlarged lymph nodes on the left side of his neck where he had previous surgery. They were quite visible and palpable. The largest one was a half inch in

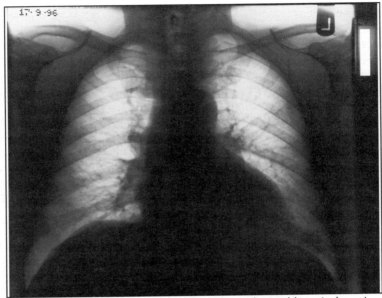

Enlarged lymph nodes on right side; enlarged heart almost touches the chest wall at lower left side.
Sep 17 terminal diagnosis X-ray a month before

diameter. He was very worried because his doctors had given him only six months, even with chemotherapy. That didn't seem worth it, so he opted for our treatment. He was extremely nervous. In fact, unwilling to believe the good news when we told him he was still basically healthy.

A glance at his blood test showed he was not at all at death's door. If we could shrink his tumorous lymph nodes and reduce his enlarged heart somewhat, he could probably get back to normal living.

His blood sugar, triglycerides, and cholesterol were not lowered yet, showing that he was still well nourished; his cancer had not yet consumed him. He was in time. But he was too anxious to believe this; he would simply have to experience it. The telltale signs of toxicity could be seen. Creatinine was a little too high, so kidney function was stressed. Calcium was too high, showing the thyroid was toxic. And potassium was slightly low.

Our testing showed two clostridium species of bacteria in his lymph nodes besides *Staphylococcus aureus*. The cause was obvious since these are dental bacteria. He must have a mouthful of bad teeth.

In addition to the usual cancer program, he was started on olive leaf tea—2 cups a day to help shrink his lymph nodes. He was also instructed to put a hot pack on his lymph nodes at the neck each day with a hot, damp towel. He was eager to comply and happy with the news, but still disbelieving.

438

His mouth was full of "restored" teeth. We tested each tooth by scraping it with an emery board, searching for copper, cobalt, vanadium, and malonates. Some of them were in very bad shape, anyway, and needed extraction. He did not object.

By October 22, the benefits of the kidney herb recipe could be seen in the blood test results, creatinine was down to 1.1. Kidney function was better. The malonate free diet and general detoxification had cleaned up his thyroid, but not yet his parathyroids, so calcium shifted from too high to too low. Malonate was still coming from his teeth, as well as copper. He could see the logic of extracting them and took the plunge. All of the uppers were removed. He felt better, instead of worse, to his surprise. In fact, there was almost no recovering to do.

By October 28, his kidneys were even better, which would, in turn, help decongest his heart.

But calcium stayed low, due, no doubt, to the toxicity of the lower teeth. His lower front teeth were pristine—he could not recall having any fillings put in them. Yet they repeatedly tested Positive for copper and malonate when scraped.

Potassium had come up enough; we could stop his potassium gluconate.

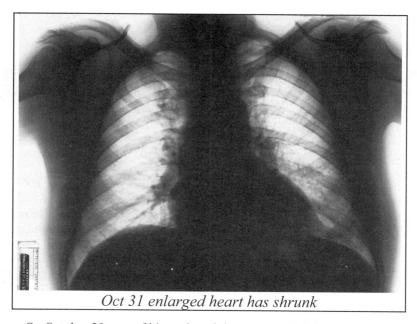

Oct 31 enlarged heart has shrunk

On October 29, one of his neck nodules was not visible and could not be felt. There were only two now. A new chest X-ray was scheduled. He was very eager to see if he could really allow himself to hope.

439

The X-ray showed great improvement along the bronchial edge of the right lung. And the heart had shrunk considerably. No wonder he was out walking now; his heart was stronger.

Each day our testing showed he still harbored cobalt and urethane, tumor inducing toxins, indicative of plastic, probably in his remaining teeth.

He decided to part with his lower front teeth, too, and make a set of dentures the solution. The very next day he felt "a thousand times better" than he had felt for a long time. It seemed unexplainable to him. He could now walk a mile. And testing was now <u>Negative</u> for copper, cobalt, vanadium, the five malonates and the plastic pollutants, bisphenol A and urethane. He finally believed he was getting well.

On November 4, after his extractions, he was Positive for urethane and malonates again! Was it leftover from when his teeth were still present? Not likely, the body cleans up a site very quickly. It was two days since the extraction. All his foods and supplements were tested. One supplement tested Positive.

It was during Bernard's stay that we found urethane pollution in the wormwood capsules. They had been provided by Self Health, our most reliable source. We typically didn't test capsules of herbs because we had never suspected them. Was it in the wormwood itself or in the capsule? Self Health provided us with samples of wormwood and several brands of gelatin capsules. The wormwood was fine, but some of the capsule brands were polluted. Self Health sent their inventory to the landfill and ordered new wormwood capsules made, using the safe brand of capsules. Meanwhile, Bernard (and everyone else) had to stop this supplement immediately. Tested capsules were filled with wormwood by hand till the safe ones were again available.

He was given D-glucuronic acid immediately in an attempt to detoxify the urethane which was showing up at his kidneys. His tests were perfect after this. No cobalt, copper, vanadium, malonates (5), solvents (3), patulin or urethane in kidneys or lungs.

His final blood test was done November 7. His iron level had not yet come up sufficiently; he was still wearing his metal rimmed glasses, a source of copper. He agreed to get them changed to plastic. And the LDH was up slightly higher than acceptable, probably due to the polluted wormwood capsules. But the calcium level was finally correct.

[*After finding urethane in gelatin capsules, we looked for other pollutants, too. A shocking number were there, including tartrazine (a yellow azo dye) and asbestos. It would be a while, however, before I discovered how damaging asbestos and azo dyes were.*]

By November 9, his new dentures were ready. We tested them for pollutants. The upper denture was safe. The lower one was polluted with all the usual toxins! (Although they were made at the same time by the same dentist in the same way!) They would diffuse out into his body if he should put them in his mouth. He was not even tempted. The dentist explained that some of the teeth used for the lower set had come from an untested lot. He made a new lower set. They tested free of all pollutants. He could put them in his mouth. It was a perfect fit. He had been worried about the appearance of his smile. But his smile was beautiful—as any smile based on happiness is.

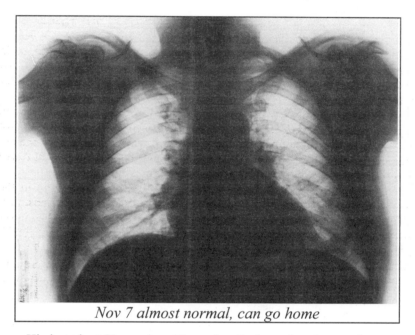

Nov 7 almost normal, can go home

His last chest X-ray, done November 7, showed no heart enlargement, ventilation was normal, lymph nodes even better than the last time. He could go home. But he was not about to leave without his precious X-rays. Fortunately, I had already sent them to be reproduced, or we would not have this story to tell.

Summary: Bernard had the patience and tenacity it takes, in a research setting, to accomplish his purpose and to leave no stone unturned. He deserved his success.

Bernard Johnson	10/18	10/22	10/28	11/7
RBC		4.44	4.67	4.63
WBC		11,300	9,7	10,1
PLT		153	143	175
glucose	120	101	95	85
BUN	14	16	13	16
creatinine	1.3	1.1	1.0	0.9
AST (SGOT)	16	14	13	13
ALT (SGPT)	13	53	18	15
LDH	142	136	144	166

GGT	36	34	49	47
T.b.	0.3	0.2	0.4	0.4
alk phos	85	94	90	91
T.p.	7.3	7.2	7.2	7.0
albumin	4.5	4.2	4.1	3.9
globulin	2.8	3.0	3.1	3.1
uric acid	4.5	3.1	4.4	4.3
Calcium	10.4	8.8	8.7	9.1
Phosphorus	3.7	3.7	3.7	3.8
Iron	76	42	65	58
Sodium	139	140	138	139
Potassium	4.0	4.3	4.8	4.8
Chloride	102	101	105	103
triglycerides	154	181	178	146
cholesterol	188	188	191	189

40   Mark Warwick   Bladder Cancer

Mark Warwick, barely in his fifties, came from Australia to avoid having a bag connected to his kidneys in place of his bladder. He had been diagnosed three years ago with bladder cancer and had twenty-eight radiation treatments for it. But now he was passing blood in his urine again. He also had pain in the lower abdomen. He couldn't sleep at night due to pain. He was very gassy and also had pain at the back of his neck on the right side (an obvious dental symptom). His surgeon at home was waiting for him to show up. Would he be able to cheat the surgeon's scalpel?

His electronic toxin test showed the usual assortment: benzene Positive (this destroys immunity so bacteria can spread); xylene Positive (this would invite tumors to the brain); malonic acid, CFC's, copper, aflatoxin, *Salmonella enteriditis*, *Shigella sonnei*, *Salmonella typhimurium*, arsenic, vanadium, all Positive, but isopropyl Negative.

He had obtained *The Cure For All Cancers* book and started on the lifestyle change two weeks ago. He also got all his dental metal changed to the recommended plastic. Now he had a mouthful of composite. He expected this to start his tumors shrinking. Why didn't it?

Note the absence of mercury and thallium in this "whole-body" test. The levels must have come down since removing amalgam. We ordered a CT of lower abdomen to show the bladder in detail.

He was started on marshmallow root tea—2 cups a day for his abdominal pain that I guessed might be coming from the bladder. This was in addition to the usual cancer program.

His first blood test showed the RBC was too high, evidence of cobalt or vanadium toxicity.

The creatinine was extremely low. The usual interpretation is "exceptionally good kidney function keeping this muscle waste so low." Because I had been testing for amino acids recently, and finding huge deficiencies in cancer patients, my new interpretation was "lack of arginine and glycine to make creatine which makes creatinine." Or "lack of methionine which makes SAM." If creatinine isn't being made, you know creatine isn't present, and creatine becomes muscle "food". Perhaps this explains the fatigue that is so devastating in tumor-bearing people.

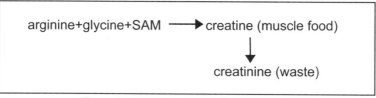

Fig. 47 requirements for creatine

We eat creatine straight when we eat meat, fowl, or fish. To get Mark's creatine up quickly, we gave him the pure compound to take: 1 tsp. a day.

The calcium was quite low, as was phosphate. When phosphate is below 3 mg/dl, there is a vitamin D shortage. This was understandable since vitamin D is activated in the kidneys, and the kidneys were part of Mark's cancer problem.

The low LDH was a nice surprise, along with the low alk phos. [*His composites were not shedding azo dyes significantly.*]

The liver enzymes, too, were exceptionally good (low)! In addition to the parasite program, Lugol's, kidney program, Mark was started on potassium gluconate powder even though his potassium level was not seriously low; it would certainly help.

The Chinese herb, Yunnan paiyao, was given to stop bleeding. And niacin, 100 mg, three times a day to make sure he had enough NAD and NADP to help his body's enzymes work.

Altogether, there was no serious deterioration in his health. Recovery should be fairly simple. Should be, that is.

By now, the fall of 1996, we had already learned that dental plastic both contained and was polluted with carcinogens. We had begun sampling the artificial teeth in each patient's mouth for testing purposes.

Only five of Mark's new plastic teeth were found to be free of copper, cobalt, vanadium and the M-family toxins. They had all been put <u>in</u> only two weeks ago! Now most of them must come out again.

A week later, he still had not begun his plastic removal. In the meantime the bleeding had stopped, leading him to think that all was well again and he might not need to make such heroic efforts.

And the second blood test, Oct. 29, showed minor improvements, supporting his idea. Creatinine had come up, the LDH had dropped a bit, liver enzymes were better, and calcium and phosphate had risen.

These were probably the rewards from going on a malonate-free diet and taking the supplements that were begun on Day 1.

By the ninth day the bleeding was back; he had not yet changed his metal glasses frames to plastic either. We started him on oral EDTA powder, ¼ tsp. once a day for five days. This would help pull the copper, cobalt, and vanadium out while he deliberated about his teeth. After all, he had just put them all in—and spent a lot of money on them.

On his tenth day (Nov. 4), the CT scan was read (not shown). It showed that his right kidney was dilated, perhaps due to a small nodule or stone, causing blockage. No stone was visible, though. A small tumor on the colon showed up! He had been unaware of it. But the bladder did not show its tumor! We recommended an ultrasound of the lower abdomen instead.

All this discomforting news persuaded him. In four days all fillings were out of his mouth. His pain level dropped so far he could sleep at night. There was only a trace of blood in his urine now.

Then I noticed Mark smelled of tobacco smoke! Perhaps he even <u>wanted</u> me to notice. He agreed immediately to switch to our "smoking herbs" that can be chewed all day to keep the mouth happy and busy.

The ultrasound arrived, showing a tumor in the kidney! The bladder had not been pictured; it was missed due to an error in communication with the radiologist. The kidney tumor measured 2.9 x 1.6 cm. What a shock.

We knew now that he had three tumor locations: the kidney, bladder, and colon. We turned our attention on the kidney tumor instead of the bladder.

In spite of getting all his plastic out, he still tested Positive for copper, cobalt, vanadium, all five M's, and urethane which we had recently discovered as another dental plastic toxin. They were all in his liver. He was still getting trace amounts, not enough to show up in his daily toxin testing at the whole body level.

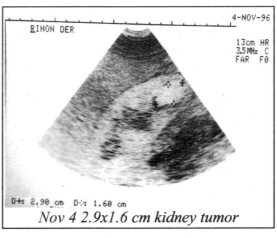

Nov 4 2.9x1.6 cm kidney tumor

There must be leftover plastic in his mouth!

We arranged for another dental appointment, this time with a dentist using a magnifying lens and a monitoring screen to see every tiny remnant left in an old cavity. Mark now reminded us that his air flight home was only a week away, and we hadn't even seen his bladder tumor yet. On November

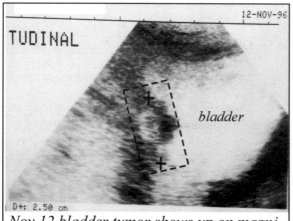

TUDINAL

12-NOV-96

bladder

D+: 2.50 cm

Nov 12 bladder tumor shows up on magnified ultrasound

12, he went for the bladder ultrasound. There it was in a magnified view, measuring 2.50 cm. He decided to extend his stay.

Even after his second dental plastic removal he still tested Positive for copper, urethane, and vanadium in the bladder.

This was just at the time we discovered urethane in a supplement's gelatin capsules—the capsules themselves. We stopped all his capsules of supplements: he was requested to use bulk supplies only. Toxic components of plastic still showed their effect in the blood test on Nov. 13. Although the RBC had come down nicely, iron and calcium had dropped, too.

This implies the continued presence of copper [*and germanium*] and malonic acid. But where from? In desperation, our entire toxin test of 80 elements was done at kidneys and bladder. Only one extra toxin was found, thulium. It was present at kidneys, bladder, and parathyroids. And we knew just where to look for it. In his vitamin C. Indeed, he was using up an old supply of vitamin C, not procured from our specially-tested stock. [*What we did not know is that lanthanides including thulium are regular components of amalgam.*]

Now his ankles were beginning to show a minor edema. But all his pain was gone. He slept well. He was still passing a trace of blood in his urine.

On November 18, there was again clear evidence of leftover dental plastic. The RBC was too high; the calcium level was down further.

A full mouth series X-ray was tried to find bits of leftover metal or plastic. Instead, several molars and one upper front tooth appeared to have large infections! Was this the clue? They were extracted immediately, and healing went well. But no dental plastic was seen in them.

A week later, Nov. 25, we studied the nucleic acid bases and amino acids in his bladder. The results were dismal.

Adenine Negative	xanthine oxidase Negative	glycine Negative
xanthine Negative	transferrin Negative	arginine Positive
guanosine Negative	DNA Negative	glutamic acid Negative
inosine Negative	RNA Negative	glutamine Positive

uridine Negative	lysine Negative	ornithine Positive
thymidine Negative	aspartic Negative	

He was requested to eat one can of sardines a day (for nucleic acid bases). He was also given: aspartic acid, glutamic acid, glycine. This proved to be insufficient to make them appear at his kidneys so amounts were doubled.

Cobalt and copper were still showing up regularly. (We could have IV-ed them out with EDTA, but this would give a false sense of security; I advised against it.)

There was only one conclusion to be reached—another remnant of plastic was present that had escaped all the dentists so far.

We sent him back to the dentist whose dental microscope and painstaking procedure would surely give him the final cleanup so much needed this time. He had only one week left before his second plane reservation.

After this final "microscopic" cleaning, we expected to see a little improvement on his blood test, but we were astonished to see his results (Dec. 2) were <u>completely</u> normal! The RBC, calcium, phosphate, and iron were all correct. He now tested Negative for copper, cobalt, vanadium, all five malonates, and urethane, at last. Was he ready to go home?

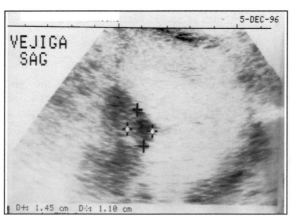

Bladder tumor has shrunk to 1.45x1.1 cm

Suddenly, a trace of bright red blood showed up in his stool! We had not paid attention to the small tumor seen in his colon on his original CT scan. What was it doing? His dental partials were made, tested, and fitted fine. His fatigue was gone. He had slightly swollen ankles. We advised him to have the colon checked to see if there was anything suspicious on the inside. But it was not done.

Instead, a follow up ultrasound of kidney and bladder was done. On Dec. 5, his new ultrasounds showed NOTHING in the kidney. Nothing at all where the tumor had been. And the bladder tumor was about half the original size. Happiness reigned for the rest of that day and he was determined to go home. But not before his cavities were filled! He had twelve empty holes in his teeth. Without authorization he got them all filled.

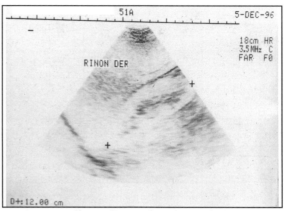

Dec 5 Kidney shown between the + signs has no trace of former tumor

On Dec. 6, we tested him one last time. He was positive for cobalt and vanadium again! And the RBC was back up.

He had obtained new temporary fillings: twelve of them. Only zinc oxide and eugenol was used; we had tested many such products and always found them pure. But had the new dentist used some "nerve protectant"? Or a faster-setting variety of zinc oxide plus eugenol? Or had unsafe plastic strips been used to contain and polish the wet cement-like mass before drying? We tested immediately. He was toxic again. He had only three days left before his flight; we could not persuade him to extend his stay to tend to his edema problem. Or his colon problem. Yet we could not let him go home with a mouthful of toxic dental fillings.

He agreed to return to the microscope dentist for complete removal again, by air abrasion; (this does not enlarge the hole). But there was no time to do another blood test and see that all toxins were gone. He rushed right over to yet another dentist for the approved zinc oxide and eugenol. Then he was on his way homeward. But too much was done too hastily. Would his edema get better or worse? Would his bladder tumor continue to shrink? Would the rectal bleeding stop or worsen?

Summary: If Mark had lessons to learn about patience, we, too, had lessons to learn. Removing plastic from teeth is not as simple as tooth-cleaning. And removing metal is also a time-intensive and demanding skill. If it is not done perfectly, it will not be good enough to save a life. It would be better to extract as many as possible, before the patient is too weak or anemic to sit in the dentists' chair.

One thing is obvious: tumors shrink rather readily. But every detail must be attended to. Nothing can be done half-way with full expectations of success.

Mark Warwick	10/24	10/29	11/4	11/8	11/ 13	11/ 18	11/ 25	12/2	12/6
RBC	4.93	5.21	4.93	4.85	4.76	5.03	4.99	4.76	4.96
WBC	5,8	8,2	7,4	7,9	9,6	7,3	8,6	7,9	8,1
PLT	206	189	258	232	208	195	236	258	211
glucose	98	93	73	153	82	73	72	106	87
BUN	19	16	17	16	9(7-21)	12	12	11	10
creatinine	0.7(0.8-1.5)	0.9	0.8	0.8	0.8	0.8	0.7	0.8	0.9
AST (SGOT)	26	17	18	16	17	18	21	22	25
ALT (SGPT)	22	21	15	19	22	20	21	12	24
LDH	163	159	145	146	141	151	167	146	159
GGT	22	18	19	18	22	24	24	17	21
T.b.	0.3	0.8	0.1	0.3	0.3	0.3	0.4	0.7	0.6
alk phos	45	48	23	26	45	50	46	48	51
T.p.	6.9	7.2	6.8	7.1	6.7	6.9	6.9	6.9	7.5
albumin	4.6	5.0	4.2	4.1	4.3	4.4	4.5	4.5	4.8
globulin	2.3	2.2	2.6	3.0	2.4	2.5	2.4	2.4	2.7
uric acid	4.7	4.7	2.9	3.9	3.8	4.2	4.3	4.0	4.0
Calcium	8.8	9.1	9.1	9.6	8.4	8.1	8.7	9.3	9.4
Phosphorus	2.4	2.7	2.8	3.1	2.9	3.7	2.7	3.0	4.5
Iron	106	29	78	65	37	48	83	90	108
Sodium	143	135	141	138	140	138	140	143	142
Potassium	4.0	4.0	4.4	4.2	4.4	4.0	4.4	4.3	4.4
Chloride	107	100	106	105	105	101	104	106	105
triglycerides	120	116	134	377	160	197	68	145	203
cholesterol	205	218	258	218	240	230	247	196	222

41   Paul Garcia   Beginning Tumors

Paul Garcia, in his early thirties, was an employee of the Diagnostic Center. Like other Mexicans in Tijuana, he had become habituated to drinking bottled water, instead of boiling it, and soda pop as a beverage. His can of pop for lunch was neatly hidden from view though. And after lunch he smelled of tobacco smoke. He had no symptoms whatever.

It was late Saturday afternoon and my plan was to search for the presence of DNA and RNA in as many healthy persons as possible, using about 40 organ slides. The pure samples of DNA and RNA had recently arrived, and I wanted to see whether they could be detected everywhere, nowhere, or at selected locations. There were still a few employees present who would be willing to "sit" for testing, besides some staff members.

The DNA and RNA samples were left in their original bottles, and simply placed on one Syncrometer plate while the organ slide was placed on the other. RNA was found to be present in all organs tested, but was normally missing in kidney and bladder. Why was there no RNA detected in the kidney and bladder? Is this normal or sick? Is it also absent in young people? These questions are not yet answered. But it seemed safe to assume that it is normal and healthy to be able to detect RNA in every organ except kidney and bladder.

But DNA was only present for 20 seconds out of each minute, and at rather low levels. Except in the ovary where it was present constantly. Even though every cell has DNA in its nucleus, it is bound to protein here most of the time. Our test-DNA was not bound to protein, a different electronic entity from the body's DNA. Being post-menopausal didn't seem to matter; DNA was still Positive at the ovary. Would it also be present in the testes of a male? We called Paul to help us discover the facts.

The test set for organs begins with adrenals and ends with uterus. When we got to liver, the circuit resonated. Several repeats gave the same answer. Paul had DNA, evidently unbound to protein, in his liver. Was that significant? Did it portend a malignancy? A growth? We continued testing in silence.

When we got to the prostate, the circuit resonated again. And again at the testes slide. We repeated these several times; there was no mistake. Did this imply a tumor or a malignancy at the prostate too? Or neither?

Paul assured us that he had no difficulty urinating, did not have to get up at night to visit the bathroom, and had no indigestion from a possible liver tumor.

Not wishing to alarm him over nothing, we scheduled a CT scan of the liver and ultrasound of the prostate for him. We would pay the bills if he did it immediately. We confessed our suspicion of some problem. Perhaps only metabolic as yet.

Being conscientious and very appreciative of our concern for his health, he did both scans promptly.

The prostate did indeed have a problem. It was much too large, so that it pushed into the bladder (large white area) above it. Furthermore, the wall of the prostate was not perfectly smooth; it was rough.

And at one edge, close to the 10 o'clock + sign and just above it, a tiny portion of the wall was missing. The missing portion appears white. (Remember, this would be black on the negative.) This small white nubbin is a small nodule, a tumor; this is what the DNA test was trying to tell us.

No tumors could be seen in the liver. A small nodule there could easily be missed by a CT scan, though. Even if there was none, there was a potential for one, implied by the DNA result.

The next question was "Is the prostate tumor malignant?" Ortho-phospho-tyrosine was tested next. It was Negative at the liver and testes, but Positive at the prostate. It was malignant. Paul was eager to correct his ways. He started the parasite killing program immediately and zapped. He promised to drink no more bottled water, soda pop, or commercial fruit juice.

449

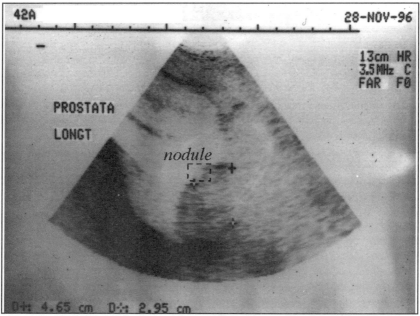

The prostate gland between the + signs has pushed into the bladder (white area).

Nov 28 radiologist spots small nodule at wall of prostate

There was not a single dental repair in his mouth! All the copper, cobalt, and vanadium in his prostate would have to come from his new beverage habit. (His childhood diet did not include these beverages.) The malonate was coming from food; he was given the malonate-free food list. The DNA-making bacteria, the clostridium family and lactobacillus, came from eating ordinary dirt in common foods [via the rabbit fluke]. Clostridium had colonized his colon. He promised to stop eating dairy foods or sterilize them; eating yogurt was another newly adopted habit.

But can a young man with no symptoms deprive himself of foods considered ordinary and safe by the public? Even an especially conscientious young man? We would see....

Meanwhile, it seemed advisable to search for early tumors in every patient, using the DNA test. If it was found, a scan would follow. More important, though, would be clearing the bacteria out of the organ involved, killing tapeworm stages, eliminating malonates [*and azo dyes*] in processed foods. Of course, killing parasites regularly and staying off the isopropyl alcohol list would come first to stop any malignancy.

More than two months passed. The clinic was in operation again at the site where Paul worked. We asked him if he had been diligent and stopped eating yogurt and drinking pop. He felt insulted. How could any intelligent

450

young man <u>not</u> stop drinking pop if it was harmful in such an important way? We apologized. Then sent him out for a new ultrasound of the prostate. In two hours he had the negative in his hands.

The tiny nodule was gone. The radiologist could not see it.

Summary: Silently this tiny malignant nodule came, and silently it went. Only the ultrasound knows the story. But Paul rose in our esteem by many feet that day. A common laborer he was, but with uncommon intelligence.

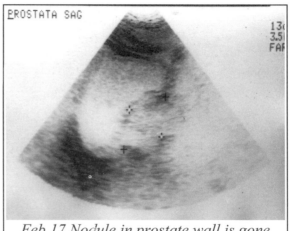

Feb 17 Nodule in prostate wall is gone

42	Victoria Boelman	Breast Cancer

Victoria Boelman, age thirty, arrived in December. She had breast cancer and was pregnant. It was called "infiltrating ductal carcinoma." Her doctor at home had recommended a modified radical mastectomy plus chemotherapy. What would happen to the fetus? No one knew. She had started herself on the parasite program one week before arriving. And she had already gotten rid of isopropyl alcohol so her tumor was no longer producing ortho-phospho-tyrosine, my marker for malignancy. But she still had benzene, wood alcohol, aflatoxin, patulin, D-malic acid, and maleic anhydride accumulation according to the whole body test. She also had freon, asbestos, aluminum, copper, mercury, and thallium. And the bacteria, *Shigella sonnei*, and *Staphylococcus aureus*. Urethane and bisphenol-A, plastic toxins, were appearing at the breast, too.

We ordered an ultrasound of the left breast and armpit. The tumor was 3.25 x 1.4 cm.

Her mouth was full of medium size amalgam fillings, fourteen in all and some plastic.

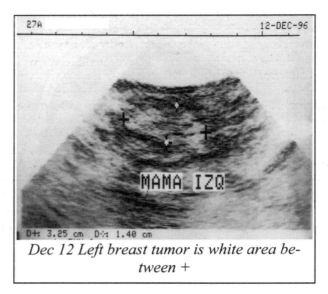

Dec 12 Left breast tumor is white area between +

Her blood test showed only the earliest effects of tumor disease, blocked urea and creatinine formation and very low calcium and phosphate levels. The presence of D-malic and maleic anhydride implied the presence of malonate before it was detoxified.

Her liver enzymes were especially good (low), as was LDH and alk phos [*implying few dye-related mutations*].

But the uric acid level was sounding a warning. It was much too low. By now, we had seen the link between bacteria and low uric acid levels. Somewhere ammonia was being produced in large amounts just when it could not be easily converted to urea. Besides, the breast would not have a large capacity for making urea such as the liver and kidney would. So nucleic acids would be used for this ignoble purpose. But only the pyrimidine variety, so that a great excess of uridine and cytidine would be produced. Both of these lead to thymidine formation, also in excess.

Somehow, the excess pyrimidines lead to insufficient purines. The purine variety of nucleic acids is absent or very, very low. And with low levels of purines, such as adenine and guanine, uric acid levels must also be low since they are derived from purines.

There are always two explanations for a low level of anything. Either not enough is made or too much is used up. If too much uric acid were used up, could this be explained by bacterial action, too? Do bacteria simply eat purines? Which bacteria were they? It was Victoria who would find the answer for us.

She was started on the usual program, and was sent to remove all metal from her teeth. Also, specific for breast cancer is wearing no bra of the regular style. Ten days later she announced that all metal was out of her mouth. A new blood test should prove this fact and was ordered.

Certainly, the WBC was lower and more normal. But the BUN and creatinine were still blocked. And the uric acid, becoming unmasked by her new procedures, indicated hordes of bacteria were still present.

The calcium level had come up and the phosphate with it, showing that the parathyroid was free of toxins at last and could make parathyroid hormone again.

A quick check at the breast and liver tissues showed glutamic acid and glutamine were Negative. Ornithine and arginine were Negative, too! Without ornithine and arginine, urea (BUN) cannot be made. Without glutamine, purines cannot be made. Without glutamic acid, glutamine cannot be made. Where had they all disappeared to? After all, she had taken these supplements that very day. A supplement check was ordered, to make sure she had them all and was taking them all. She was. Could some factor(s) in her <u>plastic</u> teeth impede progress?

DNA testing showed it was still present at the breast, as it must be when bacteria are turning RNA into DNA nonstop. I decided to search through my entire bacteria collection (the slides) for any clues to the responsible varieties.

Five clostridium species, *Lactobacillus acidophilus*, and *Staphylococcus aureus* were all still present at the breast. The clostridium family of bacteria, as well as some *Lactobacillus* varieties can make DNA from <u>our</u> RNA. The staphylococcus bacteria implied dental infection. The dentist had pointed out to her that three out of four wisdom teeth pulled a long time ago appeared to have cavitations left behind. These would house staphylococcus bacteria.

She had acquired an enlarged lymph node under her chin just recently, testimony to the streams of bacteria and toxins flowing from the mouth. And to the spread of these dangerous bacteria. Time was important. But she was reluctant to proceed with plastic removal. It was now December 23. Her family and friends wanted her home for Christmas. How would she look? So the plastic cleanup was delayed.

She returned January 3. Her first task was to see the special dentist for plastic removal by air abrasion.

When she returned from the dental visit, the breast still had all the malonates accumulated as before. A quick check showed copper, cobalt, vanadium Positive too. Had the dentist missed something?

Only two clostridium and one lactobacillus variety were still at the breast. Salmonella was also Positive at the breast. Others were Negative. Some progress had been made, but not enough. Unless the malonates and metals were removed from the teeth with meticulous care, the bacteria could not be eradicated. She was sent back to the same dental specialist to search again.

At her next visit, January 6, the results were good: copper, cobalt, vanadium, five malonates, urethane, bisphenol were all Negative at the breast. All clostridium bacteria, lactobacillus and the eight common food bacteria were Negative at the breast. She could schedule her follow-up ultrasound of the breast in ten days if this continued. A new blood test was done (Jan. 6).

BUN and creatinine were still too low, uric acid and calcium were too low, too. Perhaps not enough time had passed since the final tooth cleaning–only two days. She was started on a calcium supplement accompanied by magnesium and vitamin D.

Two days later, January 8, she passed the three month pregnancy point. Suddenly, DNA was everywhere! At the ovary, uterus, pancreas, parathyroid, breast. The magic of pregnancy was in process. The growth of the fetus could be detected through the mother.

By January 10, Victoria thought the tumor felt softer and smaller. We searched for bacteria; they were gone. We searched for DNA again. It was now Positive at adrenals, liver, lung, cerebrum, skin, thyroid, thymus, optic chiasma [*of the fetus?*]. It was still Negative at cerebellum, kidney, and stomach. What did this pattern mean? Only more research would tell. Victoria was impatient to be done. She wanted to go home. But her fourteen empty teeth struck fear in her. What if they got infected? She was instructed to floss once a day with nylon thread and brush with white iodine. But she knew her husband would be very put out. Perhaps even demand that she fill them.

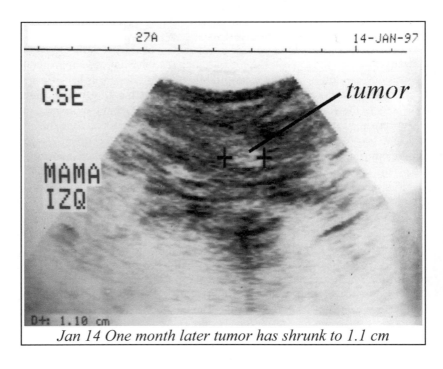

Jan 14 One month later tumor has shrunk to 1.1 cm

Would a new ultrasound show the tumor had shrunk? If it had, would this persuade her and her husband to be patient and keep the fillings open at least till the baby was born?

On January 14, she had her follow up ultrasound of the left breast. She also had a blood test done. But while on these errands panic struck and anxiety sent her directly to a dentist to put fourteen temporary fillings in her mouth.

The ultrasound was beautiful. The tumor had shrunk to 1.1 cm. No wonder she could hardly feel it.

The blood test finally showed the BUN was rising. The calcium level was the best ever. Blood fat and cholesterol were higher; she was better nourished. Uric acid though, remained very low.

The next day, January 15, only one day after the temporary fillings were put in, clostridium and lactobacillus bacteria were back in her teeth! She was devastated. We were devastated. The bacteria would reach the breast in a day. Her tumor would grow right back. The fillings were reported to be just ZOE, zinc oxide and eugenol. No Lugol's had been used to sterilize the holes before filling either. She could not bring herself to remove it all again. Her fear of the tumor was distant now. While her fear of her husband's reaction to the "open" teeth was near.

But I could not authorize her departure for home as planned. It would be a certain mastectomy and a certain death at a young age when motherhood, I felt, was her birthright. We persuaded her to extend her stay.

Two days later, January 17, depressed and anxious instead of happy and dancing, she still had done nothing. We tested at the breast again; copper was already present. We tested for copper and malonic acid in her teeth. The temporary fillings were polluted! Was the ZOE itself polluted? Not likely. But a single swipe to "coat the nerve" with any special "desensitizer" and "sealer" was probably the true cause.

How could a dentist know this? It had taken our diagnostic team two years to find the extreme sensitivity of the cancer patient to even the tiniest dose of tumorigen permanently placed in the teeth. No dentist could guess it or be blamed for applying the state-of-the-art details that make dentistry sophisticated and enjoyable. Our resolve had to be to tighten our hold on the unsuspecting patient to prevent misguided dentist visits. Only a special dentist, aware of the pitfalls of using adjunctive materials could ever be patronized in the future.

Next day, Victoria had most of the temporaries removed again. Yet she remained Positive for tumorigens; it did not all come out.

She went to another dentist with special removal methods. But the pollution remained. She would have to go back to the specialist who could do air abrasion for the third time! But she didn't go. It would cost $100. With the newly cancer-free breast all but a certainty, she did not want to spend another $100. Not even to guarantee her future. What will it hold?

Summary: A young couple have the right to expect safety in dental materials, so that they cause no harm to mother or child. Until that can be guaranteed by the dental profession, conservative treatment is best: clean the infected area with air abrasion or drilling, then keep the hole sterile by brushing with colloidal silver, white iodine, oregano oil and occasionally bleach. <u>No fillings needed</u>. As long as there is no further infection the holes cannot get larger. If infection is stopped and the holes do not get larger, why fill them?

Victoria Boelman	12/10	12/20	1/6	1/14
RBC	4.67	4.61	4.34	4.22
WBC	9.5	7.9	7.9	8.5
PLT	292	283	290	254
glucose	113	45	75	74
BUN	5.0 (5-26)	5.0	5.0	7.0
creatinine	0.7 (.6-1.4)	0.6	0.7	0.7
AST (SGOT)	17.0	17.	19.	13.
ALT (SGPT)	8.0	11	12	7
LDH	130	136	120	137
GGT	9.0	6	6	5
T.b.	0.7	0.6	0.4	0.6
alk phos	57	59	57	58
T.p.	6.8	7.0	6.7	6.8
albumin	4.0	4.3	4.1	4.1
globulin	2.8	2.7	2.6	2.7
uric acid	2.1	0.9	0.8	0.8
Calcium	8.6	9.3	8.7	9.4
Phosphorus	2.4	3.6	2.9	3.3
Iron	115	106	133	108
Sodium	139	139	137	141
Potassium	4.4	4.1	4.1	4.6
Chloride	100	97	100	100
triglycerides	84	87	83	121
cholesterol	173	174	187	200

---

43   Stacy Riley   **Lung Cancer**

Stacy Riley, forty-one, was riddled with lung cancer. She tested Positive for nickel and formaldehyde when she arrived, two serious lung toxins. She would have to clean up her home before returning to it.

She was diagnosed just half a year earlier with metastatic melanoma. But it must have begun four years earlier when a mole on her back was removed. Now she was started on interleukin at the National Cancer Institute of Bethesda, Maryland–an immune therapy. She had two sessions: 11 doses the first time and 8 doses the second time. The doctors said the cancer was advancing too rapidly, the interleukin was doing no good; she was on their high dosage already. So they told her to go home and arrange with hospice for her terminal care. That was December 22, fifteen days ago. She took the news with the stoicism of a Roman gladiator: she was given two months.

When she arrived, she was on no special medication, only Synthroid 1.25 mg. She had brought a CT scan from three weeks ago and her latest chest X-ray, made three days earlier; the lungs had a moth-eaten appearance and the report indicated 200 lung tumors, packed side by side. Only the lungs were involved. This did not seem too ominous to our staff, but Stacy did not light up with the prospect of life. She seemed resigned to her fate. We would have to pull her from the depths, not just throw her a life belt. Her family, at home, was totally against this, she said. They didn't want to spend the family assets on her wild grasping-at-straws. And we would need to work very quickly, before her sudden collapse.

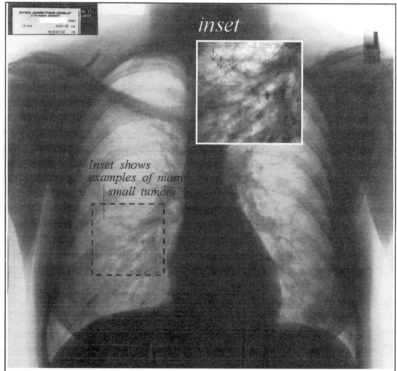

inset

Inset shows examples of many small tumors

Dec 31 about 200 closely packed small tumors (small white areas) in the lungs

We must avoid massive infection at her lungs. Would there be bleeding on a grand scale when the tumors pulled away from the thin pleura, as we had seen so often for large tumors?

Initial electronic testing at the lung showed 5 clostridium species, *Lactobacillus acidophilus*, *E. coli*, 3 salmonella varieties, *Staphylococcus aureus*, *Shigella flexneri* all Positive. Maybe *Shigella flexneri* was taking its toll on her mood; it is a depression-causing bacterium.

When so many bacteria are present, I expect a lot of growth factors to be abnormally present also. In her lungs the Syncrometer found Ca 72-4, CAA-B antigen, CAA-O antigen, alfa fetoprotein (AFP), fibroblast growth factor (FGF) very high, epidermal growth factor (EGF) very high, platelet derived growth factor (PDGF), CAA-GI, and insulin-like growth factor (ILGF). In all cases I find these are gone when the bacteria are gone!

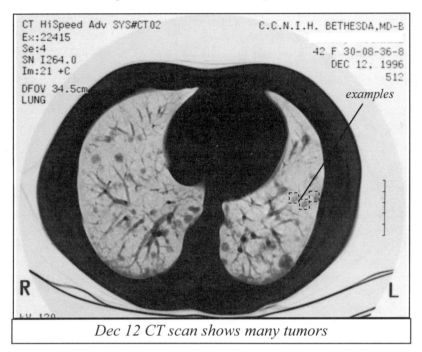

Dec 12 CT scan shows many tumors

Four amino acids were tested at the lung with these results (they should all be present): glutamic acid Positive, arginine Negative, glutamine Negative, ornithine Negative.

Lactoferrin was Negative at breast, liver, and bone marrow; it should have been Positive.

Her blood test was exceptionally good and belied her tumor-ridden lungs. Her good health and youthfulness would now be called upon to make success possible.

Neither LDH nor alk phos was elevated [*showing that damage from the azo dyes in food, hair dyes, or dental plastic had not occurred*]. The liver was still exceptionally good. But anemia was prominent and creatinine was too low. The low creatinine implied there was not enough arginine or methyl groups or glycine. Calcium and potassium were low. But her body was still well nourished.

She had been on iron tablets daily when she arrived, no doubt responsible for the excellent iron level. But it was not getting to the bone marrow to build RBCs due to absence of transferrin.

She was started on a daily enema using black walnut tincture extra strength to reduce the bacterial levels in the bowel, thereby reducing them overall.

She was told to drink raw milk, boiled 10 seconds and vitamin C-ed, to provide lactoferrin. [*More recently, in this 21-day cancer program, no milk is allowed, to avoid any possible errors in selection or treatment.*] This was in addition to the usual program of parasite killing, coenzyme Q10, glutathione, Lugol's, and other supplements.

She thought she was allergic to iodine, so peroxide was tried for dental sterilization instead of Lugol's. Her mouth was full of large fillings; she would need a lot of extractions. Later she was given homemade colloidal silver to take during dental-work days; it was definitely superior to peroxide. [*This was before our trial of diluted USP bleach, which turned out to work the best.*]

By her third day, she had extracted three teeth, but she was still Positive for DNA at the lungs. She also had maleic anhydride there, starting liquid effusion and water accumulation. And, of course, still mercury and nickel.

After one week, she had six teeth extracted by our oral surgeon. Immediately after this, her chest began hurting. Would this lead to bleeding, perhaps hemorrhaging? But we dared not slow down since time was racing her. In spite of this, DNA and the p53 gene mutation were still Positive at the lungs. Three clostridium bacteria were still Positive at the lung and one clostridium (septicum), was still Positive at the tooth location. Clostridium was also present at the parathyroids, as was the p53 gene mutation. [*The parathyroids are always targeted in cancer cases; this was pointed out by Dr. Wm. Koch nearly a century ago.*] Suspicion that parathyroids are involved occurs when calcium is too low.

Amino acids were tested. Phenylalanine was Negative at liver, lung, lymph nodes, breast, parathyroid, and thyroid. Phenylalanine is always present in our tissues in health. Why was it absent? Tyrosine, its closest cousin, was tested next. It was positive at all these locations. Evidently phenylalanine could convert to tyrosine, but not the other way around. Was the enzyme that converts tyrosine back to phenylalanine inhibited? She was taken off dairy and meat products entirely to reduce phenylalanine in her diet. This would keep tyrosine from building up. By now, *Clostridium* was eliminated from the tooth location, though it was still present at the colon.

How could we get rid of *Clostridium* in her intestine? She was started on the bowel program. [*At that time we had not discovered the magic of betaine and hydrochloric acid.*]

Her next blood test, done January 15, showed significant improvement in the RBC; she was less anemic. Creatinine was up to normal. She had been taking arginine (and ornithine) daily. Her uric acid level had fallen, revealing throngs of clostridium bacteria remaining. By making more RBCs, her iron level had dropped from 100 to 36, but then was unable to raise her iron level back to normal because of copper [*or germanium*] toxicity.

By January 16, her dental work was still not completed. But her chest pain had stopped! DNA had been Negative at the lungs for three days. Did this mean the DNA-forming bacteria (*Clostridium*) were finally vanquished?

We tested: only one clostridium species was Positive. Lactobacillus was Negative. All eight common food bacteria were Negative. The bacteria were gone both at the lungs and the parathyroids. This day phenylalanine was Positive, too; not merely tyrosine. Evidently, she could now convert it back from tyrosine. Had the enzyme block been due to bacteria?

Four days later, January 22, she had bacteria back in her lungs; it was a setback. *Rhizobium* and *Lactobacillus* were both present. So was DNA. Where were they coming from? She had benzene in her lungs! This encourages every single pathogen to multiply. The situation would be hopeless unless the benzene source was found and cleared.

The bad impact could be seen immediately on her blood test done that day. Although the RBC rose further, the LDH worsened. The benzene source must have brought with it a carcinogenic dye. [*Bursting and draining of tumors would release both*]. Would this be the beginning of a run-away trend we could not stop? But calcium and iron were coming up.

We pushed. We encouraged. We hustled. We sympathized. Finally, all extractions of teeth were done (altogether 12). A final panoramic X-ray still showed a tattoo. That would be removed at once too.

Stacy Riley	1/6	1/15	1/22	1/30
RBC	3.83	4.0	4.1	4.2
WBC	7.7	8.5	9.8	7.8
PLT	319	284	391	369
glucose	84	95	72	84
BUN	12	12	10	12
creatinine	0.8	1.2	1.1	0.9
SGOT	9	16	21	20
SGPT	8	18	9	18
LDH	143	141	181	128
GGT	5	14	20	12
T.b.	1.0	0.5	0.7	0.5
alk phos	64	76	70	58
T.p.	7.6	7.2	7.5	7.6
albumin	4.8	4.7	4.7	4.9
globulin	2.8	2.5	2.8	2.7
uric acid	2.6	1.4	3.2	0.7
Calcium	8.9	8.6	9.0	8.7
Phosphorus	4.0	3.6	4.2	4.0
Iron	100	36	72	61
Sodium	136	136	138	138
Potassium	3.6	3.8	3.8	3.8
Chloride	98	98	100	98
triglycerides	219	150	142	84
cholesterol	145	154	148	152

By January 27 she had a lot more energy than she could remember; she was sleeping better, too. Testing at her lung showed no copper, cobalt, vanadium, DNA. Besides this malonyl coenzyme A was Negative, and methyl malonyl CoA was Negative, too.

These malonyl compounds are Positive when malonic acid has been present very recently. They show how coenzyme A is harnessed for malonic acid utilization instead of allowing it to fuel the Krebs (energy) cycle.

She could tell her lungs were better and she could endure cooking odors now, like coffee. All bacteria tested Negative. She got impressions made for her new partials.

The next day she was

feeling still better. Mental clarity had returned. Appetite was better. She looked lively and alert—almost happy!

A final blood test on January 30 showed the recent improvements. The LDH was back down—way down! As was alk phos. RBC was still rising, giving her even more energy. But uric acid had dropped drastically again.

Could she have the bacteria back? Indeed she could. A quick check at the lungs showed six clostridium species Positive again. Glutathione was Negative. What caused this glutathione destruction? Searching our tumorigens, one was found in the lungs.

Ribonucleoside vanadyl complexes were Positive. These originate with vanadium. But vanadium itself was not. Could a mere trace of vanadium, as one would get sitting in traffic at the US border crossing cause this? It seemed unlikely. It remained unexplained. [*In hindsight she must have had leftover dental plastic or metal.*] She was due to leave for home in four days. A final chest X-ray was scheduled.

She returned with it next day.

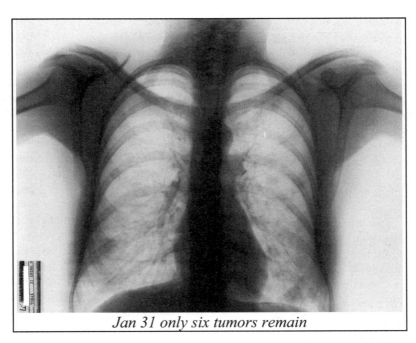

Jan 31 only six tumors remain

It was almost too beautiful to behold. The radiologist had counted only six tumors now—out of that horde of 200! The texture was beautiful too, though not yet normal.

Summary: At this rate, only one more week would surely have dissolved the remaining six. But family matters pressed. Perhaps she was just one more dental cleaning away from life-saving success. Perhaps it sufficed.

44 Jessie Healy	Lymphatic/Breast Cancer

Jessie Healy was a scientist herself with a Master's degree in biochemistry, specialized in the study of milk. This scientific bent, no doubt, explained her organized approach to all problems including her own health. She had returned to the clinic full of hope that something could be done for her creaky, painful knee and hip. This is taken from her own notes.

"January 10, first day at the clinic. Symptoms: 1) Hip pain, most important. Can't get up off chair using legs alone. 2) Right knee sore; knee pad swollen and tender. 3) Can't walk without pain. 4) Can't get out of car seat, chairs, without slow and careful maneuvering and hand pushing/lifting. 5) When in bed, painful to rest knees together to sleep on right side; painful to turn body in bed; can't rest left leg when flat on back."

Jessie had visited the clinic some years ago because of her eye disease, retinitis pigmentosa.[122] She had believed from the age of twenty, when it was diagnosed, that she would go blind eventually. And the time had come for her genetic fate to be executed. For 40 years the idea that an alternative approach was possible was branded quackery by her fellow workers, and she absorbed this disdaining attitude. But in her early sixties and about to trade her driver's license and her job for a course in Braille, she decided to investigate. To her surprise our alternative approach was entirely to her liking, being utterly scientific and begging her participation as a scientist.

Now, five years later, going blind was furthest from her mind, the disease was "in remission" and her driver's license had no restrictive clauses. She was pleased and hoped something could also be done for her decrepit condition. Personally, she believed she had done it to herself–by playing tennis–into her later years. And she was mighty proud of her athletic lifestyle. So she just took painkillers and played on. It kept her slim and trim, in touch with friends, and exhilarated with energy. I felt sorry for her as she carefully limped through the doorway.

In the first five minutes of our interview, her "arthritis" could already be explained. We tried to teach her a new kind of Bacteriology—based on Syncrometer testing. This shows that ALL PAIN IS BACTERIAL. The bacteria are streptococcus varieties. All locations in the body that have pain also have streptococcus bacteria. Streptococcus bacteria make phenol. And phenol causes pain. But that is not as important as its other effect. Phenol oxidizes you (although in regular chemistry it is considered a reducer), from top to toe, in places where you should never be oxidized. It oxidizes your vitamin C so that the molecule breaks apart to form "oxidation products", like xylose, lyxose, and threose. These cause <u>aging</u>: forming wrinkles, softening bones, making cataracts, causing diabetes. And without regular reduced vitamin C,

---

[122] Clark, H.R., *The Cure For All Diseases*, New Century Press, 1995, see chapter "Pain from Head to Toe," section "Eye Pain" for her early history.

your tissues cannot <u>heal</u>. Healing requires vitamin C. So not only did Jessie have pain in her joints, they could not heal! Bacteria can easily move around in your body, traveling from one pain location to another by swimming along in the blood. For Jessie, the clue was her painful teeth. From small colonies here, they could spread to any other location in her body that would let them gain a foothold—such as her frequently traumatized joints.

Jessie knew she had infected teeth—they were aching! But somehow this straightforward logic was easier to apply here at our clinic than by herself at home surrounded by dentists wishing to "restore" rather than extract teeth. A panoramic X-ray revealed the abscesses. But should she extract? Was there no other way? Couldn't she just try to zap the bacteria? Then a new development drove away any hesitation. When she arrived, she listed a lumpy armpit as one of her symptoms. One lump felt elongated and was about 1 inch long. Was it anything to worry about since both armpits had been "lumpy" for years?

We searched for tumors immediately. Within five minutes we had found that our DNA test was Positive at her lymph nodes and breast. She indeed had been growing tumors in both places! We scheduled a CT scan immediately, since an ultrasound could miss a very tiny tumor. (On the other hand, a CT scan can miss something that an ultrasound can catch, too.)

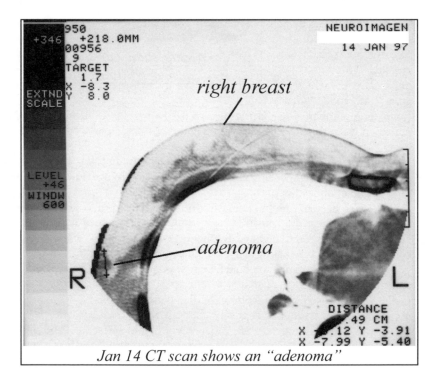

Jan 14 CT scan shows an "adenoma"

Afterwards we reviewed it together. The radiologist had marked it, measured it, and called it an adenoma. A frightening word! Arthritis could certainly take second place to beginning cancer.

To her surprise, our method of stopping tumor growth was <u>also</u> largely dental. In this case, it was clostridium bacteria hiding away under tooth fillings. The connection was rational. If tooth-infecting bacteria could also make DNA inside our cells, the infection must be cleared in a permanent way, not left to chance. Step one was to extract infected teeth (not repair them and <u>hope</u> they would not reinfect). Off she went to the dental surgeon.

These are her notes:

"January 14, extracted three teeth with large fillings showing bacteria-lines at the base, going into the teeth. (When they reach the nerve they hurt.)

"January 22, extracted two painful, dying teeth showing bacterial infection."

Between these dates, Jessie hot-packed her face for hours each day, swished with hot water, brushed with white iodine, and suddenly be-

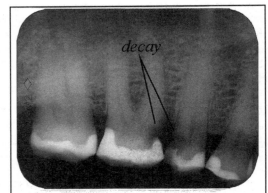

Dental periapical X-ray shows decay under fillings

came more limber. She surprised herself, getting up from a chair rather quickly now, since she was focused on her armpit and breast, not her hip and knee.

She was also hot-packing her armpit and taking the full regimen of supplements aimed at shrinking tumors. She was determined to win this new kind of game, in dead-earnest.

She also needed to remove plastic fillings, unheard of in her experience. Yet, she could hear the "positive" test results as we checked her for copper, cobalt, malonates, urethane, and bisphenol-A. Bisphenol-A, a component of composite, is described as "estrogenic", meaning 'going to the breast'! It was going to <u>her</u> breast. And the conclusion was only logical. <u>Take it out.</u> She went to see the special dentist who did air-abrasion. If a minute speck of metal was exposed at the bottom of the plastic filling, it, too, could be abraded out. But it requires dexterity.

It was Saturday, January 25, and a new problem surfaced. Tooth #9 now had a big hole on the back side. She did not care to refill it for fear of making the tumor grow. It really ought to be extracted since it was simply too damaged, but no dental surgeon could be reached on Saturday afternoon. Her flight left on Sunday.

The day her plane left she could walk normally and didn't need hands to help her out of chairs. But her focus, as well as ours, was on the tumor. Was it shrinking or would it wait on completion of the last dental work? She agreed to get another CT scan a week after her arrival at home.

Such plans go awry easily. As rational as they sound at our clinic, no doctor at "home" wants to abide by anyone else's bidding. And often do not want to listen to a patient's request. The patient is powerless in the US. The doctor is following his or her <u>own</u> agenda for the patient. Jessie kept trying to get a new CT scan but each time got "postponed" by her doctor. The effort was just not worth it. So, she simply waited to return here. Besides, she had more aching teeth and her painful arthritis was back, too. This time, though, it did not panic her. The connection between infected teeth and skeletal pain was plain to see. But had all this delay stalled her tumor shrinkage? That was the gnawing question.

She returned on March 1, half full of anticipation and half full of anxiety. These were her initial test results: mercury and thallium, both Positive at teeth, breast and lymph nodes. Obviously she had an amalgam tattoo somewhere. Rhodanese enzyme Negative at the breast, should be Positive—it is a detoxifying enzyme. Glutathione Negative at the breast. 20-methylcholanthrene Positive at the breast.

She was being challenged continuously by this endogenous carcinogen (20-methylcholanthrene)! This was due to lack of rhodanese which otherwise might detoxify it. And rhodanese was absent for lack of iron. And iron was low due to competition with copper [*and germanium*] from a tiny bit of metal or plastic left somewhere in her mouth.

With copper present, glutathione would be absent. With glutathione absent, the bacteria could thrive. So metals and bacteria could go hand in hand, anywhere. They had chosen her armpit and breast. Clostridium botulinum, Clostridium sporogenes, Rhizobium leguminosarum, Rhizobium meliloti were all Positive at the breast.

DNA was Negative at breast. At least the tumor could not be growing. This was a cherished result for Jessie. Did these bacteria not make DNA? In most other circumstances they do. What was different? Can bacteria switch on or off their DNA-making enzymes? This waits for more research.

Jessie had less than a week to stay this time; just long enough to extract, clean cavitations, and learn to drink raw milk once a week (properly sterilized) to get back the lactoferrin she was missing and long enough to get the new CT scan that was tantalizing her.

She brought it in for review, not quite believing the radiologist's Spanish comments which she thought translated to "He could not find it!" We taped it up to the window immediately. It was as the radiologist said. There was nothing there! The adenoma was gone.

Her arthritis was gone, AGAIN, too.

She accepted the idea of partial dentures with gratitude and so much joy (over the missing tumor), a little song leaped into her heart. She sang it quietly to the staff before leaving: "Not Only Smaller But Gone" to the tune of "I Wish I Were Single Again."

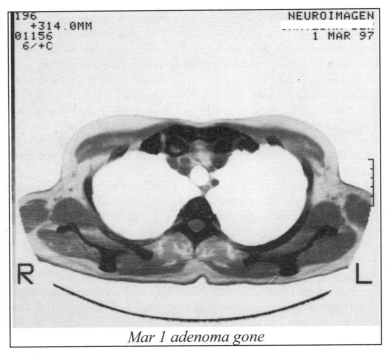

Mar 1 adenoma gone

Summary: we quietly agreed that some patients make it all worth while. The world IS waiting for a rational, that is, scientific, approach to medicine with patient input, patient-power, and an egalitarian relationship between all. This was a case of early discovery of a developing tumor, using Syncrometer technology. No blood test results were available for this case history.

45	Chris Lantz	Prostate Cancer

Chris Lantz, a civil engineer, age seventy, came from France for his prostate cancer. It was January 15, and he had already been on the herbal program for two weeks, as well as zapping.

In spite of this, he tested Positive for isopropyl alcohol when he arrived; he couldn't stop using his favorite supplements. He also tested Positive for asbestos, aluminum, cadmium, lead, mercury, thallium, and tartrazine (yellow food dye).

His symptoms actually began ten years earlier with frequent urination. In the last two years he was getting up six or seven times a night to empty his bladder. For the last three to four months he also had pain. He had been on the macrobiotic diet for two years, hoping his PSA would go down. But actually, it went up. In March last year it was 5. And in December last year it was 23.2.

The usual blood test and ultrasound of prostate were scheduled on his first day. He was given environmentally safe lodging with a restaurant nearby that could prepare malonate-free food and properly sterilized uncolored dairy products.

He had seven or eight root canals, at least four bridges, and some crowns in his mouth.

He was started on the supplements and cleanses on the first day of his stay. That very night he had no pain with urination. And there was no blood in the urine.

On his second day, January 16, we received his blood test and ultrasound. The size of his prostate was 5.1 x 6.0 cm and a small tumor was present, 1.8 cm long.

His blood test results showed he had serious under-nutrition. His triglycerides as well as cholesterol were much too low. They should have been closer to 150 and 250. We immediately stressed the importance of fat in the diet: eggs, avocados, sardines, fish, and poultry.

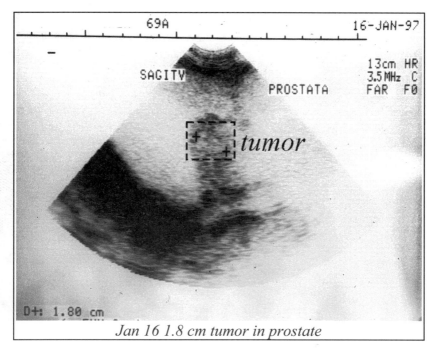

Jan 16 1.8 cm tumor in prostate

The RBC was rather low, explaining his fatigue. He had a lively personality, full of humor, but he could not express it due to low energy. His WBC was very low too, showing low immunity. Both problems stem from toxins in the bone marrow.

His LDH and alk phos were both elevated, showing there was active tumor growth [*now we know it is due to dyes*].

The calcium level was much too low, which is evidence of toxins in the parathyroid. Potassium was quite low, too, contributing to his fatigue!

But nothing was extremely high or low, and if we could improve his nutritional status while removing his body burden of toxins, he would be successful in dissolving his tumor.

He laughed with anticipation of new found health; he called the motel/restaurant his paradise, but he was happy to just rest!

On the first day too, we searched for DNA in all his tissues, to be sure there was no extra tumor growing anywhere. DNA was only Positive at the prostate (and, of course, testes).

We scheduled him for dental work to extract every tooth that had a large metal or nonmetal filling. That would leave him only three lower teeth, but he was undaunted. Onward and upward was his motto. After ten years of a failing battle with prostate cancer, switching to dentures was not a big price to pay. He would remind me during office visits: "Teeth is not importante. Only your life este importante." Then he would ask "You think you can cure this cancer?"

"Everybody else cures theirs; so can you, Chris," was my usual answer.

By January 24 he had all his teeth except three lowers removed. He was feeling extra good after the oral surgery, rather than convalescent. His mouth was not even painful.

His new blood test on January 24 showed several improvements. The RBC, WBC, and platelet count were all up, implying that toxins were reduced in the bone marrow.

And his LDH had dropped as well as the alk phos. [This showed that *Sudan Black B and DAB dyes, which are in most plastic tooth fillings* were being removed.]

His liver could now make much more protein. And the calcium level had risen to normal, showing that toxins were now out of the parathyroid. The problem had now shifted to the thyroid which can be seen in the potassium level (5.0, too high).

His triglycerides and cholesterol had come up, showing better nutritional status. He was trying to eat fat and drink milk (carefully selected and treated) for the first time in years.

He was planning his trip home as soon as new partial dentures would be ready. But first he must do another panoramic X-ray to guarantee there were no leftover bits of amalgam in his jaws and mouth tissues.

He said he felt better than in years. He walked better. There was no pain with urination, but he still got up in the night every hour! He was started on kidney herbs, a half dose on the first day, full dose on the second, and double dose after that.

Lactoferrin was now testing Positive at the bone marrow; he was drinking raw milk that had been tested for dyes and sterilized.

All toxins, as well as DNA were now Negative at the prostate. But a search at the thyroid revealed *Staphylococcus*, *Shigella flexneri*, and *E. coli*. He had not been hot packing enough and was immediately helped with this important task.

Six days later on January 30, he got a new panoramic of his teeth. It showed a large plastic filling had been overlooked in a front lower tooth. There was also a small infection in the neighboring tooth.

Nevertheless, the new blood test showed great improvements, although the RBC did not rise (3.71). The LDH dropped further, as did the alk phos. Tumor activity was definitely waning. But uric acid was extremely low, showing that clostridium bacteria were still swarming somewhere.

Potassium was normal now, showing that the thyroid had been freed. And triglycerides as well as cholesterol were still rising. His body was thriving on improved nutrition, malonate-free and safe from parasite eggs, unsanitary bacteria, and carcinogenic dyes.

On February 3, he pulled this last tooth. That night his old affliction returned, painful and difficult urination. He was crestfallen. But his airline ticket was for two days hence. Could he leave? He had been fitted for dentures and was waiting for them. Next day we tested for bacteria at the prostate, on the theory that his symptom return was due to release of bacteria from that particular tooth–the one extracted last. But no *Clostridia* were found, nor Lactobacilli, Rhizobium, or Staphylococcus.

And all tumor toxins were now Negative at the teeth. Vanadium, cobalt, copper, five malonates, urethane, and bisphenol-A—all Negative at the tooth location. He was ready to start rebuilding the prostate gland. He was given flaxseed, raw, 1

Chris Lantz	1/15	1/24	1/30	2/03
RBC	3.56	3.75	3.71	4.0
WBC	4,000	6,400	6,600	5,5
PLT	197	206	288	291
glucose	127	137	95	85
BUN	16	27	26	18
creatinine	1.2	1.0	1.0	0.9
AST (SGOT)	25	35	33	43
ALT (SGPT)	19	51	22	49
LDH	225	199	164	161
GGT	43	40	39	43
T.b.	0.5	0.7	0.6	0.4
alk phos	107	103	87	88
T.p.	6.3	7.1	6.6	6.4
albumin	4.3	4.6	4.2	4.2
globulin	2.0	2.5	2.4	2.2
uric acid	2.8	2.2	0.9	1.7
Calcium	8.6	9.2	8.7	8.8
Phosphorus	3.1	3.2	4.3	4.1
Iron	57	54	68	63
Sodium	134	133	133	138
Potassium	3.8	5.0	4.5	4.7
Chloride	95	95	99	99
triglycerides	46	59	85	200
cholesterol	100	156	157	180
PSA				19.2

tbs./day, soaked for 5 minutes first, then cooked with cereal.

It was February 5, his last day. There had been no more pain nor bleeding. His immune system had conquered the last release of bacteria. The final blood test, done February 3, was reviewed with him. At last, his red cell count had come up to 4.0. He was still anemic but much better. His kidney function was now perfect. The LDH had dropped further, but still wasn't low enough to feel totally secure. The alk phos appeared stable.

Calcium and uric acid were still too low, implying bacteria in the parathyroids; they should be searched for. He had not been doing enemas as he should. He was instructed to help his bowel function with Lugol's enemas once a day, just to get the bacterial level down. Triglycerides and cholesterol were now normal.

Only the new ultrasound remained to be seen. And the new PSA result. While he was attending to these, his new dentures were tested for tumor toxins. There were none. He arrived with ultrasound in hand! The size of his prostate was now 4.45 x 4.65 cm and no tumor was visible.

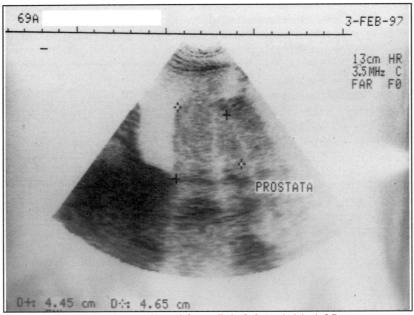

Prostate size reduced from 5.1x6.0 to 4.44x4.65 cm.
Feb 3 tumor gone, PSA dropping

He began to laugh with joy. He could hardly believe all his good fortune! His PSA result had arrived, too. It had dropped from 23.2 to 19.2 in three weeks.

But he was leaving prematurely, and he knew it. He tried on his new dentures; they needed adjustment. If the adjustment was not carefully monitored, the materials used could re-pollute the teeth. This is no small matter. Sucking on a carcinogen day and night is far more injurious than occasionally eating it. There would be no time left to re-test the teeth after adjustment. It would be wiser to leave them unadjusted. [*We now have a way of hardening "adjusted" teeth at home.*]

Summary: With the tumor gone, why wasn't his PSA down to normal, less than 4? The PSA depends on the size of the prostate, as well, and this would take longer to reduce. But he had gotten started with that, too, and hopefully, will be completely normal, soon.

46	Arlene Miller	Brain Cancer

Arlene Miller arrived on January 20 as an emergency case and was seen by the chief assistant first. She was slightly built, and only sixty-six. She had brain cancer, called "aplastic astrocytoma," and responded to all recommendations with a resounding "NO". The need for dental extractions was raised and met with further "NO", and total irrationality. But there was no time to lose, not a single day. She was on dexamethasone to control edema in the brain, dilantin to control seizures, and hydrazine sulfate, possibly to prevent emaciation, and Axid to help digestion. It was explained to Arlene's son, her caregiver, that as soon as dental extractions were complete she stood a chance of recovering, but not sooner. And in a few days it could be too late if she refused to eat or went into a coma.

Arlene had no chemotherapy, radiation, or surgery; it all happened too fast. When she began to have symptoms, her regular doctor scheduled an MRI for her—and to the family's terrible surprise, a large brain tumor was seen, too large for surgery, too large for chemotherapy or radiation. Nothing could save her, so nothing was advised.

But our chief assistant did not give up. Against all odds, she decided to try a massive dose of black walnut tincture. There was nothing to lose. Her son was instructed to give his mother: 8 tsp. black walnut tincture extra strength, 7 capsules cloves, 7 capsules wormwood, 3 to 5 whole tsp. vitamin C, 10 capsules coenzyme Q10 (400 mg each), and 30 glutathione (250 mg each)!

And if he accomplished this, to do it again, and again! She slowly became more rational, until after seven days (of the above recipe), on a Monday morning, she sat at my office desk quite lucid, though speech was garbled.

She had insight into her own case now, could understand the explanations for dental extractions, and agreed to get it done the same day. "Who cares if you eat with dentures" she said briefly, "as long as you can eat." The humor of this remark even struck her. She must have had a great personality while she was raising her family—her son was here as living proof.

She was interested in her own blood test results. There was massive infection somewhere, in her brain, no doubt; that would explain the high WBC. And perhaps a minute bit of bleeding—inside the tumor—that would explain the high platelet count.

Both BUN and creatinine were much too low; there was obviously a blockage in their formation. We should have supplemented her with urea and creatine, but in view of her great need for other things as well, I decided to wait and see first. In hindsight this was an error; urea can help the liver greatly, and the liver was already in considerable distress, judging by the elevated enzymes SGOT, SGPT, and GGT. [*Both LDH and alk phos were only slightly elevated so dye toxicity was not very intense.*]

The low uric acid reflected the imbalance between purines and pyrimidines caused by bacteria and the ammonia they excrete.

Calcium was much too low, but this was not beyond correction either. And the triglyceride and cholesterol levels were still high enough to give her an advantage in her race for survival.

She was instructed to take digestive enzyme capsules, 2 with each meal, instead of Axid. Also, hydrochloric acid drops at mealtime (10 drops of a 5% solution). She was to eat all the fat she could (eggs, avocados, cream) and take potassium gluconate powder, even though her potassium level was adequate. I suspected that as soon as better metabolism would "kick in," her body would consume potassium so fast, not even supplements could keep up.

She was given colloidal silver (home made) to take as an antibiotic before dental work and several days after. She was instructed to remove all the metal touching her; she removed all, including her two rings, without remorse. "Who needs rings?", she asked, breezily.

Then we searched electronically at her cerebrum for several more substances. Ortho-phospho-tyrosine Negative (malignancy was stopped); DNA Positive (there was still abnormal growth there); copper, cobalt, vanadium all Positive; nucleoside vanadyl complexes Positive (a mutagen made from vanadium responsible for p53 mutations); malonyl coenzyme A Positive (shows coenzyme A subverted by malonate); three clostridium varieties Positive at brain; eight food bacteria Negative; but *Rhizobium leguminosarum*, *Lactobacillus acidophilus*, *Rhizobium meliloti*, and *Lactobacillus casei* were Positive. She had numerous bacteria in her brain that could make DNA in the human manner and fuel her tumor, also *Ascaris* larvae. Would we be able to stop it all in time?

After she left, we looked at the MRI she had brought with her; a very large tumor was easy to see.

The next days were spent with the dental surgeon. Five days later, she was a new person. Eighteen teeth had been extracted. She was hot packing and hot swishing her mouth correctly. She was more alert than before, could converse about herself, could laugh when her son once teasingly called her a "dummy", and wanted nothing so much as taking charge of her own life again.

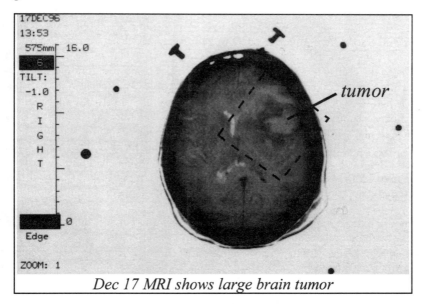

17DEC96
13:53
575mm 16.0
6
TILT:
-1.0
R
I
G
H
T
Edge
ZOOM: 1

tumor

Dec 17 MRI shows large brain tumor

The DNA, copper, cobalt, vanadium, vanadyl complexes, malonates, urethane, and bisphenol were all Negative now at the cerebrum. But *Clostridium septicum* was still Positive, the only bacterium left. Her blood test of January 31 was done just after the dental work.

The block on urea formation was removed; it was now 16. But creatinine formation was still blocked. [*We were unaware, at the time, of the huge shortages of amino acids in cancer patients, including those needed to make creatine.*]

Two of her liver enzymes (OT and PT) worsened. What could explain this? Other liver enzymes improved. Was it the anesthetic used by the dentist? Was she eating something toxic? Did she swallow a lot of mercury? No answer seemed correct. It was not explained. [*With hindsight we should have searched for lead in her drugs or supplements.*] Her iron level dropped significantly, as did her potassium, in spite of the supplement. It might have been advisable to supplement with iron.

Instead, I recommended eggs daily in her diet. All the iron tonics and syrups I had tested in the past had either solvents or mycotoxins in them. Besides, the <u>form</u> of the iron might be critically important. Some reports in the literature warn practitioners that iron makes tumors grow! Iron supplements are respected yet feared. Her potassium powder was increased to ½ tsp. three times a day.

On February 3 she was so much better mentally that she was able to comment how unhappy she was that she couldn't remember names and other things the way she used to.

On February 5, she was completely aware and alert; taking care of herself, no longer incontinent if close to bathroom. All bacteria tested Negative at the cerebrum. But she again was Positive for dental metal at her teeth (where the teeth once were). How could that be? A new panoramic X-ray of her mouth was taken. Several tattoos were visible! By February 8, two tattoos had been removed. She was fitted for dentures. At this last appointment she used no inappropriate words; her brain was healing. Her blood test now showed many improvements: her liver enzymes were going back down.

We thought she had turned the corner to health, but three days later, February 11, she was dizzy. Walking was bad again. She had definitely deteriorated. And she was very sleepy. We quickly checked for bacteria in her brain. Two varieties of *Salmonella* and *E. coli* were there. She had not been getting enough Lugol's. Nor any Lugol's enemas. Nor any black walnut tincture extra strength for a week! Both Arlene and her son thought she was "out of the woods" and could be casual with her routines. She was put back on 10 tsp. black walnut tincture extra strength plus 9 capsules cloves and 9 capsules wormwood.

She got better immediately. But three days later, February 14, she was deteriorating again. Again, she was full of *Salmonella*, *E. coli*, numerous *Clostridium* types, and *Rhizobium meliloti*, the DNA makers. Again, she was incontinent. Why was her immunity so low again? There was mercury, copper, cobalt, vanadium testing Positive, but this time at a bone location, not tooth. Evidently, there was still another tattoo embedded in her jawbone, not at a tooth location. But how could it be found?

We decided to try a new radiologist, perhaps his X-rays were of higher quality. We got his full cooperation in trying to find this tattoo. Meanwhile, we raised her supplements of arginine, glutamic acid, aspartic acid, and ornithine to ward off coma from ammonia.

The new X-rays showed nothing; we even sent them to the University of California to a dental radiologist there. But time was passing and there was very little time. Her downhill trend was obvious on the February 14 blood test. The liver was toxic.

Was she eating something toxic, accidentally, in her food or supplements? I started her on silymarin. [*I should have taken her off all supplements because this is the usual source of lead.*]

Without X-rays, a dentist is at a loss where to search for a tattoo, unless it is plainly visible. Arlene's life was hanging by a thread now. We couldn't wait for the University's results. We persuaded her dental surgeon to simply go exploring. A quadrant at a time should be surgically opened and searched for bits of leftover metal.

He found it! It was stuck in the bone.

With a clear mind again, she brought in the bone fragment like the trophy it really was. She was as happy as we were. Did he get it all this time? She was praying for this. We could now turn our attention to her high GGT. We suspected mycotoxins. Aflatoxin was positive (at liver) and zearalenone was positive (at liver), but although they were present, I wasn't convinced that was all. She agreed to do a liver cleanse that same night.

The very next day, February 18, she was much better. In fact, no sign of illness was detectable. She could walk alone. We were all amazed. But she wanted to go home. We gave her lecithin to help heal her brain (theoretically at least).

Two days later, February 20, she said she was back to her normal self; absolutely no abnormality in speech or walk or personality. She agreed to repeat liver cleanses every two weeks. She was due to leave next day. We scheduled a CT scan of the brain and a blood test. She demonstrated how well she could walk, no pain in her leg or hip anymore but she was impatient for her new dentures.

Next day, we reviewed her brain scan with her. It was easy to see the improvement. The border of her old tumor could still be seen, but the density was reduced, it was healing.

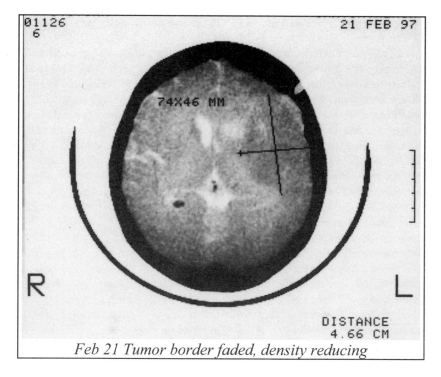

Feb 21 Tumor border faded, density reducing

She was thrilled. But the blood test results were ominous. Her GGT had doubled and evidence of bacteria (low uric acid) was still strong. The cause eluded me. Could it be due to her recent liver cleanse? Was she eating something toxic? We searched for bacteria. She did indeed again have three salmonellas and three shigellas and *E. coli* in the brain. Yet she felt so well. We lengthened our study of the cerebrum and persuaded her to lengthen her stay.

DNA Negative at cerebrum. p53 gene mutation Negative at cerebrum. 20-methylcholanthrene Negative at cerebrum (a carcinogen made from one's own cholesterol if not detoxified first by rhodanese enzymes; always associated with Ascaris parasites). Glutathione Positive at cerebrum. Tumor necrosis factor Positive at cerebrum. RNA Positive at cerebrum. rhodanese Positive. No problem could be seen.

On February 24, she slept unusually well. On February 25, she was even sleepy during the day. Yet all bacteria were Negative, as were metals and toxins. If we couldn't solve this puzzle in the next few days we would fail. Perhaps she was simply getting too much ornithine. It was stopped. And a heaping teaspoon of arginine given to wake her up. But that wasn't it. Next day, February 26, she was still asleep from the previous day! Was she sinking into a coma? Had she been getting her dexamethasone? Without this, edema fluid would accumulate in her brain and put it under pressure to the point of coma.

All office personnel were on "top-alert". If we couldn't pull her out of this emergency by the day's end, she might not come out at all and would begin her downward spiral to the infinite abyss. We prepared a urea solution (28 grams to a quart of water) to be drunk that day before leaving the office. Her dexamethasone was quadrupled. We gave special amino acids (leucine, iso leucine, and valine). We had mannitol and methylene blue on stand by. The emergency was averted. She could walk herself out of the office at day's end.

She could walk into the office next day but was still very sleepy. Obviously, the dexamethasone had not been the problem, nor done the trick.

Only one possibility remained: drug toxicity. Something was dreadfully toxic, now it was affecting the parathyroids, not just liver (calcium 7.8). She had been on dilantin and hydrazine sulfate throughout. It was an oversight. They are usually well tolerated. They were both stopped at once. We managed to feed her a cream eggnog, and a lemon oil drink for calories and nutrition in little bits throughout the day. A tsp. each of glutathione, arginine, glutamic acid (3 tsp.) and B_{12} (1 mg) and folic acid (25 mg) were her supplements, hand fed. Again, 28 grams of urea. We also gave her 1 tsp. leucine powder, 3 times a day for two days, to avert impending coma.

She was getting 2 eggs in the "shake" beverages, giving her much needed albumin. And 2 tablets of spironolactone, diuretic, since she was puffing up everywhere, even her eyelids.

After two days of force-feeding by the office staff, Arlene did not come back. I feared the worst. Her family had called from New York to ask if they should come here. I replied, <u>yes</u>.

We did not see her for six days.

On March 6, while glancing through my window, I saw her form pass by. Was it a mirage? It was Arlene, alive and well. And hale and hearty, too. She walked by herself with a strong stride. She said that even her memory was better. Her edema was gone, she was her old self. In fact, she wanted another CT scan to prove she was ready to go home. We arranged it. She had never been better. And this time she really could go home, in spite of the high GGT (1593). Perhaps her doctor at home could solve the mystery. Perhaps a change of brain diuretic was called for. She had not had any seizures either. Was she out of trouble at last? All her supplements were to be taken at half dosage for another month only at home. We reviewed her scan. It was even better than before. She said her good-byes as the vivacious person she once was. Her transformation was as amazing as seeing a butterfly emerge from its cocoon. It gave us all renewed resolve to **never take defeat**. When all is lost, try something new. Life is too precious to let it slip away from lack of initiative or plain inertia. She was a towering inspiration.

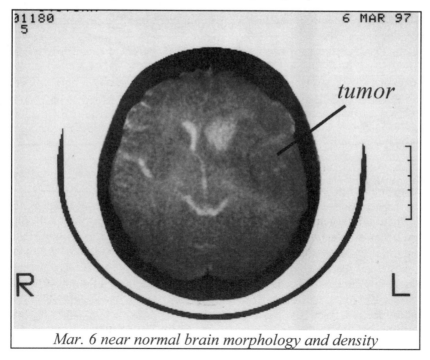

Mar. 6 near normal brain morphology and density

Summary: Some conclusions are obvious: it is much easier to shrink a tumor than to recover from toxic damage. Secondly, you must never say "it's over" until it's over. This applies to patient, caregiver, and physician alike. And one question will nag and haunt us. What was the cause of the liver failure? And what will become of it? [*With hindsight, it was probably azo dyes—escaping from the very tumor we were shrinking!*]

Arlene Miller	1/20	1/31	2/8	2/14	2/20	2/25	3/6
RBC	4.47	3.87	3.91	4.45	4.49	4.4	4.1
WBC	15,400	14,800	15,400	17,200	17,300	13,200	12,500
PLT	516,	422	495	271	379	419	403
glucose	105	115	97	144	113	86	99
BUN	6.0	16	16	16	7.0	11	17
creatinine	0.7	0.6	0.8	0.7	0.6	0.7	0.6
AST (SGOT)	47	134	53	296	123	632	605
ALT (SGPT)	93	125	70	395	476	386	755
LDH	188	156	143	178	167	220	208
GGT	399	350	230	604	1076	1219	1593
T.b.	0.3	0.3	0.5	0.5	0.8	1.0	0.9
alk phos	167	143	116	146	208	259	379
T.p.	6.5	6.0	6.5	6.7	6.8	5.9	5.9
albumin	4.1	4.0	4.3	4.2	4.3	3.8	3.8
globulin	2.4	2.0	2.2	2.5	2.5	2.1	2.1
uric acid	2.3	0.8	0.8	1.5	1.2	1.4	1.0
Calcium	8.5	8.8	8.1	9.1	8.5	7.8	8.3
Phosphorus	3.3	3.3	3.5	3.2	3.1	4.	4.1
Iron	71	33	57	28	65	62	19
Sodium	144	140	136	138	137	139	141
Potassium	4.2	3.7	4.2	3.5	3.5	3.7	4.4
Chloride	103	105	99	100	99	100	100
triglycerides	98	109	150	161	182	131	96
cholesterol	219	199	224	198	196	178	196

47   Nancy Pendergrass   Brain Cancer

Nancy Pendergrass, age seven, arrived with her parents from Australia. As she sat quietly on her mother's lap she tugged at her deep hat, pulling it down tighter over her bald head. She knew this visit was for her. Her mother told the story.

She had received immunization shots in early November of last year (it was now February 3). After this, she became ill. She had stomach pain, vomiting, cramps, loss of appetite, and hot flushes. The arm with the injection turned red. Soon afterward, by November 20, she complained of having a stiff neck. By this time, she was only urinating once a day and bowel movements had ceased. She was not getting out of bed.

One doctor thought she had encephalitis. She was taken for a CT scan and a large tumor was found in the cerebellum. It was about the size of a golf ball. She was given steroids, hoping to bring down the pressure from the tumor against the rest of the brain. The next day surgery was ordered—on November 26.

The surgery, in the neurosurgeon's opinion, was successful. However, there was a portion of the tumor, at its very base, that could not be removed. An MRI was done to see how much remained.

She was in the hospital for two weeks afterward. On December 16, she had her first chemotherapy treatment. It was given continuously, over a three day period through a "port" that was installed in her body, under her arm. After one course of chemotherapy, she became very ill. Her mother stopped it and decided to find an alternative method. The parents had been told the tumor would grow back. They decided to bring her to our office in Mexico.

She sat limply as we began our testing: DNA Positive at cerebellum (growth continuing); p53 gene (mutation) Positive at cerebellum; ortho-phospho-tyrosine Positive at cerebellum (malignancy present); isopropyl Positive (contributes to malignancy).

The parents had read the book *The Cure for all Cancers* before coming and thought that all isopropyl sources had already been removed. But she had been on a vitamin pill, untested for isopropyl pollution. It was stopped. She had already been given the parasite program (2 tsp. of black walnut tincture extra strength plus 3 wormwood and 7 clove capsules) twice, a week apart. Evidently she was reinfecting with *Fasciolopsis* stages from dairy products or meats or other sources still unknown. We would immediately give her 10 tsp. black walnut tincture extra strength plus 9 cloves and 9 wormwood capsules. She did not object and did not need to be coaxed.

This would stop the malignancy the same day. We could next focus on tumor shrinkage. Which bacteria did she have, giving her the Positive result for DNA? And what was causing her mutation of the gene p53?

Five clostridium varieties were Positive at the cerebellum. Two lactobacillus varieties were Negative. Two Rhizobium varieties were Negative. These were the only specimens in our collection that could make DNA in our cells. Clostridium is <u>always</u> found under tooth fillings, but Nancy had no tooth fillings. Perhaps she had a dead tooth, but no discoloration could be seen in any tooth. A panoramic X-ray was ordered. Her baby teeth looked beautiful and no infection could be spotted; her secondary teeth were growing as they should, in perfect order. But a tooth abscess can escape notice and a dead tooth looks no different on an X-ray than a live one.

Where were the clostridium bacteria in her cerebellum coming from if not from teeth? We searched for dental material in teeth in case one small filling had been forgotten. The tests showed: copper, cobalt, vanadium Negative at teeth; 5 malonates Negative at teeth; urethane, bisphenol Negative at teeth; mercury, nickel, thallium Negative at teeth. We concluded their memory was accurate; no dental work had ever been done.

We continued our testing at the cerebellum: thallium, mercury, cobalt, vanadium, 5 malonates, urethane, bisphenol were all Negative (note vanadium in particular). CFC's were Negative, they had already moved their re-frigerator out of doors two weeks earlier. But copper was Positive and very high; she needed to get into copper-free water immediately. At home, new plastic pipes would need to be installed before returning! They were given an environmentally safe motel room at once. Our plan was to wait three days to let the copper drain naturally from the cerebellum. If it did not, we would use EDTA by mouth to chelate it out.

A blood test was scheduled; she started on the supplement program to shrink tumors and was instructed to zap daily. She had already been zapping at home, starting two weeks ago, to get her well enough to make the trip to Mexico.

Her blood test of February 3 looked quite good. The WBC was some-what high, indicating a bacterial infection somewhere. Her liver enzymes were slightly high, particularly the SGOT, probably due to lead in the copper water pipes. The LDH was slightly elevated [*from Sudan Black B dye in foods*]. The potassium level was too high, showing that toxicity was affecting the thyroid gland.

Peculiarly, her lymphocytes (48%) were higher than neutrophils (43%), implying a viral condition. These 2 WBC varieties should be in a 20% (lymph) to 80% ratio. Could she have picked up Epstein Barre Virus or was this an aftermath of her DPT shot?

Two days later, she seemed to be in rather high spirits. She was clearly more active. But she complained of a digestive problem. We searched through our set of eight common digestive bacteria. Only *Salmonella* was Positive. She had not been getting her Lugol's iodine drops four times a day. We gave her some immediately. She drank it stoically. Best of all, her new copper test was now Negative at the cerebellum. We would not need to chelate.

Another two days later, the parents elaborated more about Nancy's past health. For two years already, Nancy had a lot of mucous in the back of her throat. She had been banged by a friend's head on her front (baby) tooth and lost it. She had frequent belly-aches for about a year. I decided to test addi-tionally for *Ascaris* next day.

The search began at the cerebellum. Five clostridium species Negative at cerebellum. *Clostridium tetani* Positive at cerebellum. (The DPT shot con-tains inactivated *Clostridium tetani*; was this somehow related?) *Lactobacil-lus casei* Positive at cerebellum. I knew these bacteria were not coming from her teeth, nor would they originate in the brain. Could they be hiding in her appendix? A quick search found the appendix Negative for all. I was at a loss, and turned my attention to *Ascaris*. Stomach aches in children are usu-ally caused by *Ascaris* or *Salmonella*, the former if chronic, the latter if ac-companied by a temperature. The test results showed *Ascaris* Positive in the "whole body" test, Negative at cerebellum, and Positive at stomach.

And all other food bacteria were Positive at the stomach too, in spite of Lugol's treatments! Evidently they were coming from the *Ascaris* worms and protected from the iodine. There was indeed a pet dog in the house (a source of *Ascaris* worms). Both parents were tested for *Ascaris*. They were both Positive. Such a parasite infection would be hard to eradicate in the whole family. They agreed to give the dog away immediately.

Nancy was given another 10 tsp. of black walnut tincture extra strength and 3 cloves plus 3 wormwood. The parents each did the same.

Had we found the source of her clostridium bacteria in the cerebellum? Namely *Ascaris* worm? The copper present would have consumed the glutathione in the cerebellum so the bacteria could multiply unchecked, and DNA would accumulate. (Just a theory.)

Three days later she was very full of energy and was sleeping much more soundly, too. She had been getting 8½ tsp. black walnut tincture extra strength instead of 10 each day. *Ascaris* tested Negative now. Her dose was lowered to 3 tsp. black walnut tincture extra strength and 3 cloves plus 3 wormwood to be taken daily, still. Both parents tested Negative to *Ascaris*, too. But would this hold up at home after leaving the clinic? All bacteria now

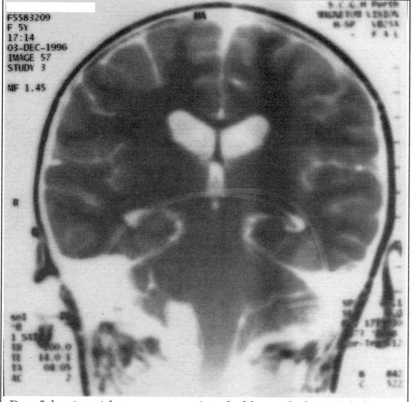

Dec 3 brain with tumor zone (circled by radiologist) left over from surgery done in Nov

tested Negative at Nancy's cerebellum. TNF was Positive there. The tumor must be shrinking.

On February 14 her MRI arrived from home, taken post-surgically at end of November 1996. The tumor remnant was actually quite large; it was probably already growing. Contrast material (white area at reader's lower left) at the surgery space is easy to identify. There is considerable displacement of the midline (not shown). The two halves are not symmetrical.

On February 17, the family was still Negative to *Ascaris*. They had been enjoying the tourist attractions and had been to the zoo!—a dangerous place for parasite-afflicted children. Nancy appeared entirely normal, climbing and jumping off our garden wall. Nobody scolded her; we were delighted to see her health return.

On February 19, a routine search for any other tumor was done (searching for DNA in 40 organs). One was Positive, the lung!

Indeed, her latest blood test showed elevation of alkaline phosphatase, implicating the lungs. [*Was she exposed to a dye unbeknownst to us?*] But a p53 test at the lung was Negative, showing that mutations were not occurring, at least not this common one. Something was growing there, though. A quick check showed all bacteria Negative at lung, but *Ascaris* larvae Positive.

We had found the problem. Fortunately, we had more than one *Ascaris* stage represented in the slide set. Were these larvae making DNA? Or was there yet another bacterium released by *Ascaris* that was not in my collection (I can't test without a sample)? And how was she getting reinfected with *Ascaris*?

Ascaris larvae were also found in the stomach now. Could there be live *Ascaris* eggs stuck in gallstones in her liver ducts to give her this recurrence? [*At that time we were not aware that raw vegetables from grocery shops carry the parasite eggs.*] Some could be killed at once (we gave Nancy 7 clove capsules, twice, 1½ hours apart), but a liver cleanse would be needed.

On February 22, her brain was free of DNA, and p53. RNA was plentiful, as it should be, but a routine check detected acetone! Acetone is the detoxification product of isopropyl alcohol! Soon isopropyl alcohol was found to be Positive, and high. A frantic search for the source ensued. Isopropyl will spur tumor growth faster than anything else—probably by leading to hCG formation. There was no time to lose. How long had it been going on without detection? Food (safe restaurant) products, our supplements were all tested immediately. It was in her hat! A new washable sun hat! It was snatched off and away. [*In retrospect this article of clothing would have given her azo dyes, too.*]

On February 26, all *Ascaris* and toxins and bacteria tested Negative. She no longer needed Lugol's iodine, she was staying clear of *Salmonella*. She could go home, <u>if</u> a new CT scan of the brain stem showed improvement. They went at once for the test.

With the trophy in their hands, just hours later, they announced that the radiologist had seen no tumor anywhere. Not even a vestige of one. Not a remnant.

Although this was a CT, not an MRI, the radiologist informed us that if there had been anything to see, he would have taken many more pictures. But there was nothing. They could schedule their flight home. A final blood test was ordered.

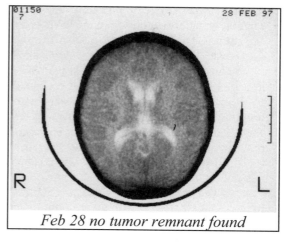

01150 7   28 FEB 97

R   L

Feb 28 no tumor remnant found

On February 28, the blood test was reviewed. It was disturbing. It wasn't perfect. The WBC was now normal, but the LDH had not gone down below 160 as it should for an adult. And the calcium level had dropped too low, implying a problem at the parathyroids.

The lymphocytes had risen again, too: lymphs 44%, neutrophils 50%.

We decided to do some more searching at the liver and parathyroid glands. Imagine our surprise at this: *Ascaris* Positive at parathyroids; *Ascaris* Positive at liver; 6 clostridium species Positive at liver; *Clostridium* and *Shigella* Positive at parathyroids! We had caught up with the infamous round-worms again. We could see there would be no end to the infestation unless bile ducts were cleared. They extended their stay for two weeks to get started with this.

On March 5, she had tried to do her first liver cleanse. But nothing could be coaxed down. Her indomitable spirit, now robust with energy, would let nothing down. Precious time was passing.

A week later, she accomplished the nasty chore, eliminating a great deal of "chaff" and one stone. She was advised to repeat the liver cleanse at home once a month. A few days later, a new blood test was scheduled. The LDH was finally normal. Some liver improvement was seen. Calcium was beginning to rise again.

But a peculiarity persisted in the electronic test results. Although all bacteria, heavy metals, solvents, and other toxins were Negative at the brain location, the nucleic acids were still not in correct amounts (inosine, uridine and thymidine were Positive, while adenine, guanosine, xanthine and cytidine were Negative). All these nucleic acid bases (or precursors) test Positive in healthy tissue. Even if they are Negative, they revert to Positive as soon as the noxious agent responsible is removed. And although vanadium was absent, nucleoside vanadyl complexes were Positive. (The complexes are only made if vanadium is present.) Were the vanadyl complexes causing interference with nucleic acid regulation? Or were there some unknown bacteria present? *Ascaris* infection brought to mind *Bacteroides fragilis*, a bacterium that also builds up in the liver. We would test. *Bacteroides fragilis* Negative at the brain. Could it be a Coxsackie virus, always found with Bacteroides? We would test. Coxsackie Virus B4, Positive, and very high!

We had found a missing link in the whole chain of events. The bacteria had been killed but the viruses lived on. Probably they had given the picture of encephalitis to her first doctors. Perhaps the DPT shot had allowed hybridization of the clostridium bacteria or lowered her immunity in other ways. Perhaps not. Steroid treatment afterward may have had some counterproductive effects too, but it was the best that could be done at the time.

Still, what was the source of the nucleoside vanadyl complexes? Was this the "trigger" for the virus? Triggers for other viruses are well known. Peanuts and other foods can trigger *Herpes* viruses. Cigarette smoke can trigger cold viruses. Was this vanadium connection keeping her Coxsackie virus activated and multiplying? [*We have since seen that the plastic used as shunts for the brain and as permanently implanted catheters shed vanadium.*]

Nancy Pendergrass	2/3	2/17	2/28	3/11
RBC	4.65	4.78	4.65	4.64
WBC	9,300	8,000	5,200	3,900
PLT	238	298	272	270
glucose	88	103	79	73
BUN	11	6.0	13	9.0
creatinine	0.7	0.6	0.6	0.6
AST (SGOT)	43	32	37	38
ALT (SGPT)	28	26	25	18
LDH	170	174	170	154
GGT	20	21	29	22
T.b.	0.7	0.3	0.4	0.4
alk phos	273	353	346	307
T.p.	6.7	7.1	6.9	6.8
albumin	4.5	4.6	4.5	4.7
globulin	2.2	2.5	2.4	2.1
uric acid	2.1	0.6	0.5	1.0
Calcium	9.5	9.4	8.5	8.7
Phosphorus	4.9	3.7	4.0	4.9
Iron	114	83	137	88
Sodium	142	139	140	137
Potassium	5.5	4.9	3.7	3.9
Chloride	106	102	104	99
triglycerides	136	103	69	34
cholesterol	222	214	230	256

It was their last day, March 14. Vanadyl complexes were still testing Positive at the brain, although the Coxsackie viruses (both B1 and B4) were now Negative. Could the vanadium source be car exhaust inhaled while crossing the US-Mexican border daily amidst a sea of traffic? There had been chronic car problems at home; could chronic pollution at home have sensitized her to vanadyl complex damage? The nucleic acids were still not correctly regulated, they tested the same as before.

They had several chores to attend to immediately when they got home to Australia.

1. Change water pipes. Use water from a hose till job was done to avoid copper.
2. Change utilities to all-electric to avoid vanadium.
3. Avoid viral triggers such as benzene (off the benzene list).
4. Give away the pet.
5. Repair the car.

Summary: Not all the questions were answered in Nancy's case. [*We had not yet learned to test for Clostridium sources at colon and esophagus (rabbit fluke). And we neglected to ask whether Nancy's teeth had ever been "sealed," this could have been the source of vanadium.*] Another MRI would be done on schedule with her doctor at home. It was a happy leave taking and a Bon Voyage to Nancy. We heard that she passed her follow-up visits with her doctor at home—no growth could be seen on her next MRI.

48	William Elliott	Brain Cancer

William Elliott was brought by his father for his bipolar depression, also called *manic depression*. He was diagnosed with it a year and a half ago. He was twenty-seven years old, a tall, sturdy, young man, and very strong. His grim look, as if teeth were clenched, suggested a powerful anger that needed constant control. Instead of lithium, he was on zoloft (100 mg/day). He chewed tobacco and also smoked cigarettes, which probably afforded some relief.

He was advised to stop using chlorinated water for all purposes—he had been an avid swimmer in childhood in heavily chlorinated pools. Chlorine "allergy" is always seen in our manic-depressive cases. This means the liver no longer detoxifies chlorine and chlorine-containing chemicals, such as bleach. It is free, then, to circulate through the body, attaching itself in different places in different people. It affects the brain in manic depression victims. He was advised to take all metal off his body including his all-metal watch, to reduce nickel absorption; nickel feeds bacteria and it becomes part of their urease enzyme.

But William was not in a mood to listen, let alone comply. His father was helpless beside his strong defiant son. I tried stronger persuasion as we reviewed his blood test together. It was essentially that of a healthy person. But his RBC was slightly elevated, showing cobalt or vanadium toxicity coming from his tooth fillings. And his alk phos was slightly high from food dyes. Surprisingly, he had a low uric acid, revealing a *Clostridium* invasion somewhere, a situation always seen in tumor conditions. Stopping these bacteria was important since their by-products would affect brain function (hence the nickel restriction).

His calcium level was too low and potassium too high, showing both a parathyroid and thyroid problem. Both conditions would cause anxiety and hyperthyroidism, favoring a manic condition but not necessarily reflected in a high thyroxine level. His iron level was too high, showing some interference with its utilization.

It is true that all these disturbances except for the uric acid were of a minor nature, yet altogether, they resembled a tumor pattern. Meanwhile, William's patience and tolerance were wearing out. In another minute he would leave, simply by walking out. He wanted no information, no instructions and no delays! In desperation to get something accomplished, I began quickly to search for toxins at the cerebrum (brain). Here are the results: Positive for isopropyl alcohol, benzene, wood alcohol, rhodanese. Negative for 20-methylcholanthrene, glutathione.

Obviously, something was using up his glutathione in the brain. Without that, metabolism would not be efficient. He must have either metal or bacteria or malonate compounds in his brain. Much better to identify these now and remove them, than to go through life as an invalid from manic depressive disorder.

Only two weeks earlier, I had received the message about a former manic-depressive patient who had committed suicide. He too had been a strong, handsome, motor-cycling young man. My memory was flooded with pain. Somehow this young man, standing before me—too impatient to sit—had to be saved. His slightly-built father could only pray and trust and search and persuade and try.

William allowed one more test; I chose DNA. It was Positive at the

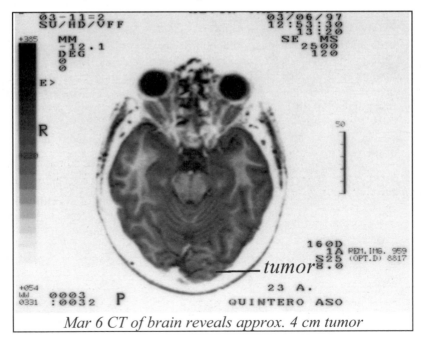

Mar 6 CT of brain reveals approx. 4 cm tumor

cerebrum. He had a tumor. I said nothing. He permitted a few more tests. They were: Positive at the cerebrum, for urethane, bisphenol-A, and for gene mutation p53.

I explained that dental plastic was getting into the brain, perhaps starting a region of poor metabolism. I recommended an MRI of the brain. Somehow his father got him to the radiologist. A few days later they arrived, negatives in hand. A tumor of considerable size was present, pressing against the meninges, the brain's protective membranes next to the bone.

We were shocked. How very fortunate…to find it <u>now</u>.

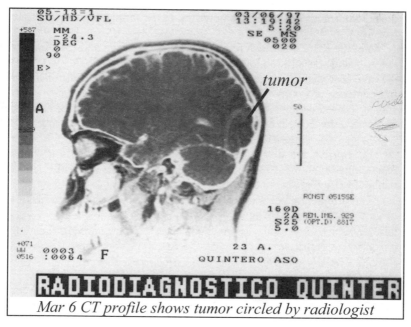

Mar 6 CT profile shows tumor circled by radiologist

He was given the cancer program now, and instructions to remove all metal and plastic from his teeth.

Ten days later he was a different young man. He had stopped using any tobacco. He made conversation with us. He had a smile. He had removed all metal-containing teeth by extraction. He was actually taking his supplements, without resistance.

His plastic fillings still needed removal to get rid of the urethane and bisphenol source. He was sent for air abrasion to remove them on March 18.

After this, on March 19, both urethane and bisphenol tested Negative. But copper, cobalt, vanadium, mercury, silver, and riboside-vanadyl-complexes still tested Positive at his bone marrow. Evidently, he still had bits of amalgam (tattoos) left in his mouth. This was reflected in his second blood test, where the RBC was still too high. All the liver enzymes plus alk phos were up slightly, too, a transient effect that I didn't understand [due to tumor drainage]. But calcium was up and potassium down, both entirely normal now, showing that toxins were out of the parathyroid and thyroid glands, a nice step of progress.

Syncrometer tests now showed DNA and p53 mutation Negative at the brain, so tumor growth and mutations had ceased.

By March 27, William said he felt "fantastic". We all noticed that he now had facial expression that had previously been missing in a mask-like appearance.

The new blood test, March 27, showed gratifying improvements. Most important were the significant drops in LDH and alk phos, suggesting no more tumor activity. (An extremely low LDH, though, can be due to cobalt toxicity.)

Yet the RBC was much too high, as were albumin and calcium, whereas the uric acid was still too low.

We searched the bone marrow, liver, spleen, and thyroid for incriminating evidence of toxins. The bone marrow search was remarkably clean. The spleen showed deficits: Negative for lactoferrin and transferrin. These should be Positive for correct handling of iron. He was instructed to drink raw milk, 1 glass per week, properly sterilized.

By April 1, his spirits were high; he was very anxious to go home and resume his home-building trade. But, obviously, there were still dental remnants of sufficient size to disturb thyroid function, and the RBC.

The uric acid level was still much too low; there were significant levels of clostridium bacteria somewhere; we must find them. The thyroid was apparently under attack so we searched there. Mercury, silver, vanadyl complexes were Negative at the thyroid. DNA, p53 gene were Positive at the thyroid. The DNA-forming bacteria must be in the thyroid, though they had vacated the brain.

Clostridium bacteria, rhizobium bacteria, and lactobacilli were Positive there. All the DNA-formers were still there. A thorough cleaning of dental tissues was called for in hopes of clearing their source.

The cerebrum, though, had already tested clear of all these, so a new MRI was ordered.

On April 7, a happy father and son arrived with their new MRI negatives. But not without some apprehension. They had learned to recognize the tumor on several frames of the first set of negatives and were unable to locate it now. But were they merely missing it, as lay persons might? No, the tumor was gone. The bulge remained where the tumor had been, but the tissue density and structure were the same as normal tissue. It was gone.

Of course, William's behavior had reflected this return to normalcy. He was his former helpful, communicative self. But could he go home? Not while the problem in his thyroid persisted.

We received the new blood test results: RBC was still much too high. We had searched the bone marrow without finding metal; we would next

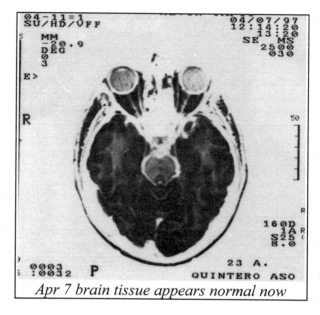

Apr 7 brain tissue appears normal now

search the spleen. Albumin was still high; but the uric acid level was now normal; calcium was back to normal; iron was being properly utilized.

A small clue came from his eosinophil count (not shown), 4%. This is slightly high, implying *Ascaris* worms. William had a dog at home so he was probably quite infested when he arrived. He would not be able to have a house pet again, being much too susceptible to *Ascaris* parasitism.

We checked for the presence of *Ascaris*. There they were, in his Peyer's patches and appendix. (Peyer's patches are lymph nodes in the small intestine.)

Then we searched the spleen for evidence of amalgam tattoos in his mouth. We found that, too. Copper, cobalt, vanadium, vanadyl complexes, and mercury were all Positive at the spleen.

He was instructed to do a high-dose of the parasite killing herbs: 8 tsp. black walnut tincture extra strength plus another 8 tsp. an hour later.

William was put on cysteine to "mop up" dead *Ascaris* worms, and in another week this could have been accomplished. He also had some tattoo searching to do. But it was not to be. He left for his job at home. He did promise to follow up in three months, and we look forward to seeing him.

Summary: It is always tempting to blame "bad" behavior on the patient if he or she is adult and "in control". Yet William's case clearly shows he was not in control. Parasites, bacteria, and metals were.

William Elliott	3/3	3/18	3/27	4/1	4/6
RBC	4.89	5.02	5.48	5.1	5.24
WBC	6.3	8.7	7.7	6.9	6.0
PLT	242	317	348	312	254
glucose	87	99	76	79	97
BUN	11	13	9	12	15

creatinine	1.2	1.1	1.3	1.3	1.1
AST (SGOT)	11	30	26	29	10
ALT (SGPT)	13	29	20	11	6
LDH	153	166	91	155	156
GGT	16	19	19	17	10
T.b.	0.7	0.6	0.6	0.9	0.4
alk phos	101	110	98	95	71
T.p.	7.5	7.6	7.9	7.4	7.9
albumin	4.7	4.9	5.1	4.6	5.3
globulin	2.8	2.7	2.8	2.8	2.6
uric acid	3.3(3.7-8.0)	1.8	2.6	2.1	6.1
Calcium	8.6	9.4	9.9	10.3	9.3
Phosphorus	4.0	3.4	3.7	3.7	3.2
Iron	153	160	147	140	81
Sodium	140	142	139	138	141
Potassium	4.9	4.3	4.6	4.5	4.0
Chloride	104	104	103	100	103
triglycerides	119	71	168	60	88
cholesterol	125	151	158	148	142

49   Maxine Naire   Brain Cancer

Maxine Naire, age seventy, came with her daughter-in-law as her care-giver. Maxine had severe memory loss, getting worse rapidly. She was very pleasant and seemed normal "until you tried to live with her." She needed help in every way except physical. Six months ago, she had replaced all her metal tooth fillings with composite; since then her mental health had deteriorated quickly. Was it a coincidence? I thought not.

An extensive search at her brain (cerebrum) gave these results: cobalt Positive, isopropyl alcohol Positive. She believed she had already removed all sources of isopropyl alcohol from her lifestyle; this was frustrating and demoralizing for her. We suggested vitamins as a source. She produced a variety of supplements she had been using. Most tested Positive for isopropyl with my Syncrometer. That finding would make the problem correctable in a day.

DNA Positive at cerebrum; was a tumor growing? p53 mutation Negative at cerebrum, Positive at bone (probably the skull). Copper Positive at cerebrum. Vanadium Positive at cerebrum. Riboside vanadyl complexes Positive at cerebrum. The Positive DNA result signified the presence of DNA-producing bacteria. The presence of excess p53 gene protein implied a mutagen. The vanadium was forming riboside vanadyl complexes to cause mutations. Copper and vanadium would consume her glutathione wherever these metals were accumulating; in this case, the brain. She would need to hurry with her treatment to stop any further bone involvement if this was a tumor.

Rhodanese Negative at cerebrum (should be positive to detoxify cholesterol derivatives). 20-methylcholanthrene Positive at cerebrum (mutagenic cholesterol derivative). Glutathione, reduced, Negative at cerebrum. Without reduced glutathione (and reduced iron), rhodanese isn't made and 20-methylcholanthrene can't be detoxified into the thiocyanate derivative.

What was happening at the spleen, bone marrow, and liver?

	at spleen	bone marrow	liver
rhodanese	N	N	N
There was considerable body depletion of this enzyme.			
glutathione	N	N	N (also very depleted)
20-methylcholanthrene	N	P	P

But 20-methylcholanthrene was only accumulating at bone marrow and liver. This whole picture suggested a beginning tumor in the brain; her memory problem might not be simply dementia or Alzheimer's. We requested an MRI of the brain.

She was instructed to do a high-dose parasite treatment (10 tsp. of black walnut tincture extra strength, plus 9 capsules cloves and 9 capsules wormwood). She was now started on the regular cancer program of supplements, including Lugol's iodine to prevent *Salmonella* invasion. All the plastic-filled teeth were to be extracted, since the holes would be too large after plastic was removed. They were eager to comply and checked into the environmentally safe motel, eating meals at the malonate-free restaurant.

Her first blood test showed no abnormality except a high RBC, implying cobalt or vanadium toxicity.

Two days later, her isopropyl alcohol was gone.

On March 31, she got her CT scan of the brain. The abnormal tissue was easy to spot. The side view, not shown, showed where it was pressing against the skull. Several frames of the top view showed how the new growth was beginning to push the midline over to the left. The triangle of abnormal look-

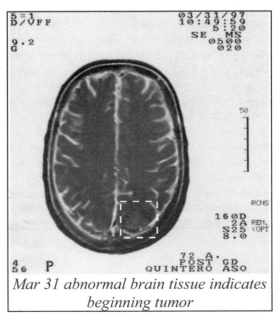

Mar 31 abnormal brain tissue indicates beginning tumor

ing tissue at lower right corner could be the beginning of a tumor.

We didn't know whether to be happy or sad; happy to have found it for Maxine so early; sad that it wasn't merely a dementia affecting her. They took the news in an accepting manner.

By April 1, thirteen teeth had been extracted. She was immediately more alert. But DNA and p53 were still Positive at the cerebrum. Cobalt and vanadyl complexes were still Positive. Glutathione and rhodanese were still Negative. Thyroid was added to her regimen, 2 grains daily.

Two days later, all her extractions were done. Her new test results at the brain showed:

Bacteria
Lactobacillus acidophilus Negative
Lactobacillus casei Negative
Rhizobium meliloti Negative
Rhizobium leguminosarum Positive (implies Ascaris presence)

Pyrimidine Bases
uridine Positive
cytidine Positive
thymidine Positive
thymidine triphosphate Negative

Purine Bases
adenine Positive
guanosine Positive
xanthine Positive
inosine Negative

Other "Bad Guys"
DNA Negative
20-methylcholanthrene Negative
vanadyl complexes Positive (there must still be remnants of dental material or another source of vanadium)

p53 Positive (still getting mutations)

Other "Good Guys"
glutathione Positive
RNA Positive
rhodanese Positive

In spite of this good news—no more tumor growth (DNA) in the brain—she was much disheartened that she still had bits of amalgam or composite left in her mouth. She wanted to let her mouth heal a bit more before searching for them. Perhaps by waiting, they would just go away.

We waited five days. On April 8, a repeat test showed: mercury Positive at brain; silver Positive at brain. Only amalgam (a tattoo) could be responsible for these.

Rhizobium leguminosarum Positive. The presence of this tumor-causing bacterium implicates left-over *Ascaris* parasites. They were tested next. Ascaris eggs Positive at brain, intestine, gall bladder, bile ducts. Other Ascaris stages Negative. [*At that time we had not yet perfected our cysteine/ozonated oil treatment for sheltered parasite eggs. Nor had we found the universal source of reinfection: raw greens and vegetables.*] We tried the 10 tsp. dose of black walnut tincture extra strength plus cloves and wormwood again. Within hours, all tests for *Ascaris* stages, their bacteria, and viruses were Negative. But even after three consecutive days of this treatment, *Ascaris* eggs reappeared at the bone marrow and spleen. Only eggs! And promptly, *Adenovirus* and *Rhizobium leguminosarum* reappeared also. We tried several doses of Levamisole, an exceptionally good drug for killing roundworms. By then the eggs had already hatched in the bone marrow. Soon they were also

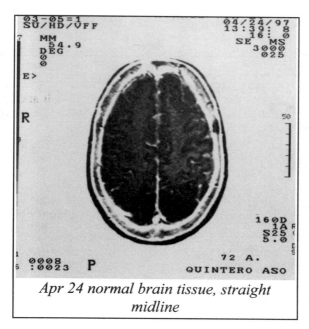

```
03-05=1                          04/24/97
SU/HD/VFF                        13:39: 8
7                                     16: 0
    MM                           SE   MS
    54.9                              3000
  DEG                                 025
    0
E>

R                           50




                            160D
                              1A   R
                            S25    (
                            5.0    [
1                                  D
  0008          P        72 A.     S
5 :0023            QUINTERO ASO
```

Apr 24 normal brain tissue, straight midline

in the gallbladder; the liver was doing its job to gather them in and try to kill them.

On April 13, she was scheduled for tattoo removal. On April 17, she arrived, triumphantly holding a little bag with cotton gauze holding a collection of tattoos. The oral surgeon had finally found them! Not one—but a half dozen!

We waited two days to see if metal or parasite eggs would return. They did not. Perhaps healing of the brain tissue was excluding them now. We scheduled her second CT scan.

On April 24 she arrived with her new scan, apprehensive and hopeful.

The news was all good; no trace of the abnormal tissue remained. It was gone. The midline was absolutely straight. She could go home. A final check showed there was still mercury present. Her last blood test showed there were still bacteria (too low uric acid). (She had three other blood tests during her stay, but none of them are shown because there was nothing else abnormal on them.) But Maxine's time was up. We would put her on some cysteine; perhaps this would detoxify the mercury and slow down its accumulation in the brain. [*This was our beginning cysteine treatment from which we learned its* Ascaris *killing ability.*]

Summary: A few weeks later, we heard from her daughter-in-law that she had gained some weight and was getting better. She was happy with her new teeth. Her memory had not improved significantly, though. Perhaps other things could be tried, now, such as a vasodilator (niacin) and herbs known to improve mental

Maxine Naire	3/27
RBC	5.1
WBC	7.2
PLT	280
glucose	135
BUN	12
creatinine	0.9
AST (SGOT)	28
ALT (SGPT)	10
LDH	98
GGT	12
T.b.	
alk phos	85
T.p.	7.4
albumin	4.5
globulin	2.9
uric acid	3.3
Calcium	8.7
Phosphorus	3.9
Iron	101
Sodium	144
Potassium	3.9
Chloride	107
triglycerides	156
cholesterol	230

function. At least she has time now to improve. They deserved it.

50	Bruce Engevik	Prostate & Bone Cancer

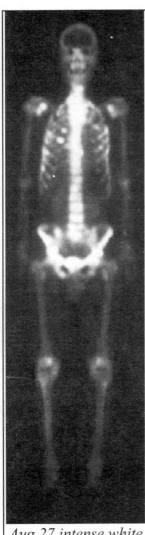

Aug 27 intense white regions show bone cancer dissolving (lysing) his bones

Bruce Engevik, fifty-five-ish, was a tall, handsome man who normally kept a twinkle in his eye, and still played tennis, racquet ball, was a swimmer, and long distance runner. Bruce had lived and worked in 80 different countries. Then his life crashed, and he was now wracked with pain. It had taken one and a half years for his doctors to diagnose his prostate/bone cancer since he also had been passing kidney stones, been extremely bloated, and suffered with stomach illnesses. When he was finally diagnosed, one year ago, it was much too late to do anything except palliative treatment; his entire skeleton was involved in bone cancer, although it had probably started as prostate cancer. His "total PSA" was 1250.0 ng/mL. It should not be over 4!

He was put on female hormone (cyproterone) at home, and was still on it (six times a day). If he missed taking this, his intense bone pains would return at once. I assured him we would not make him suffer.

He brought a total bone scan with him; the "hot spots" were too numerous to count.

He had already done ten days of the parasite-killing program before arriving, having been given *The Cure For All Cancers* as he left the hospital in Australia. He arrived on September 18. The first two days were spent getting a blood test, a panoramic X-ray of teeth, acquiring the new nontoxic body products and settling into the environmentally safe motel. His diet came exclusively from the malonate-free menu at the restaurant nearby. He was first seen by me on September 20, his shuffling gait, and stooped shoulders betraying pain.

His blood test told all; the alkaline phosphatase (780) was in the top 10% of patients I had treated. A look at the bone scan put him in the bottom one percent of "chances of recovery." His first question was, "Can you save me?" I could not truthfully answer yes, on the basis of the high alk phos. I evaded the question, but stated that we would do our best, and that he certainly stood a chance. He tried to smile, but recognized the evasion. He had come ten thousand miles for what, promises?

The staff would see to it that he was capable of following our cancer program without a single mistake. His first Syncrometer tests showed isopropyl alcohol Positive. He had not yet managed to rid himself of this elementary, and most important of all toxins. The tests also showed benzene Positive. This would destroy his immunity, including changing germanium (good organic kind that his white blood cells relied on) to toxic germanium. The benzene would also knock out a viral inhibitor that we all need. Benzene itself is detoxified by oxidation to phenol, which next oxidizes our vitamin C, cysteine and glutathione to useless items, besides causing pain.

The staff would help him by selecting his food, beverage, water, soap, shaving method, shampoo—all of it, in order to avoid benzene and isopropyl alcohol. He came prepared to extract bad teeth—not restore them. All six clostridium varieties were Positive at his teeth, bones and stomach. We started him on betaine at once.

I next searched for toxins at the vital organs where mortality is determined. By now I had realized that cancer patients do not die from their tumors, directly, but from the toxins responsible for creating them. I could then pick the sickest organs to watch most carefully. (N = negative, P = positive, asterisks denote exceptionally high values.)

	pancreas	bone	bone marrow	spleen	liver	parathyroid	thyroid	prostate	adrenals
ortho-phospho-tyrosine	N	POS	N	N	N	N	N	POS	*POS

The malignancy was not only at bone and prostate, it had begun to flare-up in the adrenal glands!

isopropyl alcohol	POS	POS	POS	POS	POS	POS	POS	POS	POS
4 isopropylidene nucleotides (probable mutations)	N	POS	POS	POS	POS	POS	POS	POS	N
4 Ascaris stages	POS	N	N	N	N	---	---	---	POS
vitamin C	N	POS	POS	POS	POS	N	POS	POS	N
dehydroascorbate	----	N	N	N	N	N	N	N	N

There was <u>no</u> vitamin C (neither oxidized nor reduced) at several tissues where a high concentration is needed, even at the parathyroids.

urethane	*POS	POS	POS	POS	POS	POS	POS	POS	*POS

His tissues were loaded with urethane, a plastic pollutant.

1, 10 phenanthroline (chelator of iron)	N	POS	POS	POS	POS	POS	POS	POS	N

ferroin (the iron chelate)	N	POS	POS	POS	POS	POS	POS	POS	N
20-methylcholanthrene	N	POS	POS	POS	POS	POS	POS	POS	N
beta propiolactone	N	POS	POS	POS	POS	POS	POS	POS	N
copper	N	POS	POS	POS	POS	POS	POS	POS	N
cobalt	N	POS	POS	POS	POS	POS	POS	POS	N
vanadium	N	POS	POS	POS	POS	POS	N	POS	N
vanadyl complexes	N	POS	POS	POS	POS	POS	N	POS	N
5 malonates	N	POS	POS	POS	POS	POS	POS	POS	N
Sudan IV dye	N	*POS	POS	POS	POS	POS	POS	POS	N
p53 gene (mutation)	----	POS	POS	POS	POS	POS	N	----	----

Note that *Ascaris* stages themselves may be living only at the pancreas and adrenals but this results in lots of 20-methylcholanthrene elsewhere in the body. Beta propiolactone is also made by *Ascaris* and had a similar pattern of distribution. The M-family (malonic acid, methyl malonate, maleic, maleic anhydride, D-malic acid) was dispersed through his body, too. Sudan IV, a carcinogenic dye was highest at bone.

The next test was to see how badly the two main growth controllers were out of kilter. Pyruvic aldehyde and thiourea should each have a one minute cycle in perfect alternation. For Bruce, thiourea, the growth stimulator, stayed on continuously (I stopped timing it after seven minutes) and pyruvic aldehyde, the "brakes" for cell multiplication, stayed off throughout this time.

The next test was for the presence of RNA which is necessary to make protein. RNA was Negative at muscle, lymph nodes, lung, joints, esophagus, diaphragm, colon, bone marrow, bone, adrenal, connective tissue, thymus, thyroid, stomach, spleen, prostate, pancreas, optic chiasma. This was a very poor showing. His body's metabolism was grinding to a halt; over half his tissues had a very serious shortage of enzymes and other proteins necessary to conduct life.

The next test was to see which amino acids (of a set of 22) were present at bone. They were all Negative, simply no trace of any, although he had been eating normally, he claimed. This is typical of the attrition that occurs in a tumor, then overtakes the tumorous organ, then affects the rest of the body. It is due, I believe, to the spread of streptomyces species through the body, releasing their numerous waste products and bacterial toxins. These include protease, streptomycin, actinomycin-D, and others. These are well studied inhibitors of protein formation. At the same time, Bruce's tissues were missing an enzyme, RNAse inhibitor, that would have protected him from digesting the proteins as soon as they were made. RNAse inhibitor was absent due to having vanadyl complexes everywhere. The streptomyces bacteria, though, are strictly dependent on tapeworm larvae and could be eliminated in a day. His RNAse inhibitor could be reinstated by getting the vanadium out of his mouth. And this was proceeding as fast as it could—dental work was already scheduled. A notable exception to the picture of absent RNA in his tissues was the skin. Here RNA remained high. Although streptomycin-like toxins could be detected at the skin, no protease was ever detected. Wherever RNAse inhibitor was missing, RNAse A had a runaway existence in his vital organs (not skin).

Parasites and bacteria were consuming his vital tissues as swiftly as caterpillars can strip an orchard tree. It had to be stopped at once.

His tests took two hours to complete. After this, his Day 1 instructions were begun. He had a lot to accomplish in the next two days, most important was killing his parasites thoroughly and getting the "restored" teeth extracted. Refilling them would run two risks: trapping clostridium bacteria again and getting a new large dose of copper, cobalt, vanadium, maleic acid, and urethane. This would terminate his life, there would be no contest. After extracting the old teeth, partial dentures could be made for him. We assured him he would look good and be able to chew. This had been discussed with him before he decided to come to our clinic. He was eager to get it all done, and was surprised to see how well he was recovering from the first extractions. He was doing the Dental Aftercare program carefully, "drinking" his food after "blending" it so that no nutrition was lost. He was water picking

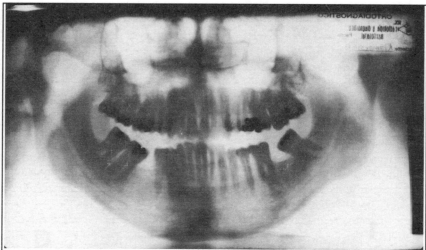

This panoramic X-ray with many "restored" teeth is typical for cancer patients

throughout the day to prevent infection since we could not risk the toxic action of antibiotics during these "final days." Final unless our program could be carried our correctly, without interference by infections or toxicity from drugs. The only additional supplement, other than the ones on the regular 21 Day Program, was zinc (30 mg per day) for his prostate.

Two days later he arrived at the office with a strong step, standing taller and with a smile. He was without pain, for the first time, although he had gone off his "estrogen" and pain killers for twenty-four hours. He was waiting for massive pain to return, but it did not. His mouth was still painful, and a spot over his left shoulder blade hurt, but this was probably liver-related, not bone.

The Syncrometer tests now showed 6 clostridium species Negative at bone; *Staphylococcus aureus* Negative at bone; 3 salmonellas Negative at bone; 3 shigellas Negative at bone; *E. coli* Negative at bone; 6 streptococcus species Negative at bone. Absence of bacteria at bone tissue explained his absence of pain. True healing is slower.

Then his parasite status was checked at the gallbladder. Stages are frequently collected here, so it is the first place to search for them. The Syncrometer test showed *Rhizobium leguminosarum* and *Mycobacterium avium* Negative at gallbladder. This negative result implies absence of all *Ascaris* and its stages.

Streptomyces and protease Positive at gallbladder. This positive result implies there are still tapeworm stages present somewhere.

Ferrous gluconate (the correct form) Negative at bone. Ferric phosphate (the wrong form) Positive and in high amounts. Inositol Negative at bone. Rhodizonic acid Negative at bone. Cysteine, methionine, taurine Negative at bone. I added inositol to his cancer program to help his metabolism make rhodizonic acid and ascorbic acid. He had a significant shortage of ferrous iron at the bones due to over-oxidation by phenol. The sulfur containing amino acids were still absent in spite of taking them. I doubled the dose.

A follow-up blood test was scheduled since it had been five days since the previous one. And an ultrasound of the prostate for the following day, September 23, 1997.

This must have been the best day in his life. From a one percent chance of survival, using our advanced method he had climbed to about a ninety percent chance of survival. His alkaline phosphatase had just dropped to one-half its starting value. In that one result, his life had been offered back to him. It was now 349. We had somehow caught and eliminated the dye that was destroying him; it was undoubtedly in some of his dental plastic. [*At this time we had not identified it as DAB yet.*]

The liver enzymes had all improved, too. His liver could make more protein, especially globulin (antibodies) which had been too low. His potassium level was adequate now. He could reduce his potassium supplement.

Testing for clostridium species showed they were all Negative now at the teeth; he had cleared them up with water picking and hot packing.

Tapeworm stages were consistently testing Negative at gallbladder, liver, and bile ducts. Was he not reinfecting? There was no way of knowing except daily testing for about five days.

Rhodizonic acid was Positive at bone and prostate. He was making it now, from the inositol supplement. In spite of these glorious achievements, there was much more to do, as the 21 Day Program progressed. We added flaxseed. He could cook the flaxseed into his cereal after ozonating the seed to detoxify any benzene.

It was time to check on his growth-regulators again: pyruvic aldehyde and thiourea. Pyruvic aldehyde had returned to its correct period: one minute being present, the following minute being absent. Thiourea was in perfect alternation with pyruvic aldehyde, as it should be. His bone tissue growth rate had normalized.

The enzymes arginase and ornithine decarboxylase were present only briefly, ten to fifteen seconds out of each minute. Spermidine was present only ten seconds out of each minute. These three substances are overproduced when a tissue is growing out of control. His were normal. It was a day of celebration for Bruce; we shared his enthusiasm for living.

The next day, he had an ultrasound (not shown) of the prostate done which he brought with him the following day, September 27. The prostate was considered normal by the radiologist, and indeed, there was nothing abnormal to be seen. The weight was estimated at 50 grams. This was hardly the gland that had produced the 1250 PSA; it had recovered considerably.

The last two pains, at the left thigh and left shoulder, were now gone though a lump could still be felt at the thigh. Clostridium species, *Fasciolopsis* flukes, and *Ascaris* were still gone, but there was evidence again of tapeworm larval stages at the bile duct. Reinfection could come simply from consuming one leaf of lettuce, a few strawberries, or a thimbleful of milk that were not sterilized. He had to learn to do this for himself. A liver cleanse with ozonated oil was advised just in case they were also stuck in his gallstones. All the amino acids tested earlier and found Negative were now Positive. RNA was now present at all organs, too.

Two days later, September 29, he exclaimed over his good appetite and lack of pain. He had done the liver cleanse and was again Negative for tapeworm larvae. We were waiting for Bruce's gums to heal over enough to permit cleaning his front teeth. Air abrasion cleaning would throw small particles in all directions. These particles would be made of alumina and baking soda, easily trapped in the gums if they haven't healed.

He was beginning to take short walks, now, on the beach. His energy was coming up.

Another four days later, October 3, he had painful spots here and there, that moved from place to place; this is the hallmark of allergic reactions and bacterial infections. He was drinking grapefruit juice exclusively and was told to stop. Tapeworm stages and *Ascaris* were again Positive at the bile ducts and gallbladder. He had reinfected again! Their toxic products were reaching the bone. He was advised to do another liver cleanse with ozonated oil. And he was started on chromium to stimulate amino acid uptake by cells, as well as sugar. Yet his next tests showed 1, 10 phenanthroline Positive at bone; ferroin Positive at bone; 20-methylcholanthrene Positive at bone; beta propiolactone Positive at bone; hydroxyurea Positive at bone; phorbol Positive at bone. He had *Ascaris* and tapeworm stages, <u>again</u>. His iron supplies had been changed to useless ferroin by the phenanthroline produced by the parasites. Tapeworm stages and *Ascaris* reinfection put him right back at "square one."

All the amino acids were again Negative, no doubt due to the protein inhibiting action of the streptomycin-like toxins. He was not sterilizing <u>all</u> his raw food. He would begin at once. But RNA was still Positive, RNAse Negative, and RNAse inhibitor Positive. Vanadyl complexes were Negative.

Three days later, October 6, he had done his third liver cleanse with ozonated oil. He looked like a strong, healthy man again, no trace of illness could be guessed. He was restless and bored. He wanted to visit somebody, somewhere or have some adventure. His latest test results were 1,10 phenanthroline, ferroin, 20-methylcholanthrene, beta propiolactone, hydroxyurea, and phorbol all Negative at bone. All amino acids were Positive, so his bones were no doubt healing.

And he was ready to get plastic out of the front teeth if there was any.

Two days later, October 8, he seemed very well; his mouth had healed and the plastic had been removed from his front teeth. The dentist had found a large unsuspected filling and extracted the tooth, rather than risk Bruce's new-found life. His weight was 70.4 kilograms now (155 lb.), he had begun to gain weight and had already gained nine and a half pounds. This was the very best sign of all, we could move him to the ninety-nine percent chance of survival category now.

His blood test on October 9, showed a brief worsening of his condition, perhaps due to the encounters with parasite reinfection, perhaps due to dental anesthetics [*or perhaps the draining of another tumor location with dye*].

Bone health had immediately suffered. His nourishment remained good, though, with higher blood sugar (glucose), higher triglycerides, and higher cholesterol. His prostate was healing, too, with a PSA of 98.

Then he left for a vacation of three days, but stayed away for two weeks, not entirely unexpected. His health had returned. He promised to be cautious, stay on his supplements and diet, and live in moderation. But that was impossible. He had faced certain death for too long. He had to celebrate somehow. As it turned out, he fell in love. And threw caution to the winds—almost. He had chosen ready made food from a health food store, instead of totally safe home-cooked food.

When he returned, he was Positive again for benzene, isopropyl alcohol, and wood alcohol. hCG was Positive everywhere, but he did not have the *Fasciolopsis* fluke, so did not have ortho-phospho-tyrosine. Nor did he have *Clostridium* invasion—there was no tooth source (his partials came just in time for his vacation). He had taken betaine religiously, so no *Clostridium* had colonized his colon. But tapeworm stages were present again, this time at the bile duct and bone. He had been eating baked cheese dishes in Mexico—they were probably not truly sterile. He was advised to do an ozonated oil liver cleanse right away, besides the parasite program.

In spite of this set back, his cell division regulators pyruvic aldehyde and thiourea were not disturbed from their normal periodicity, no bacterial amines were present to disturb them, there was no *Clostridium*.

His new blood test showed further improvement. The alkaline phosphatase was now 262. It still needed to drop to 85. We advised him to stay until it was completely normal. The LDH had dropped back down. His liver was making plenty of blood protein. His body could make urea again.

In a day his solvents were gone again, hCG was Negative, but tapeworm stages had not cleared up. He was to repeat a liver cleanse on the weekend.

Instead, he chose to repeat it at once—since his flight home was just a day away, and he wanted to leave in perfect health. Another ultrasound of the prostate was scheduled, too. On his last day, the ultrasound showed that his prostate had shrunk to thirty-seven grams and was still quite normal.

His repeat liver cleanse had done away with tapeworm stages again. I advised doing a liver cleanse every two weeks.

Summary: It was a happy goodbye. And a mission accomplished. His bone scan was not repeated since bone density does not change significantly in five weeks. The alk phos was the best monitor for his case. His prostate ultrasounds, too, could not add any information. We had missed getting an ultrasound of his prostate on the day he arrived, and by the time it was done, there were no tumors visible. The numbers tell the whole story. Numbers and physical health.

Bruce Engevik	9/18	9/23	10/9	Vacation	10/25
WBC	7.1	5.9	6.4		
RBC	4.64	4.45	4.5		
PLT	234	180	217		
glucose	77	111	98		99
BUN	8.0	19	17		18
creatinine	1.2	1.2	1.1		1.2
AST (SGOT)	19	11	19		16
ALT (SGPT)	26	11	20		22
LDH	105	96	209		93
GGT	32	23	21		22
T.b.	0.6	0.6	0.1		0.7
alk phos	780	349	444		262
T.p.	6.4	6.8	6.9		7.3
albumin	4.6	4.5	4.6		4.7
globulin	1.8	2.3	2.3		2.6
uric acid	5.8	5.4	5.3		4.1
Calcium	8.7	8.8	9.1		8.7

Phosphorus	4.4	3.2	3.4		4.0
Iron	66	76	117		78
Sodium	138	139	141		140
Potassium	4.2	4.7	4.6		4.4
Chloride	99	99	102		100
triglycerides	125	90	183		188
cholesterol	183	212	320		318
PSA	1,250		98		
prostate weight		50 gm			37 gm

51   George Hill   Brain Cancer

George was a slender boy of 15 when he arrived with a brain tumor about the size of a plum. At age 15 he missed his mother and sister at home in Peru. But he had heard his doctor say, in front of him, to his parents: "If we don't do surgery, he will die. If we do surgery, if he survives, he will be paralyzed from the waist down and his brain will be a vegetable. Neither radiation nor chemotherapy will work." He remembered each searing word. He wanted none of these choices. So the surgeon implanted a shunt (plastic tube) in his brain to drain off edema fluid and lower the pressure in the brain—he had already lost significant vision in his left eye. The diagnosis was cystic astrocytoma. His two MRIs, brought with him from home, showed the tumor was slowly growing. It was part cyst, part cancerous, with a long beak-shaped point reaching forward. Beside this was a completely calcified pineal gland; it had turned into "stone" or calcium deposits and appears black on the print.

He was here with his father. We started on his first day to search for the toxins that came from their home so it could be made ready for George's return. His "whole body" test was Positive for lead, vanadium, aluminum, thulium, formaldehyde, asbestos, isopropyl alcohol, benzene, zearalenone, aflatoxin, and all five malonates. To account for the lead, he was asked to get dust samples from each room at home. To explain the thulium, he was to get his old vitamin C bottle from home. And their sugar was to be tested for asbestos. His plastic glasses frames seeped vanadium; he was to soak and wash them, then re-test them. Other items were obvious; he had been living on "semi-food" (crackers and sandwiches, fat-free munchies), instead of meats and vegetables to avoid getting high cholesterol! All of which were laden with mold that made zearalenone. It accumulated in his skin fat and brain, there releasing benzene and phenol to lower the local immunity.

Our next search was at the brain, cerebrum. He was Positive for these mutagens: 1,10-phenanthroline, betapropiolactone, benzanthracene, hydroxyurea, cycloheximide, vanadyl complexes, 20-methylcholanthrene, and phorbol.

The tapeworm test showed five out of five types tested were Positive in his brain. It was full of microscopic eggs and cysticercus stages. He was also

Positive for *Mycobacterium avium/cellulare*, 3 streptomyces species and their products: erythromycin, protease, streptomycin, mitomycin C, and actinomycin D.

Four out of four azo dyes tested were Positive, including Sudan Black B and DAB. Urethane and inorganic germanium were Positive. The urethane must be coming from his plastic shunt since there was <u>not a single defective or repaired tooth in his mouth</u>. Our cancer marker tests showed: Ortho-phospho-tyrosine, hCG, and DNA Positive. RNA and gamma interferon were Negative. Our first task was to stop this; he was started on Day 1 of the cancer program.

Three out of three *Clostridium* tests were Positive, as well as three out of three *Streptococcus* tests. It was a daunting situation. If only there was clinical support available at every minute, day or night, in case the tumorous cyst ruptured and flooded the brain, producing such huge seizures as to stop breathing! If it went unnoticed in the night, all would be lost by morning.

The safest approach was to kill everything, detoxify, and clear everything at top speed, but without bursting the cyst-tumor. George was up to it. He swallowed and drank and mixed and sipped as never before. He was eating for dear life and was surprised to learn that I considered his "low cholesterol-cracker" diet to be non-food, hardly to be offered to roaches. He was to sign up for the special restaurant meals and consume nothing else. He would live in the environmentally safe motel with only borax water for personal and laundry chores. But he could consider himself lucky not to be on the list for dental extractions. He did. By the second day his cancer markers were corrected. And only 8 of 20 tumor tissue samples still tested Positive. Was he already showing the advantage of that mystery factor, called youth?

By the fourth day all the previous tests had become Negative that should be Negative and RNA and interferon were Positive, as they should be. Only *Streptococcus* and phenol were still Positive. And the dye Sudan Black B was still present intermittently. The cerebrum was now fairly clear. He was on 10 tsp. Black Walnut tincture daily and 2 capsules methylene blue powder daily (65 mg each). We could begin to examine the <u>tumor</u> (as distinct from the brain) electronically. First, we must identify it. It would surely still have its dyes locked inside while the neighboring brain tissues were already cleared.

Using a dye together with the cerebrum slide to specify the location where the dye was, we immediately found the tumor. Here DNA, *Ascaris* worms, zearalenone, patulin, aflatoxin, benzene, inorganic germanium, and other azo dyes were still Positive.

We next prepared his brain and liver to receive aflatoxin by giving him 30 capsules glutathione for 5 days and progressed him through Day 2 and Day 3 of the cancer program (he had been repeating Day 1 all this time). We were ready to give the tumor-opener, vitamin B_2. But it had already happened. At the cerebrum on his eighth day were all the same toxins and parasites we had originally cleared. He had a slight headache. There was no time to lose; the dyes were loose. For two days in a row he took the complete program together with 30 capsules B$_2$ each day. The cerebrum cleared up, but the cerebellum did not; would he suddenly buckle, never to walk again? Cysteine and ozonated oil were added; all items were taken at maximum dose and George made not a single complaint. Down it all went. He began to have diarrhea (from the large dose of glutathione), and strange green pea-shaped objects floated in his toilet bowl. He was getting out his liver gallstones without doing a liver cleanse! Possibly, the late evening ozonated oil was doing this.

On his eleventh day he was switched to 2 freeze dried green black walnut hull capsules 4 times a day instead of 10 tsp. tincture. This would keep up with emerging parasites more efficiently. The next day his cerebellum was clean.

The 2-week program he had scheduled at our clinic was done, and the next week father and son did their own cooking. They had learned how to select, prepare, and sterilize their food. There would be no room for error. All George's food was tested before eating. He was encouraged to enroll in the Syncrometer class so he could eventually do his own food testing. George's father cooked with absolute precision. But could he keep this up at home? What were George's chances of recovery if they left for home? Zero, I thought. They decided to stay. I estimated it could take six or more months before some reduction in size could be expected. This was not just a tumor but a cyst, also. And cysts are notoriously stable and unassailable. And dangerous because they can get re-colonized at any time. I had not attempted to shrink a cyst before, only tumors. Cysts are considered benign. But this was not benign; it was some kind of hybrid. Progress would depend on daily research.

At the next visit the entire toxic team that had once been in his brain was in his liver. He quickly did a liver cleanse; then it could all be seen at his kidneys. He drank 2 cups of parsley tea and 3 cups of the remaining kidney herb tea daily to produce 1½ gallons of urine daily. In two days the kidneys cleared.

He was scheduled for his first CT scan with us. Would the tumor-opening be apparent in some way? Even the small tumorous part of the cyst had never been clearly seen. George hoped it would

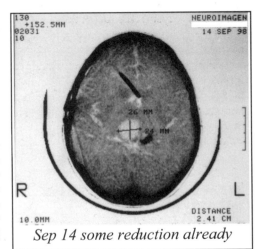

Sep 14 some reduction already

all be gone; his father hoped it was slightly smaller.

A month had passed. The CT showed that a small portion, perhaps the tumor portion was missing, leaving the large cyst intact, like a small water balloon, 24 x 26 mm in size.

He had slight pain at the front of his skull. We searched at bone to identify any lesion at his skull. Rabbit fluke and asbestos were Positive there. Was he eating this accidentally? Yet, there were no rabbit flukes in his gallbladder; they must be emerging from the cyst. As was the asbestos. They had lodged in his skull. We searched in the white blood cells of his skull; they were ferritin-coated. This lowered immunity also allowed *Streptococcus* to grow in his skull, causing pain. *Clostridium* was getting started, too. Inorganic germanium was Positive, but "good" germanium was also Positive so no p53 mutations were spotted. He was given colloidal silver, 3 Tbs. in one dose daily to reach these far away *Clostridium* bacteria. But it was a sinister development. Unless his own white blood cells could be mustered, we might lose the battle. So George gulped papain (to digest the ferritin), MSM, and powdered hydrangea.

At the next visit things were only worse; the thiourea to pyruvic aldehyde ratios were already quite disturbed. And nothing had cleared. In fact, vanadium was now added to the list of toxins accumulating in his skull interior. I believed toxins were seeping out of the cyst to gain a foothold and create a new tumor site in his skull. The ferritin was still not off his white blood cells. It was too soon. We added Levamisole to speed it up (50 mg Decaris, one a day).

A new crisis loomed. Their visas would be up and there was some problem over renewal. They needed to find temporary work, too. I suggested George enroll in school to keep his mind off gloom and doom. This idea made him happy; he was eager to study again.

Two months passed. The (new) second CT scan showed a very small reduction of cyst size, but this could be questioned due to the angle of the shot. Yet, clearly it was not growing. They could report this to the oncologist at home. Their doctor believed he had stepped off a shelf into the abyss (of quackery) when he stated he was headed for Mexico.

Suddenly he tested Positive for rabbit fluke (which brings with it *Clostridium* and *Streptococcus*). His HCl drops were missing in some of his solid foods. He corrected this.

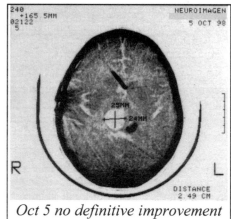

Oct 5 no definitive improvement

At each visit he was searched at the cerebrum. The plan was not to try to open the cyst for fear of cataclysm, but to simply keep the supplement protection in place to kill and detoxify everything as it slowly emerged. Fiberglass and freon emerged in large amounts; silicone and more asbestos emerged. George used to spray silicone on his glasses without taking them off first, he said, just to clean them. And more and more vanadium. They were warned never to have a fossil fuel utility again (emits vanadium).

The papain was giving him stomach aches so he was switched to bromelain.

Now three months had passed. George's WBC had dropped to 3.5, suggesting that some of the emerging toxins were going to the bone marrow. There was rabbit fluke again in his cerebrum and ferritin still coated his white blood cells there. Would the asbestos outflow never stop? Yet we dared not speed it up.

Finally, impatience struck. George and his father went to a UCLA radiologist to review all their scans. Five "cysts" were noted in the optic nerve; the diagnosis was cysticercosis. He was offered the newest tapeworm treatment and warned he could become a vegetable, but it would be done in the hospital under critical care observation. They chose to be patient again. Then we checked the optic nerve location; both *Taenia solium* and *Taenia saginata* stages were present. Four additional tapeworm stages were present at his retina. I doubled his bromelain, MSM, and powdered hydrangea to 1 tsp. 3 times a day to bolster our containment strategy. Freeze dried black walnut was increased to 3 taken three times a day. (He later told me he was actually taking more.)

The very next day the ferritin-coating came off the cerebrum white blood cells.

And in another day all the tapeworm stages were gone, as well as *Clostridium* and *Streptococcus* from the skull location.

But the pineal gland white blood cells were still ferritin-coated and the gland was full of asbestos, silicone, and azo dyes. We felt relief to know we would be getting the assistance of George's own immune system at last. To reassure George, we tested his optic nerve for our entire tapeworm collection: only one was still Positive—a composite Taenia egg collection. It was also Positive at his optic chiasma. Did we dare hope that his vision would some day return? We searched for the toxic team that had so recently left his cerebrum and pineal gland. It was at the spleen. But the spleen white blood cells were loaded up with them, obviously eating and expelling them. So perhaps all would be well.

George was now testing himself regularly and could predict what I would find at his office visit. He could shape his own research. He was a scientist at age 15, coming on 16. His birthday arrived, but no suspect food passed his lips. He could still hear his doctor's words, "You will die." And his success with us was far from assured. The spleen proved difficult to clear. Right after the toxic team arrived at the bladder, they seemed to return to the spleen. We tried 40 capsules vitamin B_2 (12 gm) in a single dose plus glucuronate (3 x 250 mg) for 4 days running to capture the dyes. It worked. They finally cleared the bladder.

His third monthly CT scan, November 19, showed no further change in size of the brain cyst. They felt defeated, but I felt glad. Glad that the 4 doses of 40 capsules B_2 had not burst open his tumor cyst and wreaked havoc and disaster.

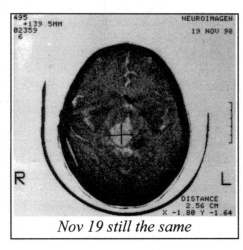

Nov 19 still the same

Meanwhile, I had obtained a made-to-order slide of the brain containing the globus pallidus. Our pathologist felt this was the true location of the tumor cyst. Perhaps now we could analyze its contents and monitor it correctly, instead of simply using the cerebrum slide. And we found the cyst at once. Even the tumor tissue types were still Positive somewhere inside. Asbestos, silicone, urethane, cobalt, vanadium, Sudan Black, and DAB dyes were all Positive. *Clostridium* was Positive, *Streptococcus* Negative. And the globus white blood cells were ferritin-coated. Zearalenone and benzene were very high, and their origin unexplainable.

George himself contributed the DNA findings, still Positive, as was *Taenia solium* cysticercus. He could find his own acrylic acid, zearalenone, and benzene, soon deducing they were all coming from the flaxseeds he was eating daily! He took himself off the flaxseed and was Negative for these a week later. He noticed that tapeworm stages regularly moved from the tumor cyst to his optic nerve. But his high doses of special supplements soon killed them here, only to be followed by another entry.

His latest blood test showed a high (nearly 1.0) ratio of segs to lymphocytes, implying a virus. It was the right time to catch Coxsackie virus on the loose. Indeed, both varieties A and B were Positive at the globus and cerebrum.

In mid-December, there was another burst of activity; his cerebrum was again full of all toxins liberated from the cyst. And the globus pallidus was now clean. Its white blood cells were not ferritin-coated.

But this only meant that most of the globus pallidus was clean. The part that was not clean had first to be identified somehow.

Christmas was around the corner and thoughts of home and mother stirred impatience. The bad job opportunity and anxiety over the upcoming CT scan contributed. His doctor at home was also impatient to hear about results. They had been in touch with him and wanted to please him. What he wanted most was a "good" MRI, <u>with contrast</u>. George asked why I would not permit contrast. "Contrast," I nearly shouted, "And get all that dye back into the cyst we have been cleaning so carefully?" Its only gadolinium, he said, prompted, no doubt, by his oncologist. It must leave quite soon. I have had several already. Could you test for gadolinium at my cyst? I hesitated, for fear he would make his point, but agreed. Shockingly, gadolinium was Positive and still very high at cerebrum, liver, and bone marrow, places that had been cleared of other toxins long ago. Gadolinium was Negative at the white blood cells of these organs. So <u>none</u> of it was being removed. He still had the gadolinium in him from his first scan with contrast, nearly two years ago. But not only gadolinium. He was also Positive for ytterbium, scandium, yttrium, terbium, thulium, and lanthanum (others not tested). Was the contrast material so impure that all the other lanthanides came along for the ride? It seemed a distinct possibility.

But why had I not discovered this sooner? This simple truth had waited for his boyish and creative mind to express itself.

I immediately noticed the disturbance in human (not *Clostridial*) DNA formation typical for lanthanides. It would start late and end even later so the total time of its production would be about 27 seconds, instead of the normal 20 seconds, as seen with the Syncrometer. This was still going on at the cerebrum and globus, but not at the spleen. At the spleen, lanthanides were Positive, but the excess iron deposits were gone. At cerebrum and globus, the lanthanides came associated with both ferrous and ferric iron deposits, as is usual. I wanted to research this further at once, but George had cold sores to attend to, needed to go home, and gone was all inclination to request a CT scan with contrast.

A week later I searched for our set of 14 lanthanide metals. <u>All</u> were present in George's cerebrum, but none were present in the cerebrum white blood cells! Yet they were not ferritin-coated. They should have been able to "eat" the lanthanides to remove them. They had one obvious abnormality; they had iron and calcium deposits. Somehow this interfered with their ability to eat toxins. We would soon see how.

At the end of his fourth month, the new CT scan (not shown) still showed no change in the size or appearance of his tumor-cyst. His cerebrum and globus (with the cyst location) were still filled with lanthanides and iron and calcium deposits, in spite of trying EDTA, a very strong metal chelator, very high doses of vitamin C, and DMSO, a penetrant. The cerebral and globus white blood cells were empty, were not eating the intruders. But a new fact had emerged. Wherever there were calcium and iron deposits the normal digestive enzyme pancreatin was missing. Could this be significant? All normal tissues were supplied with pancreatin which lasted for many hours after a meal. Normal tissues also had phosphatydyl serine, a molecule in the cell membrane that could declare the cell was ready for digestion. Calcium and iron-loaded cells did not. Yet there was no way to get the calcium deposits out.

His fifth monthly CT, January 15, again showed no change. A search of the lanthanide research literature showed that they have long been known to cause calcium precipitation inside cells. And, in fact, this normally triggers cell division. But why were they present in the lysosomes along with iron deposits? (The Syn-

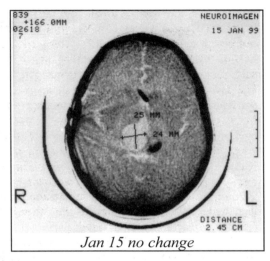

Jan 15 no change

crometer can detect the lysosomes and other cell compartments.) And why was DNA seemingly stuck to them and produced too long a time? There was a strange possibility; the lanthanides and iron could be attracting each other due to their magnetic properties. I searched the body for a susceptible spot where the DNA could be influenced using a small magnet. Indeed, the DNA abnormality could be corrected with a small "magnet patch", only 0.2 gauss, placed over the spine in a narrow (½ inch) band. We gave George such a patch, facing the North (by biological convention) side against his skin. He was taken off many other supplements since they were obviously not able to remove iron, lanthanides, and calcium deposits. But he was given pancreatin, 1 tsp. to take four times a day.

In three days most lanthanides were already out! At the globus, only thulium and lanthanum remained. A week later, there was still some thulium; even two weeks later there was thulium. Thulium sticks tightest inside cells.

Two weeks after starting to wear the tiny magnet patch, George's iron deposits had left the cerebrum as well as the lanthanides. As if by magic, the calcium deposits had left, too! And at the cerebrum all nucleosides were now gone. And in their place was ATP. A large supply of ATP! The cell-flag for digestion, phosphatidylserine, was now Positive, and with it pancreatin. Was the tumor cyst really getting digested? At the globus (his tumor-cyst) things were not as far along. In fact, nucleosides were still present, the digestion-flag was not up, and pancreatin was not there either.

But the main portions of the brain already had their immunity back. The nucleosides, iron and calcium deposits were now in the white blood cells. Was it safe enough to open the cyst? On the day we planned to try, *Ascaris* suddenly reappeared. We delayed again. Eggs and stages were everywhere. But the eggs could be seen in the brain white blood cells now. Immunity would save him. Coxsackie viruses were coursing about, but were found in the white blood cells, too, protecting him.

Days later at the globus, hydroxyurea (from some distant *Ascaris* eggs) was still Positive. We searched for them at many body organs, finding them at last in the bile ducts. Only gallstones could easily explain this; he must have the eggs in his gallstones, forever seeding his brain and cyst with them. He was instructed to do a liver cleanse—his fifth one, and the day after the cleanse to take 3 freeze-dried black walnut capsules four times a day to stamp them out.

But two days after his cleanse he still had *Ascaris* eggs in liver, gallbladder, and bile ducts. He was raised to 6 freeze-dried capsules three times a day for 3 days in a row. Surely that would snuff them out, even inside his stones. (Actually, stones can be much too hard for anything to penetrate them.) He must do weekly liver cleanses till the bile ducts came clean.

It was February 19, the date for his sixth CT scan, and a day he will remember. It showed a huge reduction in tumor-cyst size—to less than half its previous dimensions. But he did not allow himself to believe the good news. It had all happened in the last 30 days. Was it due, finally, to the presence of pancreatin? Which enzyme in the pancreatin was responsible: trypsin, chymotrypsin, lipase, amylase, DNAse, RNAse, peroxidase?

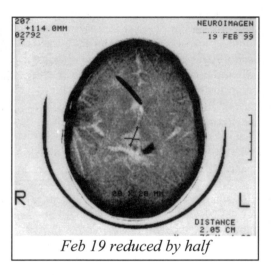

Feb 19 reduced by half

A spot could still be found in his globus pallidus that harbored *acrolein*, a fat derivative similar to burnt grease and very carcinogenic by scientific standards. Was this not being digested? Of all the pancreatic enzymes seen there by Syncrometer, only lipase was still missing, and also missing in our supplement of pancreatin. Lipase digests fat, but could it digest acrolein? We supplemented it separately (¼ tsp. three times a day) and raised his pancreatin to 2 tsp. three times a day. His daily supplements had been: vitamin B_2: 20 capsules (6 gm) to detoxify emerging dyes and benzene, Levamisole (50 mg three times a day) to prevent ferritin-coating as asbestos emerged and to help kill *Ascaris*; EDTA ($^1/_8$ tsp. in a cup of hot water) to chelate lead and other heavy metals as they emerged; freeze-dried green black walnut hull (three times a day); and vitamin C (2 tsp. three times a day).

Ten days later the acrolein was gone. Did this mean it had digested? The next scan wasn't due for another week.

The March 20 scan was also too good to be true. George had to be jolted into reality—that it was really happening for him—but still with cautious interpretation. Although the tumor-cyst was down to 9 x 10 mm, it could still easily fill up again if he were to get a dose of *Ascaris* or common food bacteria. He needed no warning. It was only on this day, seven months after his arrival, that he allowed himself to repeat the exact words of his doctor at home: You will die. Was his life scarred? I think not, for he was pursuing the hard sciences, studying

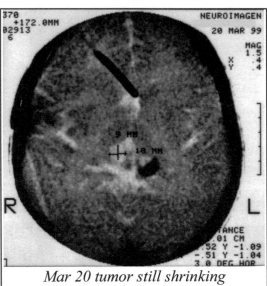

Mar 20 tumor still shrinking

English, doing very well at school, and looking forward to a university education.

April 24 brought further good news; the tumor-cyst was still smaller. But what about his blood tests? When he arrived August 3, his alk phos was clearly elevated, but was it due to his status as a young growing boy? His albumin and uric acid were slightly elevated, but nothing serious. More serious were his low triglycerides and cholesterol. His last blood test, Feb. 19, was not very different. His state of nutrition had not improved in spite of gaining height and weight. But his story was not yet done and this book must go to press.

Summary: George and his father get excellent grades. They were the first to try (and succeed) at lanthanide removal. But there is a cyst remnant remaining, a calcified pineal to rescue and, ultimately, a shunt to remove. Can it be done?

George Hill	8/3	8/10	8/24	9/7	9/21
WBC	5.3	5.5	5.9	6.4	4.9
RBC	4.67	4.81	4.97	4.53	4.94

511

PLT	173	204	240	173	212
glucose	90	75	77	86	80
BUN	13	13	21	14	11
creatinine	0.9	0.9	0.9	0.8	0.9
AST (SGOT)	18	19	18	21	21
ALT (SGPT)	11	10	10	9	12
LDH	304 (240-480)	348	301	270	301
GGT	13	14	13	13	13
T.b.	0.7	0.6	0.5	0.4	0.8
alk phos	453 (30-375)	405	434	392	400
T.p.	7.0	7.5	7.2	7.0	7.3
albumin	5.1	5.4 (3.9-5.1)	5.0	5.2	5.1
globulin	1.9	2.1	2.2	1.8	2.2
uric acid	6.2 (2.4-6.1)	5.5	4.5	3.6	4.3
Calcium	9.2	9.6	9.1	8.9	9.6
Phosphorus	5.0	5.3	5.6	6.0	5.3
Iron	101	174	68	110	187
Sodium	136	138	136	136	141
Potassium	4.0	4.1	3.9	4.3	4.3
Chloride	98	108	102	104	104
triglycerides	68	66	110	165	73
cholesterol	137	142	121	128	148

George Hill	10/5	10/28	11/19	12/8	2/19
WBC	4.7	3.5	7.6	6.0	6.1
RBC	4.87	4.8	4.9	4.55	4.62
PLT	191	—	—	194	175
glucose	112	101	96	98	74
BUN	19	12	11	12	18
creatinine	0.9	1.0	1.0	0.6	0.8
AST (SGOT)	20	22	25	24	14
ALT (SGPT)	15	12	13	12	7
LDH	300	356	400	163 (71-210)	173 (120-230)
GGT	11	13	14	11	22
T.b.	0.7	0.7	0.9	1.1	0.5
alk phos	391	400	418	291 (30-375)	300 (35-125)
T.p.	7.5	7.7	7.5	8.1	6.5
albumin	5.3	5.3	5.3	4.9	4.3
globulin	2.2	2.4	2.2	3.2	2.2
uric acid	4.0	2.9	2.7	4.1	2.6
Calcium	9.2	9.8	9.4	9.2	9.1
Phosphorus	5.4	3.7	4.3	4.3	4.6
Iron	69	80	96	105	69
Sodium	136	141	137	144	141
Potassium	3.8	4.6	4.1	4.8	4.0
Chloride	96	101	102	109	106
triglycerides	65	72	63	133	75

cholesterol	138	—	140	146	125

52   Katherine Morales (continuation)   Bone Cancer

It was three years since we had last seen Katherine Morales. Her story begins at the start of this chapter. We begged her to visit us. Finally, she agreed. It was April 3. Katherine walked in rather breezily for an earlier bone-cancer case. She had no cane or walker, and my impulse was to grab her before she might fall. But her family seemed unconcerned. This was a follow-up visit, solely for the record. She was not ill in any way. She was not on any pain medication—and not in pain. She had gained back 30 lb. and now weighed 110 to 112 lb. We had agreed to meet at the clinic's malonate-free restaurant. She was eager to talk and get updated on all developments. There was no hint of developing mental impairment, although she was eighty-five now. She walked with ease; in fact, she had fallen recently at home without the slightest injury—contrasting with the frequent breaks she used to endure in the past. What was her secret? Was she on a special supplement? Eating something special? Her answers were <u>no</u> and <u>no</u> again.

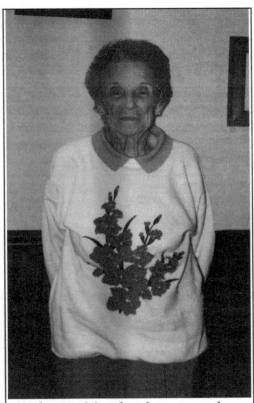

Katherine Morales three years later

She had agreed to a follow-up bone scan even though bone density does not improve enough to show decisively on an X-ray, after bone cancer clears up. I thought that surely a <u>little</u> improvement in bone density would be visible, though.

Here are some of the questions I asked and answers I got.

Q. Are you on any supplements?

513

A. No, except vitamin C. I take ¼ tsp. powdered vitamin C in my water at meal time, not too much, just enough to give it a taste. (Her forthright, precise answers surprised me.)

Q. Are you on any medicine? Weren't you on heart medicine long ago?

A. Oh heavens, NO. I'm not taking any medicine.

Q. May I take your pulse, then? (It was a perfectly regular 72.) Why are you so healthy now? What's your secret?

A. I don't have any secret. Except that I zap every day. I haven't missed more than five days since I came to see you.

Then we left the restaurant to meet at the office. There I did some Syncrometer testing. I searched for all the amino acids in her brain, since she seemed so young in attitude. (As organs begin to fail in our bodies, they have fewer amino acids.) Twenty-two amino acids Positive at brain. This was most unusual. And without a supplement! NAD and NADP both Positive at brain (good). NADH and NADPH both Negative at brain (good).

She was oxidizing extraordinarily well at the brain. No hint of a respiration block such as begins to affect us as we age. She had indeed been on a shark cartilage supplement for one and a half years. She had been on rhodizonic vials for at least half a year. But this was all in the past. Did this have a long lasting effect?

I tested further. Rhodizonic acid Positive at cerebrum (brain); she was making her own, normally. Vitamin B_2 (riboflavin) Positive at cerebrum. Coenzyme Q10 Positive at cerebrum. Without taking these as supplements, she had these oxidizers in her tissue! I tested for phenol—our nemesis of aging. There was none at the brain, but it was Positive at her joints. She had no pockets of streptococcus bacteria throughout her body to make phenol: only in her joints were they Positive. Without phenol, she would not oxidize her vitamin C into the "aging" causers, threose, xylose, lyxose. I tested her state of reduction at the brain.

L-ascorbic acid Positive	L-threose Negative
dehydroascorbic acid (oxidized) Negative	D-threose Negative
glutathione Positive	L-xylose Negative
glutathione (oxidized) Negative	D-xylose Negative
ferrous gluconate Positive	L-lyxose Negative
ferric phosphate (oxidized) Negative	L-cysteine Positive
iron sulfide FeS Positive	L-cystine (oxidized) Negative
iron sulfide FeS_2 (oxidized) Negative	

She was not over-oxidized! Was she not aging at all? In fact, getting younger somehow? But she had no magic answers for my questions. Finally, in frustration, I asked Katherine, "Well, what <u>are</u> you eating? What do you eat over and over, nearly daily?" "Chicken soup," she said. And there was the magic. Surely she was benefiting from this diet the way our patients benefit from the chicken broth that is part of their 21 Day Program. Some factor, perhaps RNAse inhibitor, perhaps not, was allowing her to have all the amino acids present in her tissues for whatever task her cells wished to accomplish. We wished her well and said our good-byes.

Next day, we received her new bone scan. The radiologist noted some regions of osteoporosis, nothing suggestive of cancer. We can see the reduced intensity of former hot spots. Especially along the back of the head and neck and upper spine; the bone appears entirely normal.

Summary: Katherine worked hard to recover from the bone cancer that gave her painful lesions, too numerous to count three years ago. But other patients did, too, without so much success. What was the difference? I believe Katherine had several advantages. She had dentures—she was not burdened with the extra toxicity of metal, plastic, or infections of the jaw that come with numerous restorations. Besides this, the extra high doses of rhodizonate she took initially surely would have detoxified the food dyes accumulated in her body. We knew nothing about them at that time; we now accomplish this with co-enzyme Q10 and vitamin B_2. She did not use hair dye—another lucky break. After overcoming her bone cancer, she not only became well, but extraordinarily well. What was responsible for this? She had two unusual habits: zapping daily

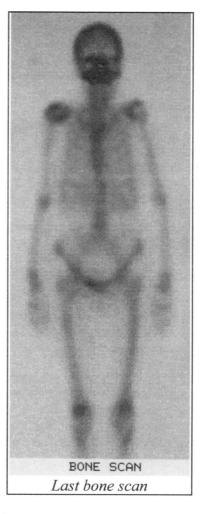

BONE SCAN

Last bone scan

for three years and a diet rich with chicken soup. (She even saved chicken stock for use in cooking many other dishes during the week.)

Katherine kept us inspired through the three years we were developing the 21 Day Program. Thank you Katherine.

Long Term Follow Up

Curing yourself of mosquito bites or the common cold is not a serious challenge but it can be quite a frustrating task; they often last and last. Eventually, they are gone. Do you then heave a sigh of relief and say, "Great job, now they will never be back?" Chances are that a year later you will have them again.

Parasite or pathogen-caused diseases are bound to come at you again and again, so a long term follow-up by itself makes little sense.

The malignancy, being parasite-caused could come back at any time. The tumor growth, being part parasite, part bacterial, and part environmental toxin, could also return. The whole concept of Long Term Follow Up for cancer is faulty and should be abandoned. A follow up of <u>parasitism</u> and <u>infection</u> plus <u>tissue levels of heavy metals</u>, <u>solvents</u>, <u>dyes</u> and our <u>sulfur reserves</u> makes more sense.

But this is far from discouraging news! Seeing that cancer in all its forms has external causes and is not due to "degenerative disease related to aging" brings back hope. And I hope you got a good sense of how to accomplish the "impossible," and in some cases, how easy it can be!

Food Rules

1 tsp. (teaspoon) = 5 ml = 5 cc	1 tbs. (tablespoon) = 3 tsp. = 15 ml
1 cup $\cong$ 240 ml	1 pint = 2 cups $\cong$ 500 ml
1 quart = 4 cups $\cong$ 1 Liter	1 Gallon = 4 Quarts = 3½ Liters
1 ounce = 30 ml	1 pound = 454 gm $\cong$ ½ kg
°F = (°C x $^9/_5$) + 32	°C = (°F - 32) x $^5/_9$

Safety is our main concern. Safety from live parasites, safety from harmful bacteria, safety from solvents, carcinogenic dyes, and mold. Safety from asbestos. And from silicone (defoamer) and acrylic acid which turns into acrolein.

Yet making tasty food is important so you can truly enjoy it. To achieve this with ease and efficiency, you will need to equip the kitchen with:

- A stainless steel pressure cooker and glass bowls with lids to fit inside.
- A blender; an additional juicer/extractor is optional.
- An ozonator.
- A bread maker.
- A microwave oven for sterilizing (optional).
- Plastic cutlery.
- Glass or enamel pots and pans (not metal).
- Glass jars and bowls for food storage (not plastic). Some should have lids and fit inside the pressure cooker.

To <u>cook</u> use glass or enamelware, not metal. To <u>fry</u> use glass or enamelware; occasional (once a week) use of Teflon or Silverstone is allowable. To <u>bake</u> use glass, enamel, or Teflon-coated ware. Do not use special sprays to grease; they contain silicone, which I detect in tumors. Use lard, butter, olive oil, or coconut oil which do not turn into acrylic acid. To <u>microwave</u> use low-wattage (600w) with a rotating plate.

> The principles to observe are:
> 1. Avoid asbestos, heavy metal, and silicone contamination.
> 2. Detoxify dyes, benzene and mycotoxins.
> 3. Sterilize everything.
> 4. Don't overheat unsaturated fats

All fruits and vegetables were grown in soil that was fertilized and had filth in it. Dust and dirt made contact with the food. This explains why the Syncrometer finds rabbit fluke parasites on all of it. *Ascaris* eggs as well as tapeworm eggs and hosts of bacteria are all present. All meats, poultry and fish are similarly contaminated. Even chicken eggs, though shielded by bacteria-proof shells, have rabbit fluke within!

Only a few fruits are so safe they don't need extra caution: watermelon, cantaloupe, and honeydew melon. The thinner-peeled fruits, including bananas, avocados, and citrus require careful sanitizing.

Yet simple ways have been found to make food safe. Not merely cooking and baking the old-fashioned way. These fail to kill rabbit fluke and *Ascaris* eggs, although they do kill many pathogens. Not merely pressure-cooking, which kills more, but still fails to kill *Ascaris* eggs in hard foods. Not microwaving with its uneven temperatures. But with simple **stomach-like** chemistry!

Canned food is not safe either. The dust and dirt on the food prior to canning did not get sterilized. Even canned meat did not get sterilized, the temperature stayed too low. Roasted meats or turkey, even if oven-baked, are not safe; the temperature did not go high enough. Although the temperature may have been set at 400°, the food in the oven is considered done at 185°F and lower! Nothing goes beyond boiling point as long as water is present. Although microwave temperatures go much higher, it does not heat evenly.

Nothing presently employed in the art of cooking reaches the 250°F (121°C) that is considered minimum in a hospital to sterilize bandages or instruments.[123]

But an ordinary child can sterilize all the food it eats! Without heat or equipment and, while eating with dirt-laden hands, the food is sterilized. The stomach is left with no more bacteria than there were before eating; about 10 bacteria per teaspoonful of stomach juice. The amazing chemical is simple **hydrochloric acid**. It is called muriatic acid when it is used by plumbers to dissolve lime deposits. Plumbers must use this very carefully or it will dissolve sink, stool and cement! It could dissolve your teeth! It all depends on its concentration.

A child's stomach has 1000 times more hydrochloric acid (HCl) than most adults over 50 years old (pH 2 versus pH 5; every pH number smaller represents 10 times more acid).

It is not surprising, then, that 2 drops of hydrochloric acid kills all the rabbit flukes, *Ascaris* eggs, tapeworm stages, and bacteria in one 8 oz. cup of 2% milk. The HCl must be USP Grade diluted to 5% in strength (a little stronger than vinegar). And although one drop is sufficient, I prefer to err on the side of safety by doubling this. This is chemical sterilization at its finest—duplicating the body's very own chemistry.

Would it not be wiser, though, to stimulate the stomach's own production of HCl rather than adding it belatedly? Indeed it would. But a way of doing this must first be discovered. This discovery would surely be the closest to the "fountain of youth" ever imagined.

Meanwhile, we can make sure that we stop eating filth with our food for the first time since humans domesticated animals. Yet we must not dissolve our teeth nor disturb our body's acid/base balance by using too much HCl.

Our chloride levels and bicarbonate or carbon dioxide levels are regularly included in blood tests. If you are getting too much HCl, you could expect the body to be too acid; the chloride or

---

[123] Murray, P., Baron, E., Pfaller, M., Tenover, F., Yolken, R., Eds., *Manual of Clinical Microbiology* 6th ed., ASM Press, 1995, p. 240.

CO_2 levels would be too high, while bicarbonate is too low. We easily see there is <u>no</u> tendency for chloride to creep upward after three months of use at the level of 45 drops daily, besides what was used in cooking. Nor did the urinary pH reflect greater body acidity; it remained at 6.0. Evidently, this amount of chloride (2.62 mEq) is negligible out of a blood total of over 500 mEq. In spite of this assurance, however, I recommend that you do <u>not exceed</u> 45 drops daily, not counting the drops used in food preparation before serving.

Just how to prepare each food and be sure it is sterilized is given in the table that follows. The rules are:

1. If it has asbestos contamination, peel it, or wash thoroughly and core widely.
2. If it has molds, dip in HCl water (2 drops per cup).
3. If it has dye or benzene (pesticide) contamination, add vitamin B_2 powder. Only a pinch is needed, and you may add it to the HCl wash, if appropriate.
4. If it has dust or filth, as all vegetables must, cook them twice. After cooking the first time, cool for 10 minutes. This seems to be the trigger that forces parasite eggs to hatch, making them vulnerable. Then bring to a boil again for 5 minutes to kill all the newly hatched larvae. Always use salt in cooking to raise the boiling point. Since salt, except pure salt, needs sterilizing itself, be sure to add it before you finish cooking.
5. If it has a hard center, like rice or beans, dried peas and lentils, use a pressure cooker to kill *E. coli* and *Shigella* bacteria that also survive regular cooking at the center. After a 15 minute cooling-off period, cook them a second time. Again, cooking the first time merely hatches(!) the *Ascaris* eggs and cultures(!) bacteria deep within these foods.
6. Nearly all supermarket produce has been sprayed to retard sprouting or mold growth or wilting, or to give better color, or as pesticide. All, including bananas and avocados must be soaked in hot water twice for one minute each time, drying both times. This removes spray wax,

asbestos, dyes, lanthanides, and benzene altogether. If you soak longer, they re-enter the food.

7. Finally, when adding HCl to food, add two drops per serving of each item on your plate, unless otherwise noted (e.g. 2 drops on potatoes, 2 drops on green beans, etc.). Don't sterilize water or Lugol's water.

Common Food Rules

	has asbestos	has dye	has benz (pesticide)	has mold	dip in HCl (2 d/ cup water)	add HCl (to serving)	add B$_2$
Fruits			Yes or No				
Apples, kiwi, pears, peaches. Soak twice in hot water for 1 minute, dry, cut out stem and flower ends deeply.	Y	Y	Y	N	Y	Y	Y
Avocado, banana. Soak twice in hot water, dry.	Y	Y	Y	N	N	Y	N
Canned fruit	Y	Impossible to remove asbestos. Avoid.					
Cherries and most berries.	N	N	Y	Y	Y	Y	Y
Coconut, fresh. Remove brown skin from pieces.	N	N	N	N	Y	N	N
Currants, raisins, other dried fruit.	Y	Can't be washed off. Avoid.					
Grapes, strawberries		Avoid, too moldy.					
Grapefruit, lemons, pomegranates. Soak in hot water twice and dry.	N	Y	Y	N	N	Y	N
Pineapple. Wash and drain. Peel very thickly so no "eyes" are left.	N	N	Y	N	N	Y	Y
Plums, kumquats, nectarines. Soak in hot water twice for 1 minute, cut out stem and blossom widely.	Y	N	Y	Y	N	Y	Y
Grains							
Breads	N	Y	Y	Y	N	Y	N
Buckwheat, Kamut, oats, quinoa, millet, cornmeal, cream of wheat, grits, rice. Wash three times and drain to remove asbestos. Cook twice.	Y	Y	Y	Y	Y	Y	Y
Flaxseed	N	N	Y	Y	Y	Y	Y
Flour, white and bleached.	N	N	N	N	N	N	N
Sunflower seeds	Y	Too difficult to remove asbestos. Avoid.					
Wheat berries	Y	Too difficult to remove asbestos.					

Vegetables

Artichokes. Cook twice.	N	N	Y	Y	Y	Y	Y
Beets, radishes (raw). Wash, dry. Peel the top half first so no dirt or fingers touch clean part. Wash hands, turn beet to finish peeling.	N	N	Y	N	Y	Y	Y
Canned vegetables	Too many chemicals. Avoid.						
Chilies, peppers; hot soak twice.	Y	N	Y	N	Y	Y	Y
Corn in husk, cut away tip if exposed.	N	N	N	N	N	N	N
Dried beans, incl. Adzuki, pinto, soy, garbanzo, split peas, lentils. Wash several times to remove asbestos. Use pressure cooker; cook twice.	Y	Y	Y	Y	Y	Y	Y
Eggplant, cucumber; hot wash twice, peel.	N	Y	Y	N	N	Y	N
Cooked greens, incl. beet tops, cauliflower, collards, cabbage, kale, Swiss chard, green beans. Wash twice in hot water. Cook twice.	Y	Y	Y	N	Y	Y	N
Raw greens, incl. lettuce, spinach, parsley. Soak in hot water twice, shaking between soaks. Sterilize in cold HCl-water.	Y	Y	Y	N	Y	Y	N
Mushrooms	Too difficult to sterilize, don't use.						
Nuts, in the shell only. Remove brown skins.	Y	N	Y	Y	Y	Y	Y
Onions, garlic, leeks. Peel apart. Hot soak twice; then HCl-water.	N	N	Y	N	Y	Y	N
Peanut butter	N	Y	Y	Y	N	Y	Y
Potatoes, red and white. Hot soak twice. Peel carefully.	Y	Y	Y	Y	Y	Y	Y
Potatoes, brown	Has too much zearalenone throughout. Avoid.						
Squash, incl. acorn, butternut, zucchini. Soak in hot water twice and dry. Peel if possible.	N	Y	Y	N	N	Y	N
Tapioca	?	Y	Y	Y	Y	Y	Y

Dairy (HCl is added **while** stirring)

Butter. Let butter soften in a bowl. Add B$_2$ and HCl, whip. Refrigerate.	N	Y	Y	N	N	4 per ¼ lb.	Y
Buttermilk	N	Y	Y	N		4/ cup	Y
Cheese. Melt. Add vitamin B$_2$ and HCl, stirring well or cook twice.	N	Y	Y	N	N	4/2 oz.	Y
Eggs, wash and dry first; soak in HCl-water or Lugol's (1 drop per quart)	N	N	N	N	N	1/egg	N
Half 'n half	N	Y	Y	N		4/ cup	Y
Milk	N	Y	Y	N		2/ cup	Y
Whipping cream	N	Y	Y	N		6/ cup	Y
Yogurt, plain	N	Y	Y	N		6/cup	Y

Sweets

Flavoring, incl. maple, vanilla, lemon.	N	Y	Y	Y	N	Y	Y
Maple syrup. Bring to a boil first.	N	N	Y	Y	N	Y	Y
Sweet baked goods	Y	Impossible to remove asbestos, avoid.					
Sugar, incl. white, brown, confectioners, raw, fructose.	Y	Too difficult to get asbestos out. Only manufacturer's sucrose and Paraguayan organic sugar was safe.					
Honey (commercial)	Y	Too difficult to get asbestos out; avoid.					
Honey (local), sterilize	N	N	N	N	N	Y	N

Other foods

Coffee, boil twice; then filter twice. Sterilize	Y	Use double paper filter.					
Herbal teas, boil twice.	N	Y	Y	Y	N	2/cup	Y
Meat, fish, fowl. Cook regular way first; then microwave to sterilize, or cook twice, cooling between.	N	Y	Y	N	Y	Y	Y
Olive oil, coconut oil, lard.	N	Y	Y	N	N	2/cup	Y
Pasta	N	N	N	Y	Y	Y	N
Spices, salt; sterilize	N	Y	Y	Y	N	Y	Y

Public Food

If you are not in control of the kitchen, you must make your own safety rules **at the table**:

1. Eat nothing sweetened. Unless maple syrup was used, it will certainly have asbestos. Add HCl to honey.
2. Eat nothing fried; it will certainly have acrylic acid.
3. Dust all food with vitamin B_2 powder from a capsule or bring your B-C salt-shaker (see *Recipes*). A very light dusting is sufficient to detoxify traces of benzene, azo dyes, and acrylic acid. Mix slightly with fork.
4. Add 3 drops HCl (5%) to each serving on your plate, including beverages, except water.
5. Add 4 drops HCl to foods that are hard, gummy, or impenetrable like beans, meats. Mix as well as possible on your plate. Even salt (except pure salt) needs sterilizing.

A cancer patient should always carry these items in purse or pocket: a few vitamin B_2 capsules, an HCl dropper bottle, closeable salt shakers for potassium gluconate and B-C salt, a squeeze bottle of locally produced honey or maple syrup for sweetening. Also a very small ethyl alcohol dispenser to clean fingers (and under fingernails) before eating, and a dropper bottle of Lugol's.

If you are eating in a restaurant, ask a favor of the server <u>after</u> your food arrives: to microwave your loaded plate for three extra minutes. This includes the salad which will now be limp, but still tasty with oil/vinegar dressing. Then distribute 18 drops HCl (this is a few more than with home cooked food) over it all, except in water. Remember to take the Lugol's at end of your meal.

Kosher foods are an exception

Most foods labeled Kosher had no asbestos, azo dyes, lanthanides, heavy metals, acrylic acid, or urethane. They did not even have rabbit fluke! Does this reflect on superior sanitation or quality control? Or some mystery-method? How do they do it?

Going Shopping

Shop for Kosher foods whenever possible. Search for these symbols: Ⓤ, K, ☆. This still does not <u>guarantee</u> their safety. Any processed food could still have a solvent residue; that is why the cancer patient is advised to eat home-cooked food. Kosher food must still be properly prepared and sterilized.

Organic produce has much less <u>dye</u> and <u>pesticide</u> pollution (benzene) than regular produce. But <u>asbestos</u> tufts adhering to the outside of foods is just as severe a problem. When I tested some farmers' market produce, it was free of asbestos. Search for <u>organic produce at farmers' markets</u>. Next best might be a small corner grocery store.

None of these recommended foods is safe, though, unless cleaned up with hot washes and later sterilized. Do not buy a spray that removes spray, either; the one I tested had more solvents than the original sprayed food.

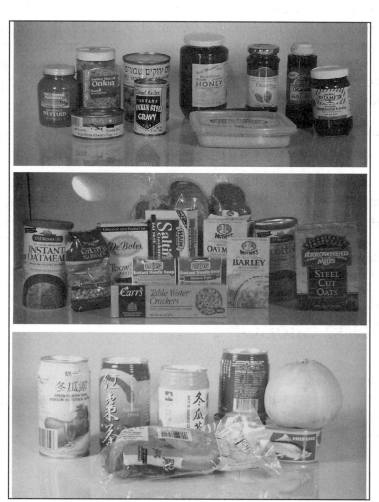

Fig. 48 Kosher and Asian foods superior

Sterilize for Storage

Food will keep much better if given a sterilization treatment before putting it in the refrigerator.

Eggs should be washed and dried with a paper towel before storing. Throw away the carton; it is full of *Salmonella*.

Greens, vegetables and fruits can be soaked for 1 minute in HCl-water (2 drops per cup) or Lugol's-water (1 drop per quart) before storing.

Microwaving to Sterilize

Microwaving is especially useful for meats (fish and fowl).

Although 3 minutes of microwaving kills many parasite eggs and larvae left over after the food has been baked, it is still not as reliable as double-boiling. Meat that is boiled till totally soft, cooled, and boiled again for at least 10 minutes is safe. Many primitive cultures cooked this way!

Stay away from the microwave oven while it is on. How far should you stay? The distance the electromagnetic field reaches, as measured by a field meter (see *Sources*). It is easy to use and rather educational, costing less than $150.00 (U.S.).

Old, powerful units may spew the hazardous field up to 15 feet! Walk out of the kitchen if you have one of these. Newer, small units, 600 watts, spew only a few inches around the seams. Some spew nothing. Having food in the oven while it is on greatly reduces the field that is spewed out. Never have it on when empty.

I have not done extensive food testing for safety after microwaving. These experiments await the future. In preliminary tests of microwaved oil and water, I did not observe them in my immune system minutes later. I did observe the destruction of organic "good" germanium which is essential for a strong immune system and the appearance of bad (i.e. oxidized) germanium. So, caution is advised. Use it for sterilization of food, not as a convenience.

Sterilize Hands

Do not let human hands touch your food, unless they have been freshly sterilized. Even a few bacteria, that would not harm a healthy person, will seek out your tumor and prevent shrinking. You cannot trust restaurant food to be untouched. Simply touching the toast, a piece of pie or fruit to nudge it onto the plate contaminates it.

Your own hands are just as important. Nails should be very short to facilitate sterilizing them. They must be sterilized before eating and after bathroom use. (If you are bedridden, use a spray bottle.)

Leftovers

Do not eat leftovers unless they are re-boiled as in the beginning. All food picks up bacteria while it is open to air and then stored in the refrigerator. After a few days these few have increased their numbers to a dangerous level for a cancer patient. Re-heating the food without actually sterilizing it only cultures (increases) them; soon there are many more.

Although it is extra work to select food and cook it, these Food Rules will save your life!

Recipes

These are the minimum items an advanced cancer patient needs. Many more items are discussed in my other books.

Staples

Use <u>pure</u> salt only (see *Sources*), like for laboratory use. Store salt could have additives and often has *Ascaris* eggs and mold.

Two to One Sodium-Potassium Salt

2 cups pure salt
1 cup potassium chloride

Mix. Store in tightly closed glass jar with rice added to absorb moisture. Label. Use in a salt shaker without a metal lid. If you don't mind the taste, a one-to-one mixture is even more beneficial.

B-C Salt

The easy way to get B_2 and vitamin C into all your food.

½ cup pure salt or sodium-potassium salt
1 capsule vitamin B_2
½ tsp. vitamin C (ascorbic acid) powder (also try 1 tsp.)

Shake together in closed jar. Pour into closeable non-metal salt shaker. When using salt in cooking, don't wait until the end to add it. It needs to be twice-cooked itself, besides raising the boiling point of the food to be cooked.

Your diet will be very low in sodium salt because in the 21 Day Program you need to consume your daily potassium gluconate first, which you "salt" your food with. This is beneficial

529

because sick tissues become overloaded with sodium. Pulling the sodium out of them with potassium in the diet (or cesium as a medicine) helps them recover.

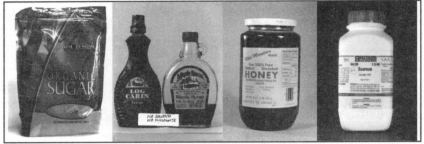

Organic sugar, maple syrup, locally produced honey, and sucrose.
Fig. 49 Safe sweetening

Sweetening

Use honey and maple syrup. All granulated forms I purchased at grocery stores or health food stores had asbestos fibers in them(!) except for the organic variety shown; it is imported from Paraguay. Sucrose purchased from a chemical supply company also did not.

Preserves must be homemade:
1 cup fruit
1 tbs. water
sweetening

Soak twice for 1 minute each time in very hot water and dry; this removes wax-spray and dye. Peel. Heat to boiling in water, stirring with wooden spoon. When done, add half as much sweetening as fruit and bring to boil again. Add HCl drops at point of use (2 drops per cup).

Variations: add lemon juice for extra zip.

Nearly Butter

10 oz. coconut oil
2 oz. olive oil

½ capsule riboflavin (vitamin B$_2$)
$1/_8$ teaspoon pure salt or sodium-potassium salt (to taste)

If coconut oil is solidified, melt it first by warming. Then add oils together in jar. Most oil contains *Ascaris* eggs and must be sterilized. Add HCl drops, 2 per cup. Shake until uniformly mixed. Add riboflavin and salt. Shake again. Pour into mold or butter dish. Refrigerate. Remove from mold with hot water.

Note about colors: coenzyme Q10 gives a butter-yellow color. Riboflavin gives lemon-yellow color. Turmeric is another safe yellow colorant. You may use these other colorants as long as a pinch of B$_2$ is added to detoxify any benzene.

Water

Use cold tap water only, never bottled water. The bottling process adds traces of antiseptic and solvents which includes isopropyl alcohol, xylene, and toluene. Let your faucet run in the morning until one gallon has been lost. This flushes possible overnight accumulations of pipe material.

Do not use ice cubes. If you like cold water, store it in a glass container in the refrigerator, but do not drink it if it is over a day old.

Do not purchase water from dispensers (again, because of sterilization contaminants). Carry your water in glass bottles. Plastic exudes plasticizers while allowing bacteria to permeate and culture in it. Do not drink out of personal dispenser bottles—they are immediately contaminated with bacteria. Sterilize your water while in foreign countries by boiling twice and later adding HCl.

Bread

According to Syncrometer tests, homemade bread has beta-glucans, known to stimulate Natural Killer cell activity (immunity).

Make homemade bread using cake yeast. Ask your grocer to order it. Keep refrigerated. (Granulated yeast had residues of solvents and petroleum products.) All the flours on the super-market shelves tested free of aflatoxin. Use water instead of milk for the recipes during a dairy-free period.

White bread purchased at a bakery is safe if ¼ inch is trimmed off the bottom where petroleum grease (bringing benzene) was used in the bread pan. Here, also, you would find silicone being used as a "non-stick agent."

Eggs

Since eggs carry rabbit fluke, internally, they must be sterilized. This is easy to do while in the liquid, raw state but impossible after cooking. Add 1 drop HCl to each raw egg used. Beat or mix well. After serving add 2 drops per egg.

Beans, Dried Peas, Lentils and Rice

These foods have hard centers even after regular cooking. *Shigella* bacteria and *Ascaris* eggs not only survive there, they are helped to multiply. The eggs hatch into larvae on a massive scale during the cooling down period, ready to invade. But once hatched, they are vulnerable and can be killed by boiling briefly again. Refried beans or rice and twice cooked peas and lentils are safe. Pressure cooking these foods until very soft speeds up the process, but still does not kill everything at first. After a 10 minute cool-down (adding cold water shortens this to 5 minutes), bring to boil again for 5 minutes. They must still be sterilized at time of serving.

Meats

Cook, bake, poach or fry them the usual way first. Then scoop it all into a plastic "cooking bag" and microwave until meat falls apart (one serving typically takes three minutes). On the plate add HCl, three drops per serving. If meats have been cooked, as in soup or stew, a second boil sterilizes them, too.

Vegetables and Fruit

Most are sprayed with combinations of wax, dye, pesticide, anti-sprouter, anti-mold, etc. Fast green (Food Green 3) is present on most and brings with it the lanthanide elements. This dye, plus lanthanides are water-soluble and penetrate the food deeply. But double soaking in hot water for 1 minute removes it. Even organic bananas, pears, grapefruit, and potatoes must be double soaked this way.

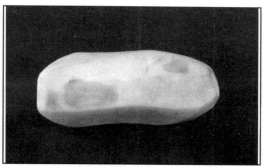

Fig. 50 mold hidden in potatoes

Peel all vegetables and fruit that <u>can</u> be peeled. It is true that the peel contains beneficial nutrients and roughage. But safety is more important. And since you are now returning to an "all natural" diet, your nutrition will already be much better. Peeling lets you see fungus (mold) invasion that is otherwise invisible. The mold in potatoes produces zearalenone. Stick to Red and White varieties that have far less mold.

Lugol's Food Sanitizer

1 drop Lugol's iodine solution
1 quart/L water

Fill sink or bowl with the measured amount of water. Draw a line here, so future treatments do not require measuring the water. Add Lugol's (1 drop per quart). Dip lettuce and spinach so leaves are well wetted for one minute! Rinsing is optional. Do not save the water for later use—it will lose its potency.

Cysteine-Salt Food Sanitizer

$^1/_8$ teaspoon cysteine powder
$^1/_8$ teaspoon salt
1 quart/L water

Stir to dissolve. Immerse produce for five minutes. No need to rinse.

When cysteine-salt is used to sterilize a beverage, such as milk or juice, it soon becomes sulfurous, so use beverage immediately.

HCl Food Sanitizer

1-2 drops per cup water

Agitate food well. Let stand several minutes.

Better Digestion

Cancer patients have been parasitized in the liver. The liver is the seat of digestion. It controls appetite, too. Even though parasites are dead, and heavy metals, solvents and food dyes are gone, a weak digestion is still present. We must select food and a style of cooking that makes digestion easier.

Ascaris parasites block pepsin and acid secretion in the stomach. The stomach may have suffered for years in this way. Although they are gone, we must still focus on food that is kind to the stomach. Taking pills at mealtime is certainly not soothing either. But raw beet juice helps in several ways, besides HCl drops, vinegar, and digestive enzymes.

Raw Beet Cocktail

several medium size red beets
HCl-water
white vinegar

Peel the beets before washing or rinsing them. Avoid getting dirt on the freshly cut surfaces. It does not wash off, nor will the surface allow sterilization. Peel one half first. Then rinse one hand and hold the peeled half. Finish peeling. Drop into HCl-water to sterilize. Remove and cut in quarters. Add an equal volume of water to blend. "Liquefy" in blender for one minute or until smooth. Add half as much vinegar and blend again. Store in refrigerator. Serve 2 tbs. of beet cocktail just before each meal, adding 1 drop HCl.

Variations:
1. Add 1 tsp. sweetening per serving.
2. Add cysteine supplement (it is "covered" by beet flavor and sterilizes at the same time).

Beet Juice

Extracting the juice and discarding the pulp makes a stronger potion for anti-phenol (better digestion) action. If you have extreme pain or very bad digestion, choose beet juice as your cocktail. Peel, wash, and sterilize as before. After juicing add 1 tsp. vinegar per 2 oz. serving, and two drops HCl when served.

Variations: add fruit juice in small amounts; increase vinegar to suit taste; sweeten or spice in other ways.

Complete Nourishment Feeding

When a meal is missed, weight is lost and the body is stressed. If you are a caregiver and your patient is refusing food, and cannot be given IV-feeding for whatever reason, you can make a drinkable "feed" that will protect their life and health temporarily. Coax your patient to try at least one of these meal replacement drinks.

Quick Vanilla Drink

1 egg
1 tbs. coconut oil
1 tbs. sweetening
¼ tsp. vanilla
pinch of vitamin B$_2$
potassium salt to taste
water to make 1 cup total

Quick Almond Drink

1 egg
1 tbs. sweetening
1 tsp. coconut oil
pinch of vitamin B$_2$
potassium salt to taste
almond milk (see Beverages) to make 1 cup total

Blend together, add 4 drops HCl when serving, stir well.

Lemon-oil Drink

Soak one lemon twice in hot water, drying each time; peel thinly; blend it whole, rind, seeds and all. Strain and discard pulp. Add 1 tbs. olive oil and enough honey and water (1½ cup) to make it tasty. Read the label on the lemon-packaging; avoid those that have been sprayed. Ask your grocer if that information is not obvious. Sterilize with 2 drops HCl.

Beverages

Moose Elm Drink

We use this drink to soothe upset stomachs and intestines.

1 tbs. moose elm powder (also called slippery elm)
1 cup water
potassium gluconate or sodium-potassium salt
1 tbs. sweetening
2 drops HCl to sterilize

Variations: use half 'n half instead of water when dairy is permitted.

Make a paste with the herb and 3 tbs. water. Stir paste into remaining water as if making cocoa. Add remaining ingredients. May be drunk hot or cold.

Alginate Intestinal Healer

2 tsp. sodium alginate powder
1 pint water or soup stock
$^1/_8$ tsp. potassium gluconate or sodium-potassium salt
4 drops HCl

Blend all together till smooth and clear. Add HCl in last few seconds.

For intestines that are sore from surgery, blockage, or inflammation this will soothe, as it finds even the narrowest passageway and keeps it open to counteract blockage. The alginate is not meant to be digested; it forms a gelatinous ribbon right through the intestine, giving bulk and absorbing toxins along the way. Consume 1 cup a day in tablespoon amounts that you add to soup, stew, pudding, pie, broth or moose elm drink.

You may combine moose elm and alginate beverages.

Almond Milk

1 cup almonds with brown skins on
Potassium gluconate or sodium-potassium salt

Soak almonds for two days in water, changing the water several times. This loosens the skin. Or pour boiling water over them and let cool. Slip skins off by hand. Blend, adding water to drinkable consistency. Add $^1/_8$ tsp. salt per pint. Sterilize with 4 drops of HCl per cup.

Variations: add vitamin C and sweetening to taste; add half n' half when dairy is allowed. This is very nutritious; helps gain weight.

Melon Lemon

1 peeled lemon (wash twice with hot water first)
1 honeydew melon, peeled and cleaned
sweetening

Blend or juice. Add 2 drops HCl per cup. Variation: use 2 lemons and call it "lemon melon."

Watermelon Banana

One watermelon
6 to 8 bananas soaked twice in hot water for 1 minute and dried before peeling to draw out Fast Green food dye and lanthanide metals.

Peel the watermelon so thickly that only the juicy red part is used. Discard all seeds. Blend and refrigerate. To serve, put one cup back in blender with ½ banana. Add 2 drops HCl per cup when served.

Honeydew Ambrosia

One honeydew melon

Peel honeydew so thickly that only the sweet flesh is used. Discard all seeds. Liquefy in blender or put through juicer. Sterilize with HCl when serving.
  Variation: Add almond milk in equal parts.

Chicken Broth

One whole chicken
½ white onion, peeled apart and soaked in B_2-water
1 bay leaf
5 peppercorns
¼ tsp. pure salt per quart water

Cover chicken with water. When coming to a boil, skim off foam repeatedly. Then add other ingredients. Cook about 2 hours adding water to keep the level up. Or pressure cook 30 minutes. Pour off the broth. Do not throw away the fat. Pack it into a "butter tub" for use in frying.
  The chicken itself makes a meal, but is not yet safe for a cancer patient. It may be cooked a second time, waiting ½ hour to

cool first, or microwaved, preferably in a cooking bag to retain moisture and flavor. Meat should fall apart when done. Finally, add HCl before serving. <u>Turkey</u> and <u>Cornish hen</u> can be similarly prepared.

Coconut Milk

meat from one coconut, carefully washed and brown skin removed
3 cups water

Place chunks in blender to liquefy. Strain. Save pulp for toppings and desserts. Add sweetening to taste and 2 drops HCl per cup when serving to kill bacteria from handling.

Variation: add pineapple juice in equal amounts; add 1 egg, 1 tbs. sweetening, $^1/_{16}$ tsp. salt per cup to make another "feed"; add ½ banana to 1 cup liquid and blend.

Supplement Recipes

Raw Bitters

Especially for liver improvement.

one small handful foraged greens
½ cup water
1 tbs. black cherry concentrate (see *Sources*)
1 pinch vitamin B_2
2 drops HCl to sterilize

To forage greens, you must find an area that is away from traffic; do not forage near a parking lot or street. Get a book from the library to identify edible varieties. Poisonous plants, like mistletoe or jimson weed or morning glory are rare. If you can't find a book, start with dandelion-like plants, thistles of all kinds, lettuce-like and spinach-like plants. Wild mustard is easy to identify, as are common "weeds" like plantain, chicory, shepherds' purse, cheese plant, lambs quarters. Choose the most perfect leaves, near the top, and also the growing tip. Two leaves, a growing tip, and a flower give you four specimens. Five plants give you the handful you need. Sterilize in plastic bowl with Lugol's or HCl-water, stirring well to open any air pockets. Place in blender. Add water. Blend. Add cherry concentrate and B$_2$ and blend again. Add 2 drops HCl and drink at once.

Variations: add a capsule of ginger or turmeric for flavor.

Raw Liver Cocktail

Especially for liver improvement.

¼ slice raw beef liver (about 2" x 2") freshly purchased
$^1/_{16}$ tsp. pure salt

Blend with ½ cup water. Strain. Add 4 drops HCl. Drink at once. Additions:
1. An equal volume of cherry concentrate.
2. 2 tbs. vinegar.
3. 2 drops wintergreen oil.
4. Raw garlic juice.

White Iodine

88 gm potassium iodide, granular

Add potassium iodide to one quart or one liter cold tap water. Potassium iodide dissolves well in water and stays clear; for this reason it is called "white iodine." Label clearly and keep out of reach of children. <u>Do not use if allergic to iodine.</u>

Lugol's Iodine Solution

It is too dangerous to buy a commercially prepared solution for your internal use. It is certain to be polluted with isopropyl alcohol or wood alcohol. Make it yourself or ask your pharmacist to make (not order) it for you. The recipe to make 1 liter (quart) is:

44 gm (1½ ounces) iodine, granular, USP
88 gm (3 ounces) potassium iodide, granular, USP

Dissolve the potassium iodide in about a pint of the water. Then add the iodine crystals and wait till it is all dissolved. This could take a few hours with frequent shaking. Then fill to the liter mark (quart) with water. Keep out of sight and reach of children. Do not use if allergic to iodine. Be careful to avoid bottled water for preparation or you may pollute it yourself with isopropyl alcohol!

Lugol's Iodine Potion

6 drops Lugol's iodine solution
½ glass water

This is specific for *Salmonella* in your body. It can be taken at any time. If taken at end of meals, it helps to sterilize the food just eaten. Do not take with other beverages. Do not take throughout (except in restaurants) or before meals or with vitamins since these will become over oxidized. Do not use daily as a supplement. Keep out of reach of children. If the problem has not cleared up in two days, you are reinfecting.

Vitamin D Drops (professional use only)

1 gram cholecalciferol (see *Sources*)
10 cups olive oil

Mix in a non-metal container. It may take a day of standing to dissolve fully. Refrigerate. Use within a year. Ten drops contain 40,000 IU. This recipe is enough for 50 people for a year, each getting 50 cc. (10 tsp.)! The dosage for adults during dental work or with bone disease is ten drops (no more, no less) daily, placed on tongue or on bread, for 10 days only. After this, use ten drops twice a week only. The 21 Day Program recommends 25,000 U daily, about half this dosage, but twice as long. You can get too much of this; don't exceed dosage.

Bone Healer Tea

Irish moss (*Chondrus crispus*)
Comfrey root (*Symphytum officinale*)
Mullein leaf (*Verbascum thapsus*)
Burdock root (*Arctium lappa*)

Combine herbs in equal amounts. Add one half cup of the combined herbs to three cups of water. Let stand at least three hours or overnight. Bring to a boil. Turn burner down to low; cook for 20 minutes. Strain and let tea cool. Boil again for 5 minutes. Add sweetening and two drops HCl per cup at time of serving. Drink ½ cup with each meal.

Lung Tea

Comfrey root (*Symphytum officinale*)
Mullein leaf (*Verbascum thapsus*)

Combine herbs in equal amounts. Prepare the same way as bone healer herbs. Garlic belongs with this recipe but can be eaten separately: 1 small clove, raw, with each meal.

Shark Cartilage

Recipe #1
1 tbs. shark cartilage
¼ cup cold water
1 capsule fenuthyme
1 tbs. vinegar

Recipe #2
1 tbs. shark cartilage
2 or 3 capsules betaine
¼ cup cold water
½-1 tsp. turmeric
1 tbs. vinegar

Recipe #4
1 tbs. shark cartilage
1 tsp. honey
1 capsule fennel
1 capsule ginger

Recipe #5 (if dairy allowed)
2 tbs. shark cartilage
2 capsules fennel
½ cup buttermilk

Recipe #6 (if dairy allowed)
2 tbs. shark cartilage

Recipe #3
1 tbs. shark cartilage
¼ cup beet juice or puree
1 tbs. vinegar

2 capsules fennel
½ cup milk
1 tsp. vitamin C

Shark cartilage tastes awful to me, so here are six different ways to take it. If you are taking papain, which tastes (actually, smells) even worse, you could combine it also, on the theory that bad tastes neutralize each other!

Shark cartilage should be sterilized to kill bacteria. <u>Add 2 drops of hydrochloric acid to each recipe just before drinking</u>. Stir until smooth. Increase water or vinegar to taste.

Flax Seed

whole flax seed or linseed

Throw away damaged seeds. Rinse 1 tbs. flax seed in HCl-water and drain. Set to soak in fresh HCl-water for 10 minutes or till soft enough to chew. Add to cereal, salad or, later, to cottage cheese.

Back to Dairy Foods—After 21 Days

All dairy foods come from one source—milk. And since milk is contaminated with bacteria and their spores, parasite eggs and stages, and the ubiquitous rabbit fluke, it is understandable that the Syncrometer detects all these in cheese, yogurt, ice cream, etc. Pasteurization kills some, boiling kills more, pressure cooking kills even more, yet the rabbit fluke and *Ascaris* eggs survive. But a few drops of hydrochloric acid kills them. Stir in drops according to the table below, and let stand 2½ minutes or more. It takes this long to kill tapeworm stages.

Dairy Food	5% hydrochloric acid (HCl)
Milk, one cup	2 drops
Buttermilk or yogurt, one cup	4 drops

Melted cheese, half cup	4 drops
Half 'n half, one cup	8 drops
Whipping cream, half cup	6 drops
Cottage cheese, half cup	6 drops, stir well

But this is not all. Dairy foods are polluted with dyes that cause mutations. Fortunately, they can be detoxified by **adding vitamin B$_2$ powder**. A mere pinch is sufficient. This simple treatment does not guarantee that the treated dyes are harmless. For this reason, cancer patients are totally off dairy foods for the first 3 weeks.

Most Kosher dairy products had none of these pollutants or parasites but must be treated like other varieties to avoid all risks.

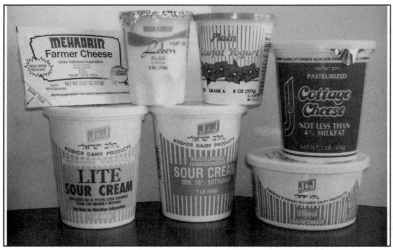

Fig. 51 No azo dyes in <u>these</u> Kosher dairy products

Body Care Recipes

All the commercially produced body care products are contaminated with highly toxic antiseptics. Traces of these, in addition to dyes and silicone, put into or onto the body numerous times a day amounts to a toxic overload for a cancer patient. (They are not good for healthy people, either.) Cancer patients have lost much of their immune power and ability to detoxify foreign substances. These accumulate in the vital organs, as well as the tumors. "Health" or "natural" brands use the same antiseptics!

Take care of your personal needs using <u>only these recipes</u>.

It's very tempting to buy "safe" shampoo or body lotion, especially if the company is listed in *Sources*, or the salesperson "guarantees" it meets my high standards for purity. <u>Do not!</u> No one can check every bottle for every possible pollutant. After your tumors have shrunk you can take these small risks again. For now, avoid them.

Borax Liquid Soap and Shampoo

An empty 1 gallon plastic jug
1/8 cup borax powder
Plastic funnel

Funnel the borax into the jug, fill with <u>very hot</u> tap water. Shake a few times. Let settle. If it is all dissolved, add more borax until there is some left to settle. In a few minutes you can pour off the clear part into dispenser bottles. This is the soap!

Use it for all purposes: laundry (see instructions on box), dishes (use in granular form to scour), dishwasher (2 tsp.), and shampoo.

Shampoo: Borax liquid should feel slippery between your fingers; if it does not the concentration is too low; start over, using a heaping tbs. in a plastic container and enough <u>very hot</u> water to dissolve. To rinse, use <u>citric acid</u> (see *Sources*). Remove traces of benzene (petroleum residue) from citric acid by microwaving the entire box for 1 minute first. Ascorbic acid and lemon juice or vinegar are not strong enough to rinse out borax. Put ¼ teaspoon citric acid in a plastic container like a cottage cheese carton. Add about 1 cup of water to it while under the shower when done shampooing. Leave rinse in hair for one minute while showering your body; then rinse out lightly. After rinsing, your hair should feel silky. If it does not, perhaps you did not use enough citric acid.

Baking Soda Liquid Soap

1 tbs. baking soda (Remove traces of benzene by microwaving a 1-pound box for 1½ minutes.)
1 cup <u>very hot</u> water

Place both in a plastic container and stir with your fingers until dissolved. This is the soap. To <u>shampoo</u> scoop it up over your hair by hand; if you pour it, too much runs off. Rinse very thoroughly with ascorbic acid or other acids. Leave rinse in hair 1 minute. To add sheen to hair, wash a whole lemon twice in hot water; then press lemon against hair.

Hand Sterilizers

Food grade alcohol: make up a 70% solution. Food grade alcohols are grain or cane (ethyl) alcohol. Only the large size Everclear bottle (750 ml or 1 liter) is free of isopropyl or wood alcohol contaminants. Purchase at a liquor store. Next, find a suitable dispenser bottle. Pour 95% grain alcohol (190 proof) to the half-way mark and add half as much water. If using 76% alcohol, use it straight. Use alcohol for general sanitizing purposes and for personal cleanliness. Before leaving bathroom, sterilize hands by pouring a bit in one palm; put finger tips of the other hand in it, scratch to get under the nails, repeat on other hand.

Lugol's iodine solution, one drop in a glass of water. Pour onto napkin and wipe hands to kill surface bacteria. This is easy to do in a restaurant. For deeper sterilization, like if you are going to put your hands in your mouth to floss, put three drops in a glass of water and wash thoroughly. Unless nails are short, though, the hands will still be contaminated and infectious.

General Sterilizers

Use chlorine bleach for the toilet, except with lung cancer. When lung cancer or other lung disease is present, use povidone iodine (available at pharmacies, it doesn't stain).
Use alcohol for the rest of the bathroom, and kitchen area.

Moist Towelettes

Always keep a few in a zippered baggie in your pocket or purse. Cut paper towels in quarters and stack. Place in heavy duty plastic zippered bag. Pour ethyl alcohol or Lugol's sterilizer solution (1 drop per cup) over the towels. Zip shut.

Deodorant

Sweating removes toxins from the body. It should be encouraged. A cancer patient should use no chemicals for any purpose in the armpits (not even baking soda). Simply wash (without soap).

Dental Bleach

The chemical name for bleach is hypochlorite. There are different grades. The grade used for laundry is not good enough for internal use. Purchase "USP", which means food grade. You, or your health food store, will need to order it (see *Sources*). Just because you are using an acceptable grade doesn't mean you can use any quantity you want. Bleach is very powerful stuff. It must be diluted before you can use it without harm. Please follow these directions carefully.

1 tsp. (5 ml) regular bleach, USP grade (5% hypochlorite)
1 pint water (500 ml)

Use a plastic teaspoon to measure and mix. The result is 1/100 as strong, or .05% hypochlorite. This is only a quarter as strong as the .2% solution recommended by Bunyan (page 79), but is strong enough.

Combine in glass pint jar with tight-fitting, non-metal lid. Use a plastic sheet under metal lid or to tighten the fit. KEEP OUT OF REACH OF CHILDREN. You may add a cayenne capsule to make it distasteful and safer from accidental use. **If accidentally swallowed, give milk to drink.**

Make sure you are starting with 5% hypochlorite solution (same as household strength); do not use this recipe if you can not verify this. If you start with some other strength, get an expert, like your pharmacist, to help you make the correct solution.

Flossing Teeth

The purpose of flossing is to open the gum spaces so colloidal silver or other antiseptic can run down them to reach bacteria. Use fishing line (2 to 4 pound test). Rinse under tap. Double it and twist for extra strength. Floss gently, not to cut into the tooth base or cause bleeding. Commercial floss has been soaked in toxic antiseptic; the waxed or flavored kind has been dipped in petroleum products. In an emergency, use strips torn from a shopping bag. Remember to brush after flossing.

Brushing Teeth

Buy a new tooth brush. Wash in borax water first to remove dyes and antiseptic.

Use oregano oil to kill *Clostridium* bacteria, even in crevices. Pour 1 drop in plastic spoon. Barely dip toothbrush into it. (If you use more, it may burn your tongue for hours.)

Colloidal silver is also effective for killing *Clostridium* bacteria but does not penetrate crevices. Buy a colloidal silver maker (see *Sources*). Use 4 or 5 drops on toothbrush.

Hydrogen peroxide, food grade, and plain salt water are also good antiseptics.

Dental bleach is safe for mouth contact. It must not be swallowed. Do not use it daily unless recovering from dental work. It introduces too much chlorine into your body. Keep eyes closed while brushing to avoid spatter.

Cleaning Dentures

Dentures that acquire gray or black discoloration are growing clostridium bacteria! Kill them by brushing with colloidal silver and letting them stand without rinsing until the discoloration is gone.

Or soak in dental bleach overnight.

Denture Adhesive

1 rounded tsp. sodium alginate
1 cup water
5 drops wintergreen
3 drops hydrochloric acid
2 tsp. grain alcohol

Bring water to boil. Add alginate, stirring till all dissolved. To make it thicker, boil longer. Add wintergreen and HCl. After cooling add grain alcohol.

Don't keep partials or dentures in your mouth at night. Sterilize them. Salt water, colloidal silver, or dental bleach are satisfactory. Rotate these for more effectiveness.

Mouthwash

Mouth odor is usually caused by *Clostridium* bacteria! Don't cover this up with mouthwash or fragrances. See a dentist! Search for a hidden infection. After clearing it up, floss and then brush teeth with oregano oil or colloidal silver; they serve as a mouthwash at the same time.

Lip Crayon

Use this to replace "chap sticks" and "vaseline." Pour warmed coconut oil (with vitamin B_2 and 1 drop HCl added) into the caps of ball-point pens. Cover any holes with tape. Stand them upright in holes made by a sharp pencil in a tissue box. After filling, refrigerate. When hard, release them under the hot water tap. Store in closeable baggie in refrigerator. Wrap each in a small piece of paper towel.

Commercial chap sticks, like most cosmetics, contain silicone and acrylic acid, not to mention the antiseptic and petroleum residues.

Suppositories

The coconut oil molded in pen caps can be used as a suppository. If treating hemorrhoids, add one teaspoon brewer's yeast for every ten suppositories.

Skin Lotion

3 tsp. pure cornstarch (see *Sources*)
1 cup water

Boil starch and water until clear, about one minute. Cool. Add a pinch of vitamin B_2 powder. Pour into dispenser bottle. Keep refrigerated.

Shaving Supplies

Switch to an electric shaver to avoid all chemicals.

After Shaves

A quarter teaspoon vitamin C powder dissolved in 1 pint water. Keep refrigerated.

Lipstick

A stick of raw red beet cut like a "French fry" is more convenient and useful than any recipe. Store in plastic bag in refrigerator. Use also on cheeks for rosier complexion.

Black, Red and Brown Henna Hair Dye

Henna is an herb traditionally used for dying hair. You can buy the herb in bulk, or you can purchase the herb pictured, packaged specifically for hair. There are other henna hair dye preparations, often with other added chemicals and dyes, so I can not stress this point enough: use only bulk henna herb (by the pound), or the brand shown!

A young person's hair turns black with this black dye. But older hair turns slate-blue. (To get a brown color, mix red and black henna, using 2 parts red to 5 parts black powder.)

The instructions given with the box work well but take rather long. This recipe is a shortcut. It takes ½ hour (to prepare the dye) plus 50 minutes in contact with hair.

The recipe given is enough for short hair. For medium length, double the quantities. It will not stain the bath tub. After dying is complete, you will need to shampoo it out of your hair, so regular shampooing supplies, either borax plus citric acid or baking soda plus vinegar are also necessary.

½ cup distilled white vinegar
½ cup tap water
7 heaping teaspoons Dalia Black Henna (see *Sources*)

This recipe is very sensitive. The smallest deviation could cause failure of the dye to "take". Please be extra careful to observe details.

Heat water in open, non-metal saucepan until near boiling. Turn off burner. Add vinegar. Allow to cool until just a wisp of steam is still seen coming from the saucepan. Remove 2 tablespoons to a different container, to use later. Then add henna powder. Stir with plastic spoon. It will bubble and rise at first.

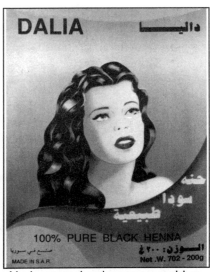

100% PURE BLACK HENNA

MADE IN S.A.R.   Net .W. 702 - 200g

No isopropyl or benzene residue,
nor synthetic dyes or metals.
Comes in red and black.

Fig. 52 safe hair dye

When thoroughly stirred, the consistency should be like thin gravy. If too thick, use up some of the solution set aside or hot water. If too thin, add more powder. Cover and let stand in warm place such as oven or microwave for twenty-five minutes. The dye is being extracted.

Meanwhile, prepare the bathroom. Fold a long piece of paper towel (three sections) in half lengthwise, and then again in half to make a long neck-band. Get ready an 8½ x 11 plastic food storage bag to cover hair later, and two more single paper towels. Set comb and shampoo supplies nearby, also within reach from shower.

After exactly twenty-five minutes, stir the henna one more time. Take the saucepan to the shower and dip the solution over your hair by hand in small amounts. Get all the hair roots wetted before the long hair. Keep it out of your eyes by keeping them closed. Then wash your hands and dry with the single piece of towel. Poke a hole in the end of plastic bag to let it breathe. Then stretch it by pulling it at the rim until it fits over your head. (Practice this beforehand.) Tie the long paper "scarf" around your neck, tucking in the ends. Wipe up drips with the last paper towel. Note the time.

Leave it all intact for fifty minutes to one hour. During this time some dripping must occur. Wear old clothing. If your hand or finger nails have turned slightly bluish or brown after the application you already know the dye will take.

Finally, wash the henna out under the shower until no little particles can be felt on your scalp. Then shampoo and rinse, or merely rinse. Leave rinse in your hair until you finish your shower, at least one minute, this softens and adds gloss to your hair. Then lightly wash out rinse under shower.

After stepping out of the shower, comb hair first—straight back. Dry hair before the rest of your body. Dry by pressing with towel in a straight-back direction about a dozen times. This puts curl in your hair. Never rub hair with towel or change the direction. For extra gloss, rub your hands with a washed lemon; then pat hair with hands in same direction. Let air dry, or sun dry, or hang hair over an electric radiator. Keep warm.

Follow the recipe exactly. If the water for dye extraction is too hot or too cold, it will not work. If the time for extraction is too short or too long, the product changes. If the mixture is too thin it will run off your hair. If it is too thick it will spatter without good contact. But the time to leave it on your hair can be made longer—and probably helps it darken. Don't give up until you have tried several times.

Experiment using other combinations of dyes and other kinds of herbs. Keep notes. Please contribute your tips to the publisher!

Eyebrow Color

1 capsule freeze-dried green black walnut hull
2 drops Lugol's iodine
¼ tsp. Everclear alcohol (in 750 ml or 1 L size bottle)

Dissolve all in a plastic spoon. Apply carefully. Keep eyes closed. Do not apply dye of any kind to eyelids or eyelashes.

Recipes for Household Products

Carpet Cleaner

Whether you rent a machine or have a cleaning service, don't use the carpet shampoo they want to sell, even if they "guarantee" that it is all natural and safe. Instead add these to a bucket (about four gallons) of water and use it as the cleaning solution:

Wash water
1/3 cup borax

Rinse water
¼ cup grain alcohol
2 tsp. boric acid (see *Sources*)
¼ cup white distilled vinegar or 4 tsp. citric acid
1 bottle povidone iodine (optional)

Borax does the cleaning; alcohol disinfects, boric acid leaves a pesticide residue, and the vinegar or citric acid give luster. Povidone iodine kills parasite eggs. If you are just making one pass on your carpet, use the borax, alcohol, boric acid, and iodine. Remember to test everything you use on an unnoticed piece of carpet first.

Health Improvement Recipes

One of the most important items is **black walnut hull tincture** extra strength. Although I included this recipe in every other book I wrote, I am not including it here because usually an advanced cancer sufferer can not wait until the black walnut trees are in season. I suggest you purchase it immediately, but only from the sources listed. The tincture must be greenish to be useful (and, of course, free from pollutants).

Bowel Program

Bacteria are always at the root of bowel problems, such as pain, bloating and gassiness. They can not be killed by zapping, because the high frequency current does not penetrate the bowel contents.

Although most bowel bacteria are beneficial, the ones that are not, like salmonellas, shigellas, and clostridiums are extremely harmful because they have the ability to invade the rest of your body and colonize a trauma site or tumorous organ. This will prevent tumor shrinking after the malignancy is stopped.

One reason bowel bacteria are so hard to eradicate is that we are constantly reinfecting ourselves by keeping a supply on our hands and under our fingernails.

- So the first thing to do is **improve sanitation**. Use 70% grain alcohol in a spray bottle at the bathroom sink. Or Lugol's iodine, one drop per cup water. Sterilize your hands after bathroom use and before meals.
- Second, take **Lugol's** solution, 6 drops in ½ cup water 4 times a day. This is specifically for *Salmonella*.
- Third, use **turmeric** (2 capsules 3 times a day). This is the common spice, which I find helps against *Shigella*, as well as *E. coli*. Expect orange colored stool. Increase to 6 capsules (1 tsp.) 3 times a day for serious problems.
- Fourth, use **fennel** (same dosage as for turmeric).
- Fifth, take **hydrochloric acid** (5%). Put 10 drops in a glass of water. Drink between or with meals. ONLY ONCE A DAY. This restores natural pH to the whole intestine.
- Sixth, use **oregano oil** (*Oreganum vulgare*), 10 drops in an empty capsule. If spilled on sides, wash capsule before swallowing. Eat bread with it if stomach is sensitive. Take 3 times a day.
- Seventh, if you are constipated, take **Cascara sagrada,** an herb; Start with one capsule a day, use up to maximum on label. Take **extra magnesium** (300 mg magnesium oxide, 2 or 3 a day), and drink **a cup of hot water** upon rising in the morning. This will begin to regulate your elimination.

With this powerful approach, even a bad bacterial problem should clear up in two days. If it doesn't, you are reinfecting. Throw out all the food in your refrigerator. It has been touched by hands. Keep your own hands sanitary. Eat only sterilized food. Keep fingernails short. Do not put fingers in mouth. Your tummy <u>can</u> feel flat, without gurgling, and your mood <u>can</u> be good. Remember, cancer is <u>not</u> the cause of your bowel problems.

But it may take all the remedies listed. Afterward, you must continue to eat only sterilized food, until your natural immune power is restored.

Enemas

If you should fail to have a bowel movement in a <u>single</u> day it is a serious matter. An ill person cannot afford to fill up further with the ammonia, and toxic amines that bowel bacteria produce. But the purpose is even greater: to eliminate parasites, and toxins drained from your tumors. Fortunately, enemas are very easy to do. Do an enema before going to bed.

There are several kinds of enema equipment available in pharmacies; most important is NEVER to use anyone else's equipment, no matter how "sterilized" it is guaranteed to be. Get your own. Do not use the equipment used by a professional bowel-cleanser. It is impossible to completely avoid cross-contamination. You must completely avoid it.

A Fleet™ bottle, obtained at your local pharmacy, will do for a start (other equipment, like shown below, is available, see *Sources*). This is a squeeze bottle with a plastic applicator for insertion. Dump the contents since you are unable to test it for toxins. Refill with <u>very warm</u> tap water. Water that is too cool causes cramping and inability to hold it.

The lubricant can be made in 5 minutes.

4 level tsp. cornstarch
1 cup water
1 pinch vitamin B_2 (to detoxify possible benzene)

Bring this to a boil and cook for about one minute. Set in the refrigerator to cool quickly. Pour a tsp. or more on top of a plastic bag for convenience in use. The only other lubricants are olive oil and coconut oil, also treated with vitamin B_2 and a drop of Lugol's or HCl to sterilize.

For many of us, the rectum has ballooned out into a pocket due to past times of constipation. This is called a *diverticulum*. It is just a few inches from the anus so it is quite accessible by enema.

The diverticulum walls are weak due to constant over-stretching. But in just a few weeks of daily cleansing, the pocket will shrink and may even disappear. As soon as the 21 Day Program is completed and if natural evacuation is possible, stop taking enemas: Hemorrhoids can be made worse by them.

To avoid hemorrhoids, do not strain and always cleanse your bottom with wet paper, not dry paper. Wet a bolus of paper with hot water. Apply a dab of cornstarch lubricant before wiping. Wipe at least 6 times. At last wipe, push hemorrhoid back inside. If hemorrhoid is large, use a gloved finger (cut fingers off thin plastic gloves; wear one at a time on middle finger, lubricate with cornstarch; push hemorrhoid as far in as possible). If hemorrhoids are internal, use suppositories (page 550). **To relieve pain apply honey.**

Lugol's Enema

(Not for persons who are allergic to iodine.) Add ½ tsp. of Lugol's iodine to 1 pint of very warm water; pour into cup-size Fleet™ bottle (giving yourself 2 doses), or enema apparatus. Administer enema slowly and hold internally as long as possible.

Black Walnut Hull Extra Strength Enema

Add 1 tsp. of green black walnut hull extra strength tincture to 1 pint very warm water. Repeat as above.

Plain Enema

If you have none of the other solutions available, use plain salt water, 1 tsp. per quart. In the absence of salt, use plain water. Remember, you must move your bowels or cleanse at least once a day.

Coffee Enema

Although this has profound effects that are beneficial, you must take special precautions due to asbestos pollution of all coffees tested. They also contain *Ascaris* eggs and Sorghum mold (the variety that causes purpura and strokes). Use 4 heaping tbs. regular coffee in 1 quart/L water, boil 3 minutes. Let cool 10 minutes. Then bring back to boil 5 more minutes. Filter through a double (Mr. Coffee) filter to remove asbestos. Sterilize with 1 drop Lugol's per cup. This also destroys mold. Especially useful to reduce pain. Kills *Ascaris* stages all over body; stimulates bile production.

Giving Yourself The Perfect Enema

Any drop you spill and everything you use to do the enema will <u>somehow</u> contaminate your bathroom. Yet you must leave it all perfectly sanitary for your own protection. So follow these instructions carefully.

Spread a large plastic trash bag on the bathroom floor. Place a plastic shopping bag beside it and a paper plate on it. Set a chair nearby, too. The trash bag is for you to lie on. Lie on your back if you have nobody to help you.

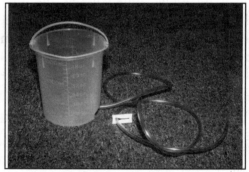

Fig. 53 Enema container, tube, pinchcock

Instructions on commercially available enema bottles advise you to be on your knees. This may be workable for the small squeeze-bottle of ready-made solution you can purchase. Other instructions tell you to lie on your side. It is quite impossible, though, if you are elderly, have painful knees or are simply ill and must try to take in a whole pint.

Test the apparatus first, in the bathroom sink to see how it works. Wipe away the grease that comes with it on the applicator; it is sure to be a petroleum product and be tainted with benzene.

Pour a tablespoon of oil onto the paper plate for the lubricant (sterilized with 1 drop HCl per cup).

After filling the container with the enema solution, run some through the tubing until the air is out of it and close the pinchcock. Place it on the shopping bag.

Insert the applicator tube as far as you comfortably can. Then lift the container with one hand while opening the valve with the other. The higher you lift it, the faster it runs. Take as much time as you need to run it in. You may wish to set the container on the chair. Very warm liquid is easier to hold. Don't force yourself to hold it all. At any time you may close the valve, withdraw the applicator, and place it on the shopping bag.

Cleaning up the apparatus, the bathroom, and yourself: This topic is seldom discussed, but very important. Notice that some bowel contents have entered the container by reflux action, which is unavoidable. Consider the whole apparatus contaminated. For this reason you must never, never use anybody else's apparatus, no matter how clean it looks.

First, wipe the applicator tube. Then fill the container and run it through the hose into the toilet. Repeat until it appears clean; this is appearance only; you must now sterilize it. Fill it with water and add Lugol's iodine or povidone iodine until intensely red in color. Place the end of the tube in the container to soak. Empty and wipe the outside of the tube with paper. Empty container. Do not dry the container. Store in a fresh plastic bag. Throw away the trash bag, shopping bag and paper plate. Clean the sink with straight alcohol or Lugol's. Then wash your hands with skin sanitizer. Be sure to include fingernails.

If all went well, you may risk taking the next enema on your bed. If not, take a shower and stick to the floor location.

Kidney Cleanse

It takes a lot of liquid to "wash" the inside of your body. Taking it in the form of herbal teas gives you extra benefits. And extra enjoyment if you learn to make them with variations—especially if you need to produce a gallon of urine a day!

Any edema or "water holding", whether in lungs, arms, or abdomen, also requires strengthening of kidneys with this recipe.

When kidneys or bladder are actually involved in the cancer, gradually increase the dose to <u>double</u> the regular amounts. Be sure to <u>start</u> just as slowly though to avoid feeling pressure in the bladder. You will need:

½ cup dried hydrangea root (*Hydrangea arborescens*)
½ cup gravel root (*Eupatorium purpureum*)
½ cup marshmallow root (*Althea officinallis*)
Black Cherry Concentrate, 8 oz
Pinch vitamin B_2 powder
4 bunches of fresh parsley (obtained at supermarket)
Goldenrod tincture (leave out of the recipe if you are allergic to it)
Ginger
Uva Ursi
Vitamin B_6, 250 mg
Magnesium oxide, 300 mg
HCl drops
Sweetening (optional)

Previous versions of this recipe included vegetable glycerin. Recently I have been unable to find a source free from asbestos and silicone. Omit it.

Measure ¼ cup of each root and set them to soak, together in 10 cups of cold tap water, using a non-metal container and a non-metal lid (a dinner plate will do). Add vitamin B_2 powder. After four hours (or overnight), heat to boiling and simmer for 20 minutes. Add black cherry concentrate and bring back to boiling. Pour through a bamboo or plastic strainer into glass jars. Drink ¾ cup by sipping slowly throughout the day (stir in two drops HCl first). Refrigerate half to use this week, and freeze the other half for next week.

Other versions of this recipe allowed reboiling the roots when your have finished your first batch. Although this saves a few dollars, advanced cancer sufferers should use new roots each time. You need to do the kidney cleanse for six weeks to get good results, longer for severe problems.

Find fresh parsley at a grocery store. Soak it in HCl-water (1 drop per cup) with a pinch of vitamin B_2 in it for 2 minutes. Drain. Cover with water and boil for 1 minute. Drain into glass jars. When cool enough, pour yourself ½ cup. Add 2 drops HCl. Sip slowly or add to your root potion. Refrigerate a pint and freeze 1 pint. Throw away the parsley. Always add HCl at point of consuming even after pre-sterilizing.

Dose: each morning, pour together ¾ cup of the root mixture and ½ cup parsley water, filling a large mug. Add 20 drops of goldenrod tincture and any spice, such as nutmeg, cinnamon, etc. Then add a pinch of B_2 and 4 drops HCl to sterilize. Drink this mixture in divided doses throughout the day. Keep it cold. Do not drink it all at once or you will get a stomach ache and feel pressure in your bladder. If your stomach is very sensitive, start on half this dose.

Also take:

- Ginger capsules: one with each meal (3/day).
- Uva Ursi. $^1/_8$ tsp. (one capsule worth) in the morning, and ¼ tsp. (two capsules worth) in the evening.
- Vitamin B_6 (250 mg): one a day.
- Magnesium oxide (300 mg): one a day.

Take these supplements just before your meal to avoid burping. You do not need to duplicate the B_6 and magnesium doses if you are already on them.

Some notes on this recipe: this herbal tea, as well as the parsley, can easily spoil. Reheat to boiling every third day if it is being stored in the refrigerator. Add HCl drops just before drinking. If you sterilize it in the morning you may take it to work without refrigerating it (use a glass container).

When you order your herbs, be careful! Herb companies are not the same! These roots should have a strong fragrance. If the ones you buy are barely fragrant, they have lost their active ingredients; switch to a different supplier. Fresh roots can be used. Do not use powder.

Liver Herbs

Don't confuse these liver herbs with the next recipe for the Liver Cleanse. This recipe contains herbs traditionally used to help the liver function, while the Liver Cleanse gets gallstones out.

6 parts comfrey root, *Symphytum officinale* (also called nipbone root)
6 parts tanner's oak bark, *Quercus alba* (white oak bark)
3 parts Jacob's staff, *Verbascum thapsus* (mullein herb)
2 parts licorice root, *Glycyrrhiza glabra*
2 parts wild yam root, *Dioscorea villosa*
2 parts milk thistle herb, *Silybum marianum*
1 part lobelia plant, *Lobelia inflata* (bladder pod)
1 part skullcap, *Scutellaria lateriflora* (helmet flower)

Mix all the herbs. Add 1 cup of the mixture to 2 quarts of water. Bring to a boil. Put lid on. Let sit for six hours or overnight. Bring to a rolling boil. Strain and add sweetening. Also add a spice to your liking. Sterilize with HCl. Drink two cups a day for six to eight weeks. Put the strained herbs in the freezer and use them one more time.

Liver Cleanse

Cleansing the liver of gallstones dramatically improves digestion, which is the basis of your whole health. You can expect your allergies to disappear, too, more with each cleanse you do! Incredibly, it also eliminates shoulder, upper arm, and upper back pain. You have more energy and an increased sense of well being.

Cleaning the liver bile ducts is the most powerful procedure that you can do to improve your body's health.

But it <u>should not</u> be done before the parasite program, and for <u>best results</u> should follow the kidney cleanse.

It is the job of the liver to make bile, 1 to 1½ quarts in a day! The liver is full of tubes (*biliary tubing*) that deliver the bile to one large tube (the *common bile duct*). The gallbladder is attached to the common bile duct and acts as a storage reservoir. Eating fat or protein triggers the gallbladder to squeeze itself empty after about twenty minutes, and the stored bile finishes its trip down the common bile duct to the intestine.

<u>For many persons, including children, the biliary tubing is choked with gallstones</u>. Some develop allergies or hives but some have no symptoms. When the gallbladder is scanned or X-rayed nothing is seen. Typically, they are not in the gallbladder. Not only that, most are too small and not calcified, a prerequisite for visibility on X-ray. There are over half a dozen varieties of gallstones, most of which have cholesterol crystals in them. They can be black, red, white, green or tan colored. The green ones get their color from being coated with bile. Notice in the picture how many have imbedded unidentified objects. Are they fluke remains? Notice how many are shaped like corks with longitudinal grooves below the tops. We can visualize the blocked bile ducts from such shapes. Other stones are composites–made of many smaller ones–showing that they regrouped in the bile ducts some time after the last cleanse.

At the very center of each stone is found a clump of bacteria, according to scientists, suggesting that a dead bit of parasite might have started the stone forming.

As the stones grow and become more numerous the back pressure on the liver causes it to make less bile. It is also thought to slow the flow of lymphatic fluid. Imagine the situation if your garden hose had marbles in it. Much less water would flow, which in turn would decrease the ability of the hose

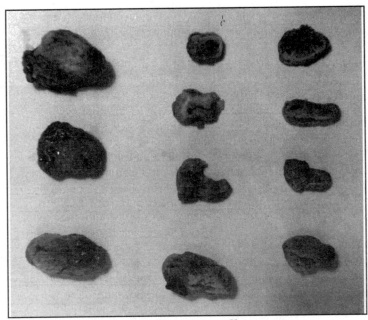

Fig. 54 These are gallstones.

to squirt out the marbles. <u>With gallstones, much less cholesterol leaves the body, and cholesterol levels may rise.</u>

Gallstones, being porous, can pick up all the bacteria, cysts, viruses and parasites that are passing through the liver. In this way "nests" of infection are formed, forever supplying the body with fresh bacteria and parasite stages. No stomach infection such as ulcers or intestinal bloating can be cured permanently without removing these gallstones from the liver.

For best results, <u>ozonate</u> the olive oil in this recipe to kill any parasite stages or viruses that may be released during the cleanse.

Preparation

- You can't clean a liver with living parasites in it. You won't get many stones, and you will feel quite sick. <u>Zap daily the week before, or complete the parasite killing program before attempting a liver cleanse.</u> If you are on the maintenance parasite program, you are always ready to do the cleanse.

- Completing the kidney cleanse before cleansing the liver is also <u>highly recommended</u>. You want your kidneys, bladder and urinary tract in top working condition so they can efficiently remove any undesirable substances incidentally absorbed from the intestine as the bile is being excreted.

Ingredients

Epsom salts	4 tablespoons
Olive oil	half cup (light olive oil is easier to get down), and for best results, ozonate it for 20 minutes. Add 2 drops HCl.
Fresh pink grapefruit	1 large or 2 small, enough to squeeze 2/3 cup juice. Hot wash twice first and dry each time.
Ornithine	4 to 8, to be sure you can sleep. Don't skip this or you may have the worst night of your life!
Large plastic straw	To help drink potion.
Pint jar with lid	
Black Walnut Tincture, any strength.	10 to 20 drops, to kill parasites coming from the liver.

Choose a day like Saturday for the cleanse, since you will be able to rest the next day.

Take <u>no</u> medicines, vitamins or pills that you can do without; they could prevent success. Stop the parasite program and kidney herbs, too, the day before.

Eat a <u>no-fat</u> breakfast and lunch such as cooked cereal, fruit, fruit juice, bread and preserves or honey (no butter or milk). This allows the bile to build up and develop pressure in the liver. Higher pressure pushes out more stones.

2:00 PM. <u>Do not eat or drink after 2 o'clock.</u> If you break this rule you could feel quite ill later.

Get your Epsom salts ready. Mix 4 tbs. in 3 cups water and pour this into a jar. This makes four servings, ¾ cup each. Set the jar in the refrigerator to get ice cold (this is for convenience and taste only).

6:00 PM. Drink one serving (¾ cup) of the ice cold Epsom salts. If you did not prepare this ahead of time, mix 1 tbs. in ¾ cup water now. You may add 1/8 tsp. vitamin C powder to improve the taste. You may also drink a few mouthfuls of water afterwards or rinse your mouth.

Get the olive oil (ozonated, if possible) and grapefruit out to warm up.

8:00 PM. Repeat by drinking another ¾ cup of Epsom salts.

You haven't eaten since two o'clock, but you won't feel hungry. Get your bedtime chores done. The timing is critical for success.

9:45 PM. Pour ½ cup (measured) olive oil into the pint jar. Add 2 drops HCl to sterilize. Wash grapefruit twice in hot water and dry; squeeze by hand into the measuring cup. Remove pulp with fork. You should have at least ½ cup, more (up to ¾ cup) is best. You may use part lemonade. Add this to the olive oil. Also add Black Walnut Tincture. Close the jar tightly with the lid and shake hard until watery (only fresh grapefruit juice does this).

Now visit the bathroom one or more times, even if it makes you late for your ten o'clock drink. Don't be more than 15 minutes late. You will get fewer stones.

10:00 PM. Drink the potion you have mixed. Take 4 ornithine capsules with the first sips to make sure you will sleep through the night. Take 8 if you already suffer from insomnia. Drinking through a large plastic straw helps it go down easier. You may use oil and vinegar salad dressing, or straight honey to chase it down between sips. Have these ready in a tablespoon on the kitchen counter. Take it all to your bedside if you want, but drink it standing up. Get it down within 5 minutes (fifteen minutes for very elderly or weak persons).

Lie down immediately. You might fail to get stones out if you don't. The sooner you lie down the more stones you will get out. Be ready for bed ahead of time. Don't clean up the kitchen. As soon as the drink is down walk to your bed and lie down flat on your back with your head up high on the pillow. Try to think about what is happening in the liver. Try to keep perfectly still for at least 20 minutes. You may feel a train of stones traveling along the bile ducts like marbles. There is no pain because the bile duct valves are open (thank you Epsom salts!). **Go to sleep**, you may fail to get stones out if you don't.

Next morning. Upon awakening take your third dose of Epsom salts. If you have indigestion or nausea wait until it is gone before drinking the Epsom salts. You may go back to bed. Don't take this potion before 6:00 am.

2 Hours Later. Take your fourth (the last) dose of Epsom salts. You may go back to bed again.

After 2 More Hours you may eat. Start with fruit juice. Half an hour later eat fruit. One hour later you may eat regular food but keep it light. By supper you should feel recovered.

How well did you do? Expect diarrhea in the morning. Use a flashlight to look for gallstones in the toilet with the bowel movement. Look for the green kind since this is proof that they are genuine gallstones, not food residue. Only bile from the liver is pea green. The bowel movement sinks but gallstones float because of the cholesterol inside. Count them all roughly, whether tan or green. You will need to total 2000 stones before the liver is clean enough to rid you of allergies or bursitis or upper back pains permanently. The first cleanse may rid you of them for a few days, but as the stones from the rear travel forward, they give you the same symptoms again. You may repeat cleanses at two week intervals. Never cleanse when you are ill.

Sometimes the bile ducts are full of cholesterol crystals that did not form into round stones. They appear as a "chaff" floating on top of the toilet bowl water. It may be tan colored, harboring millions of tiny white crystals. Cleansing this chaff is just as important as purging stones.

How safe is the liver cleanse? It is very safe. My opinion is based on over 500 cases, including many persons in their seventies and eighties. None went to the hospital; none even reported pain. However it can make you feel quite ill for one or two days afterwards, although in every one of these cases the maintenance parasite program had been neglected. This is why the instructions direct you to complete the parasite and kidney cleanse programs first.

CONGRATULATIONS

You have taken out your gallstones <u>without surgery</u>! I like to think I have perfected this recipe, but I certainly can not take credit for its origin. It was invented hundreds, if not thousands, of years ago, THANK YOU, HERBALISTS!

This procedure contradicts many modern medical viewpoints. Gallstones are thought to be formed in the gallbladder, not the liver. They are thought to be few, not thousands. They are not linked to pains other than gallbladder attacks. It is easy to understand why this is thought: by the time you have acute pain attacks, some stones <u>are</u> in the gallbladder, <u>are</u> big enough and sufficiently calcified to see on X-ray, and <u>have</u> caused inflammation there. When the gallbladder is removed the acute attacks are gone, but the bursitis and other pains and digestive problems remain.

The truth is self-evident. People who have had their gallbladder surgically removed still get plenty of green, bile-coated stones, and anyone who cares to dissect their stones can see that the concentric circles and crystals of cholesterol match textbook pictures of "gallstones" exactly.

Freon Removal Program

Freon accumulates in the diaphragm and skin in healthy persons. In sick persons the Syncrometer detects it in the weakened organ. Freon in your body can be ozonated to render it capable of detoxification. One to three glasses a day of ozonated water mobilizes it toward the liver.

- 1-3 glasses ozonated water. Ozonate water about 5 minutes. Make sure the tip of ozonator tube is sterile by dipping in HCl-water or Lugol's-water.
- 1-3 cups liver herb tea. Drink one cup tea for each glass of ozonated water drunk. This helps the liver detoxify the freon so it can move toward the kidney.
- Kidney herbs, 1¼ cups daily. This helps the kidneys pull it into the bladder for excretion.

It takes about 6 weeks to remove freon from your body. Be sure to get a freon-free refrigerator before you begin.

Amino Acid Mixture

Essential Amino Acids
1 part isoleucine
1 part leucine
1 part lysine
1 part valine
1 part methionine
½ part phenyl alanine
½ part threonine
½ part tyrosine
½ part cysteine
⅓ part arginine
⅓ part histidine

Non-essential Amino Acids
1 part glycine
1 part taurine
1 part glutamic acid
1 part alanine
½ part aspartic acid
½ part ornithine
½ part proline
½ part serine

Note that tryptophane is missing in the recipe. That is because it is not generally available. Note also that arginine and cysteine are in very small amounts. It is assumed that you will be taking much larger amounts of these, separately, and thus avoid crowding out the remainder in this combination recipe.

Mix them all together (or as many as you can find) and take them in teaspoon amounts with meals or as described in the 21 Day Program. Don't let the name fool you: the "non-essential" ones are necessary, too!

Ferritin Fighter

When white blood cells contain asbestos, they become coated on the <u>outside</u> with ferritin. This ruins their immune function. Their outside surface has <u>receptor sites</u> that must be able to "see" and "feel" enemies of your body. Removing this ferritin restores their immune functions. The drug Levamisole (available in Mexico) can do this (50 mg, take 3 a day), but here is an over the counter recipe that works also.

1 tsp. bromelain (3000 mg) 600 GDU/gm, or papain
½ tsp. methyl sulfonyl methane (MSM)
½ tsp. powdered hydrangea
1 capsule fennel for flavoring
½ cup water, milk, or buttermilk
2 drops hydrochloric acid to sterilize

Mix everything together and drink. Take this dose 3 times a day. For convenience, you can mix larger quantities of the dry ingredients ahead of time (this reduces the odor). Cut dosage in half after a week. Do not take with meals to avoid consuming enzymes with food. Continue for a month.

The bromelain or papain will digest the ferritin off your white blood cells, enabling them to remove asbestos, dyes, bacteria, and plastics from your tissues again. But ferritin will return to coat your white blood cells if you continue your exposure to asbestos. The MSM is a strong reducing agent, returning ferric to ferrous iron. The powdered hydrangea is a source of organic germanium to replace that lost by oxidation. Combining them is for convenience only.

In advanced cancer use bromelain <u>plus</u> papain <u>plus</u> Levamisole for <u>two</u> weeks, before reducing dosage.

Benzoquinone (BQ) (for clinical use only)

500 mg benzoquinone powder (not hydroquinone). (One size 00 capsule filled with powder, by hand.)
500 ml (1 pint) cold tap water that has been run for a full minute. Such water is safer than the regular water "for injection" since water for injection often has antiseptic contamination.

This should be made and supervised by a physician. Empty the BQ capsule into water, stirring with a plastic spoon until completely dissolved (about one minute). Further dilute this as follows: ½ ml BQ solution as prepared above is added to a second pint of water. All quantities can be approximated, since the final concentration should be one part per million but need not be exact. After the second dilution, the BQ solution must be used within 20 minutes. If there is further delay, the solution must be made up from the powder again. A dose of one cc (2 cc for persons over 100 lb.) is given in the muscle (IM) in the hip after cleaning skin with ethyl alcohol. This is 1 mcg. Give the shot slowly to reduce burning. Patients may exclaim over their improvement by the time the needle is out.

The BQ solution is thrown out when it is twenty minutes old. All containers are new glassware and to be used only for this purpose. Before use, it is rinsed with tap water to remove any adhering antiseptic. It is only rinsed and drained—never chemically cleaned.

Castor Oil Pack

This can be used to give pain relief on any area. It can also be placed over large lumps in the abdomen to speed shrinkage. It is actually an immune stimulant of ancient renown. Use for three days in a row; then rest for four days and repeat as needed.

white flannel cloth or soft cotton (cheese cloth will do)
plastic sheet
hot water bottle
bath towel
two safety pins (optional)

Protect bedding with plastic sheet (such as large trash bag). Prepare cloth by washing in borax and drying before first use. For abdominal application, it should be ¼" thick when folded and measure about 10 inches wide by 14 inches long. For smaller areas, fold this over.

Put a small plastic sheet under cloth and pour castor oil onto the cloth. Make sure the cloth is well saturated. It should be wet but not drippy.

Lie down and apply the cloth to the abdomen or other area being treated. Place the small plastic sheet over the soaked flannel cloth. On top of that, place a hot water bottle. Wrap a towel, folded lengthwise, around the entire area. You may fasten it with safety pins.

The pack should remain on the treated area between one to two hours.

You may clean your abdomen afterwards, by using one quart of water mixed with 4 tbs. baking soda (pure variety only, or microwave to remove benzene).

Keep the flannel pack in a resealable plastic bag for your future use.

Topical Tumor Shrinker

Use this <u>at the same time</u> as the 21 Day Program.

For Skin Growths
1 drop vitamin A (retinyl acetate or palmitate) 50,000 U
1 drop wintergreen oil (not synthetic, not distilled)
1 drop DMSO, a penetrant
1 pinch freeze dried green black walnut hull powder
1 pinch vitamin B_2 powder

Stir all together with plastic knife. Scoop up with your fingers onto skin growths. Immediately tape over with masking tape or cellophane tape to make a tight seal to skin. Leave undisturbed for three days. If edges fray, add more tape. Leave in place during showers. Do not use soap, except borax, on your skin. Do not use cosmetics, except homemade. Do not use lotions or oils intended to soften or lubricate skin.

Renew the application after three days. At the same time, take 1 to 3 drops vitamin A (50,000 U per drop) by mouth daily.

High doses of vitamin A are necessary to dissolve the growths. The neighboring area may become red with a burning sensation; also, the outer layers of skin may rub or peel off. This is exactly the effect desired for your skin cancers. But you may slow down the action by treating less often if desired.

Caution: continuous use of this dosage of vitamin A will cause hypervitaminosis A (rash, headache, redness, itching, flaky skin). Weigh this disadvantage against any gains you are seeing. One method might be after six days, rest for six days to let symptoms abate, then repeat.

For tumors under the skin but close enough to the surface to be felt, like breast or armpit lumps, you still have a good chance to reach them with this topical tumor shrinker. You will need to make a larger batch.

Apply the mixture to the skin surface with your finger. Tape over tightly and securely. Use an ACE bandage or athletic bra to keep it in place. Do not wear a regular bra or tight clothing over it. For larger areas, use:

1 tsp. vitamin A (1.5 M U/gm)
1 tsp. DMSO
1 tsp. wintergreen oil
1 capsule vitamin B_2 (300 mg)
1 capsule freeze dried green black walnut hull (see *Sources*)

Place all ingredients in a small glass jar, shake or stir with finger. After applying, place a plastic sheet over the area and tape down securely at edges (the corner of a plastic bag is suitable for the breast). Do not remove to shower. After three days, peel open at top edge to add more salve or replace entirely.

Read caution above regarding hypervitaminosis A.

For Oozing Tumors

When skin is broken, there is danger of infection. You may use Lugol's iodine or dental bleach to disinfect. Other disinfectants are not strong enough. Use a square of toilet paper. Place over oozing area. Drip Lugol's iodine, drop by drop, onto the paper till completely coated. You may also use diluted dental bleach (1 part dental bleach to 10 parts water) and apply. Then drip oregano oil over the paper, drop by drop, till wetted again. Expect some burning. Test your skin surface first with both types of application to see if they are tolerable. Leave treated wound uncovered by clothing. The paper will keep it dry, draining and aerated.

Heat, namely, a hot water bottle in the armpit and on the breast, is healing, in a similar way to Dental Aftercare. Tumors can be "drawn" to the surface, which is a much better place to drain them than internally. The heat also brings in arterial blood with greater immune power. But when oozing through the skin has begun, the area should be kept dry to assist healing.

If tumors that are treated topically do not shrink, but grow larger instead, you are continuing to infect with food borne parasites and bacteria, and to take in toxins such as asbestos, isopropyl alcohol, and benzene. There are no exceptions. You must search for a source of these in food and dentalware. **Be sure to consult a physician.**

Curing Dentures

Various kinds of dentures, including colored, can be hardened using this recipe. This means they will not seep to a detectable level, releasing acrylic acid, urethane, bisphenol, metals or dyes. This was tested with a Syncrometer by soaking dentures of various kinds and colors in water for many hours and sampling the soak-water. Since you will not be able to test, I recommend repeating this denture-cure three times.

Denture Hardening

candy thermometer or other easy to read thermometer

small metal sauce pan, teflon coated is okay.

Practice run: find the 150° and 160° F marks on the thermometer. Fill saucepan 1 to 2 inches with cold tap water. Place on burner set at lowest heat. Place thermometer in water, being careful that it could not accidentally tip out and fall on burner.

Note the time. Check the temperature of the water every few minutes. It should reach 150° F in 20 minutes, <u>not sooner</u>. If it went too fast, throw out the water, set burner lower and start over. When the right speed of heating is reached, you are ready to cure your denture.

Place denture in saucepan, add cold water from tap to previous level. They should be well covered. Heat as before.

When 150° F is reached, turn burner off, leave denture in water for another 10 minutes; water temperature should eventually reach 160° F.

Pour off water and cover denture with fresh cold water. Rinse. Denture is ready.

Note:

1. If something went wrong during your first try, simply repeat the whole procedure.
2. Your mouth should have no reaction, no redness, no burning, no odd symptoms from wearing your dentures. If symptoms occur, repeat the hardening recipe.

Syncrometer Biochemistry

It is invitingly simple to study your body's manufacturing processes, called **metabolism**, using the Syncrometer.® You merely need to purchase the smallest amounts available of the chemicals you wish to study.

If you already know the main metabolic pathways, you could study glycolysis, the pentose phosphate shunt, and the Krebs cycle, as well as fat formation and amino acid interconversions.

Even without this background knowledge you could study basic processes such as the appearance (resonance) and disappearance (no resonance) of vitamins or amino acids or waste products in your organs.

You will be able to find metabolic blocks or missing enzymes in hours, not years as in regular biochemistry. I routinely find such blocks in the presence of a particular parasite or toxin.

For example, if you have retinal disease and find a toxin or parasite specifically in your retina, you could be quickly led to a plan of action. If you found *Toxoplasma* in your retina you could learn about this pathogen off the Internet or a biology book. Finding that it comes from cats, you would test your house dust for its presence, next. If this were positive you might give your cat away, dispose of the litter box, replace carpets, and thoroughly clean the house. This would at least halt ongoing reinfection. Or perhaps you could find a breed of cat that did not have it!

Since *Toxoplasma* is shed in dog and cat feces, you might further search in ordinary garden soil. If present, you might suspect raw vegetables as another source since they have soil clinging to them. By sterilizing your raw vegetables in addition to killing parasites, you might control your infection, reduce symptoms and improve your vision.

It is assumed that you have basic training or are self taught with the Syncrometer as described in *The Cure For All Cancers*. There are courses and a training video available (see *Sources*).

The experiments chosen here are a <u>sample</u> of a much larger set (*Syncrometer Biochemistry Laboratory Manual*, New Century Press, 1999). These are some of the most interesting.

Please note these precautions when doing Syncrometer biochemistry:

1. Some test substances are toxic, but there is no need to open <u>any</u> test substance bottles; simply use the material in original sealed bottle.
2. Don't do such research in the presence of children.
3. Keep your test substances locked up, labeled with poison signs so no accident could <u>ever</u> happen.

Exp. 1 Finding Ascaris

Purpose: to find the source of *Ascaris* and other parasites.

Materials: prepared microscope slides of *Ascaris megalocephala* (available from Southern Biological Supply, see *Sources*), *Ascaris lumbricoides*, *Ascaris eggs*, *Ascaris* (lung stage), *Leishmania*, *Toxoplasma* (Carolina Biological Supply Company). HCl, cysteine, pure salt, Lugol's iodine, povidone iodine (Spectrum).

Methods: make samples of the dust in your home. Collect a dust sample from bedroom furniture with a damp piece of paper towel, 2 inches by 2 inches (5 cm x 5 cm), and place in a reclosable baggie. Collect a dust sample off carpets. Sample the food in your refrigerator, as well as canned goods. Prepare samples of lettuce, cabbage, strawberries, and other raw foods.

Search each sample for all four *Ascaris* slides. (You put the dust sample on one Syncrometer test plate, an *Ascaris* slide on the other test plate, and test for resonance. Then repeat with other slides and dust samples.) Note that *Ascaris* is present in the dust or carpet only when a pet lives there or a pet once lived there. Note that *Ascaris* is always present in raw foods, even after thorough washing, and in bottles of oil, many canned vegetables, and your dinner.

Compare the effectiveness of plain washing, HCl-soak, cysteine-salt soak and iodine in treatment of vegetables. Use one drop Lugol's iodine in a quart of soak water. Retest after one minute. Soak raw foods in solution of ¼ teaspoon cysteine powder plus ¼ tsp. salt in one quart of water for five minutes. Soak other raw foods in HCl-water (1 drop per cup water). Treat oil, canned goods, and your dinner with HCl drops.

Try to sanitize the carpet and clear the dust of *Ascaris* eggs. Use povidone iodine in the water while shampooing the carpet. (Test carpet for staining first). Sample carpet dust again, later.

Note that cysteine sterilization alone does not kill *Toxoplasma* or *Leishmania*. These are also present in dirt. To kill these, table salt must be added to the cysteine soak. Lugol's solution kills all, as does HCl-water.

Exp. 2 Finding Tumors

Purpose: To find a growing tumor.

Materials: DNA, ortho-phospho-tyrosine (Sigma), *Clostridium tetani*, *Clostridium botulinum*, *Clostridium sporogenes*, *Clostridium septicum*, *Clostridium perfringens*, *Clostridium acetobutylicum* (Wards), a set of tissue slides like adipose tissue human sec, bone dry ground human CS, colon human sec, human kidney sec, human skin white v.s., liver human sec, mammary gland inactive human sec, prostate young human sec, red bone marrow human smear, thyroid gland human sec, tongue general structure sec, tooth in situ ls, urinary bladder collapsed human sec (Wards), spleen human sec, testis human fetus (Carolina Biological), ovary sec (Southern Biological), white blood cells (home made, see *The Cure For All Cancers*).

Methods: Search in all your organs for the presence of DNA.

Although DNA is present in all cells with a nucleus, it is in the free state (like the test sample) during cell division. DNA

579

only tests <u>continuously</u> Positive in ovaries or testes. DNA may also test Positive in a healing tissue such as bone after a tooth extraction, or the tongue after you burned it accidentally with hot food. Note that it disappears in a few days from these "healing" locations. In other tissues DNA only tests Positive for 20 seconds out of each minute.

If you find DNA <u>continuously</u> Positive in an organ like your liver, breast, or colon, you can infer that some part of this organ is growing much too rapidly—a tumor. What is your next step? Search for ortho-phospho-tyrosine to find out if the tumor is malignant. Also search for clostridium bacteria because they are the source of the extra DNA. If you find them in your teeth, you confirm the need for immediate dental work. Till then, brush teeth with oregano oil.

Exp. 3 Finding Mutations

Purpose: to search for tumor-related mutations.

Materials: p53 probe, bcl-2 probe, bax probe, (Calbiochem), nucleoside vanadyl complexes (Sigma), vanadium pentoxide atomic absorption standard (VWR Scientific Products), clock with a second hand, tissue samples listed in Experiment 2.

Methods: p53 is a good gene, present in everyone's DNA. But the Syncrometer typically does not detect it, I think because it is not loose in the cell's cytoplasm. So if the Syncrometer does detect p53, that is abnormal, and indicates a problem.

Search for the presence of p53 using all your tissue slides. If one is positive, search for vanadyl complexes there, followed by vanadium. I always find these present. You should also find, once the vanadium is gone (by eliminating gas leaks, metal glasses frames, plastic or metal teeth), that the p53 mutations are gone, too.

Next, in the same p53-positive tissue, search for an imbalance between bcl-2 and bax gene products. Using the clock, test continually for bcl-2 until it comes ON, namely resonates. Continue testing until it goes OFF. Repeat for bax. They should be ON for 30 seconds out of each minute, in perfect alternation. Find your time ratio. Find an organ that does not show the presence of p53 mutations. Repeat all tests. Is the ratio correct now?

Conclusion: vanadyl complexes cause p53 mutations, but can be corrected by cleaning up the environment. P53 mutations cause bcl-2/bax imbalances, but these, too, can be easily rectified.

Exp. 4 Effects Of Isopropyl Alcohol

Purpose: to find metabolic effects of isopropyl alcohol.

Materials: 5,6-isopropylidene L ascorbic acid, 2',3'-o-isopropylidene guanosine, 2',3'-o-isopropylidene cytidine, 2',3'-o-isopropylidine adenosine, 2',3'-o-isopropylidene inosine, human chorionic gonadotropin (hCG) (Sigma), acetone, isopropyl alcohol (Spectrum).

Methods: search for these compounds in your tissues. They should not be present. Repeat for a person who has just eaten a "fast-food" item and is positive for isopropyl alcohol.

Conclusion: we have been taught that isopropyl alcohol is detoxified by the body to acetone. No doubt you will find this also. But <u>before that happens</u> isopropyl alcohol will do other damage! In just a few minutes after accidentally eating a trace of this antiseptic in food or beverages you can see some of the new, potentially harmful, compounds.

5,6-isopropylidene-L ascorbate is formed almost instantly. I suppose you could regard this as a good thing, that our valiant vitamin C can also help out to detoxify isopropyl alcohol, but should we be using up our precious vitamin in this way? Would this not give us a novel kind of scurvy in spite of taking large amounts of vitamin C as a supplement? Consider, also, the possible toxicity of this new compound.

I also detect isopropyl alcohol / nucleoside combinations, i.e. 2',3'-o isopropylidene guanosine, 2',3'-o isopropylidene cytidine, 2',3'-o isopropylidene adenosine, 2',3'-o isopropylidene inosine. Surely, this could cause a flurry of mutations. Perhaps such a mutation could result in the excessive production of hCG. The Syncrometer detects hCG widespread in the body when isopropyl alcohol is present. hCG has been implicated in cancer for decades. In fact, it was formerly used as a cancer marker. Perhaps, if we consumed a lot more vitamin C, our nucleic acids would be protected from isopropyl alcohol. What becomes of the nucleoside adducts (combinations)? Are they toxic?

Exp. 5 Brakes And Accelerator

Purpose: to find toxic amines made by bacteria and observe their effect on pyruvic aldehyde (the "brakes" for cell division) and thiourea (the "accelerator").

Materials: tissue samples used in Experiment 2, 1,5-diaminopentane, agmatine (Acros), tyramine (Spectrum), diaminopropane, guanidine, ethylene diamine, cysteamine (Sigma), six clostridium species used in Experiment 2, *Rhizobium leguminosarum*, *Streptomyces albus*, *Streptomyces venezuelae*, *Streptomyces griseus* (Wards), *Mycobacterium avium/cellulare* (no current source), *Streptococcus pyogenes*, *Streptococcus mitis*, *Streptococcus lactis* (Wards), *Streptococcus alpha*, *Streptococcus beta*, *Streptococcus faecalis*, *Streptococcus pneumoniae* (no current source), *Staphylococcus aureus* (Wards), pyruvic aldehyde, thiourea (Sigma).

Methods: search for any of these bacteria in an organ that is severely handicapped such as underactive or overactive thyroid, ovary with cyst, breast with lump, prostate with hypertrophy, etc. Then search for amines in organs (both with and without bacteria). Then compare length of time pyruvic aldehyde is present (resonant) with time thiourea is present in organs with and without amines.

Conclusion: *Clostridium* causes <u>all</u> amines to be present while other bacteria cause <u>some</u> to be present. A few are present even without bacteria there. In handicapped organs (that have amines) pyruvic aldehyde may be "on" only briefly (one minute) while thiourea is "on" for many minutes. In healthy tissues (without bacteria, without amines) pyruvic aldehyde and thiourea are "on" one minute each, in perfect alternation.

Exp. 6 Restoring Bases

Purpose: to compare purine and pyrimidine bases in normal and tumorous organs.

Materials: four purines (guanosine, adenine hydrochloride, xanthine monosodium salt, inosine), three pyrimidines (cytidine, uridine, thymidine) (all from ICN except thymidine from Sigma), six clostridium species used in Experiment 2, tissue samples used in Experiment 2.

Methods: Test for all bases (or derivatives) at a normal, handicapped, or tumorous organs. Test for *Clostridium* presence in the same organs.

Conclusion: when clostridium bacteria are Positive, all four purines are absent while pyrimidines sound exceptionally high. (Remember, though, the Syncrometer cannot make quantity measurements). When clostridium species are gone, all seven bases are present. Try eating sardines (one can a day) to supply the missing bases. Does it work?

Exp. 7 Inositol Benefits

Purpose: to observe vitamin C and rhodizonate being formed in the body after eating inositol.

Materials: L-ascorbic acid, rhodizonic acid potassium salt, inositol (Spectrum), dehydroascorbate (Sigma), tissue samples used in Experiment 2.

Methods: find an organ, possibly your handicapped organ, that has neither ascorbic acid nor dehydroascorbic acid and is negative for inositol and rhodizonate, also. This establishes the situation <u>before</u> eating inositol. Eat ½ tsp. inositol dissolved in

½ cup water. Immediately search for ascorbate, dehydroascorbate and rhodizonate again. Continue testing for 5 minutes.

Conclusion: ascorbate and rhodizonate both appear simultaneously, while inositol soon disappears. Dehydroascorbate stays Negative the whole time, so it's safe to say that the ascorbate was not derived from it.

Exp. 8 Finding Azo Dyes

Purpose: to identify azo dyes in your body, clothing, food and common bleach, and observe their association with "bad" (non-organic) germanium.

Materials: germanium and thulium atomic absorption standards (Spectrum), a set of azo dyes including Sudan IV ("scarlet red," color index [CI] 26105, CAS 85-83-6, Sigma #S-8756 or Spectrum #SU120), p-dimethylaminoazobenzene ("DAB" or "butter yellow" CI 11020, CAS 60-11-7, Sigma #D-6760), Sudan Black B (practical grade, CI 26150, CAS 4197-25-5, Sigma #S-2380), Fast Green FCF (C.I. 42053; Food Green 3), pure sodium hypochlorite (bleach) (Spectrum), regular bleach from grocery store, tissue samples used in Experiment 2.

Methods: search for the presence of each dye in spleen, liver, kidneys, pineal gland, bone marrow, your handicapped organs, and then in the adipose (fatty) portion of these by placing the adipose slide on the same test plate. Also search for "bad" germanium. Next search for these dyes in new clothing before and after washing in borax. Repeat washing of clothing, using bleach, ⅛ cup per load, and test again for dyes.

Search for azo dyes in your two bleaches. The laboratory hypochlorite should have none, the grocery store brand may have several. Now search for azo dyes and laboratory bleach in food, especially dairy products.

Conclusion: highly carcinogenic azo dyes are in our new clothing, food, and household bleach. Dyes can generally be washed out, but DAB sticks tightly to clothing even after washing. However, washing in bleach, even bleach that contains dyes, gets DAB out! In food, numerous dyes appear together (or are absent together) suggesting they were not added individually. Foods containing azo dyes also test Positive for pure sodium hypochlorite. Foods that are Negative for dyes, also are Negative for hypochlorite. Could regular household bleach, used in manufacturing to sterilize things, be the source of widespread pollution with azo dyes? But Fast Green is associated with lanthanide metals such as thulium. Search for these on citrus and other fruit.

Once azo dyes are in our body, you always find "bad" germanium in the same place. Are azo dyes responsible for oxidizing "good" germanium to "bad" germanium?

Exp. 9 Freeing WBCs

Purpose: to observe the behavior of white blood cells (WBCs) in an organ containing asbestos, silicon, or "fried food" compounds.

Materials: toothpaste, corn oil or canola oil (grocery store), asbestos (water outlet gasket for car engine, automotive store; place a chip in small glass bottle, cover with water), silicon, acrylic acid (Spectrum), ferritin (horse spleen, Calbiochem), tissue samples used in Experiment 2.

Methods: search for asbestos in your tissues. Then search for asbestos in the tissue WBCs by placing the WBC slide on the same test plate. Be sure to include kidney and bladder tissues. If it is present in these excretory organs, we could conclude asbestos is being actively excreted. A further test of excretion would be searching in urine for the presence of asbestos (remember to dilute with water).

Next, search for ferritin in the WBCs of asbestos-containing tissues and in tissues that do not have asbestos. Normal tissues have WBCs that do not show ferritin to be present continuously. But asbestos-containing tissues have WBCs that do show ferritin to be present continuously. According to scientific reports,

WBCs are often "coated" with ferritin in cancer patients. We have seen that the cause is asbestos lodged in the tissue.

Next, search the immune-disabled <u>organ</u> for silicon and acrylic acid. If present, search the WBCs of that organ. If the WBCs are not "eating" these toxins, what will become of them? Where would silicon come from? Test your toothpaste, furniture polish, and the bottom of a bakery roll. Where would acrylic acid come from? Test your cooking oils. Also test foods that harbor *Ascaris* stages. These foods also have acrylic acid and acrolein! Does *Ascaris* make them?

Conclusion: healthy people may have asbestos in their organs, but it is also in their kidneys and bladder, indicating excretion ability. Advanced cancer sufferers always have asbestos, but never in their kidneys or bladder. It is accumulating in the tumorous organ because the WBCs there have stopped "eating" it. They have become ferritin-coated.

Ferritin coating is known to disable WBCs. Now we see asbestos is the real cause.

Exp. 10 Tumor Shrinking

Purpose: to observe (electronically) a tumor regressing.

Materials: DNA and tissue samples used in Experiment 2, various types of tumor tissue like acute granulocytic leukemia, acute monocytic leukemia, acute myelomonocytic leukemia, adenocarcinoma of breast, adenocarcinoma of colon, carcinoma of colon, fibroadenoma of breast, fibrocystic disease of breast, hemolytic anemia, hepatoma of liver, Hodgkin's disease in spleen, Hodgkin's granuloma, malignant melanoma of skin, mesothelioma, metastatic carcinoma of liver, oat cell carcinoma, villous adenoma of colon (Carolina Biological Supply), acute lymphatic leukemia, breast carcinoma, hairy cell leukemia, kidney carcinoma, lung carcinoma, lymphatic leukemia, metastatic-liver cancer, myeloblastic leukemia (acute), myeloblastic leukemia, spleen human cancer, uterus fibroid tumor (Wards), tumor causing toxins like copper, cobalt (atomic absorption standards from Spectrum), vanadium (from Experiment 8), organic germanium (use hydrangea root), inorganic germanium (from Experiment 3), malonic acid, urethane (Spectrum), asbestos , ferritin, acrylic acid (from Experiment 9), and the tumor causing bacteria (six clostridium species used in Experiment 2).

Methods: find a growing tumor using the DNA test substance and tissue specimens. Then search for resonant tumor-tissue types at that organ. Pick one or two tumor tissue types and search for tumor causing toxins and bacteria in both the tumor tissue and the associated organ. Finally, search for ferritin in the organ's WBCs. You will probably find the organ with the tumor tests Positive to most of the types of tumor tissues, but the organ does not test positive to the toxins and bacteria. The tumor tissue, however, will probably test Positive to all the toxins and bacteria! This indicates the organ has the tumor, and the tumor has the toxins.

Now comes the exciting part. Start the 21 Day Program. It will digest away the ferritin, "reduce" iron and germanium (turn them into good forms) with MSM, kill parasites, remove *Clostridium*, and keep pathogens away by instructing you to sterilize all your food with HCl. Repeat your testing once each day. Stay on the Program for all 21 days, even if you test Negative to DNA much sooner.

Conclusion: hours after you kill clostridium bacteria, DNA will test negative, indicating your tumor has stopped growing. After toxins test Negative (environmental and dental work is done), within twenty-four hours your tumorous organ will test Negative for all types of tumor tissues, indicating mutations are cleared up. But later toxins and pathogens will start testing Positive in your tumorous organ, indicating the tumor is opening and releasing its poisonous load to the surrounding tissue. Meanwhile, by day five of the 21 Day Program, ferritin will be gone, leaving white blood cells free to do their "immunity jobs."

Test each day to see which toxins are left.

As is emphasized throughout this book, you should do scans and blood tests as you go through the 21 Day Program. These should confirm your electronic observations.

If you are not sick, you can choose to experiment more scientifically by focusing on just one part, like cleaning up *Clostridium* while you monitor DNA.

Note: Stopping tumor growth is not tantamount to tumor shrinkage. Yet it often occurs. Just how it happens is further elucidated in later experiments.

Sources

This list was accurate as this book went to press. <u>Only the vitamin sources listed here were found to be pollution-free, and only the herb sources listed here were found to be potent</u>, although there may be other good sources that have not been tested. The author has no financial interest in any company listed.

Note to readers outside the USA:

Sources listed are typically companies within the United States because they are the most familiar to me. You may be tempted to try a more convenient manufacturer in your own country and hope for the best. <u>I must advise against this</u>! In my experience, an uninformed manufacturer <u>most likely</u> has a polluted product! Your health is worth the extra effort to obtain the products that make you well. One bad product can keep you from reaching that goal. This chapter will be updated as I become aware of acceptable sources outside the United States. Best of all is to learn to test products yourself.

When ordering chemicals for internal use, always specify a <u>food</u> grade.

Item	Source
Amino acid mixture, liquid for IV use and other IV liquids in glass bottles	Abbott Laboratories; Mexican pharmacies
Amino acids	Spectrum Chemical Co.; Seltzer Chemicals, Inc.
Baking soda (sodium bicarbonate)	Spectrum Chemical Co.

Betaine hydrochloride	Seltzer Chemicals, Inc.
Biotin	Spectrum Chemical Co.
Black cherry concentrate	Bernard Jensen Products; health food store
Black Henna	See Hair dye
Bleach (Chlorine) 5%, called sodium hypochlorite	Spectrum, be sure to get USP (#SI304).
Borax, pure	Grocery store
Boric acid, pure	Spectrum Chemical Co.; health food store; pharmacy
Butyrate, sodium	Mallinckrodt Baker
Calcium hydroxide	Spectrum Chemical Co. (#CA150)
Calcium carbonate	Spectrum Chemical Co.
Cascara sagrada	San Francisco Herb & Natural Food Co.
Chemical Supply Companies (research chemicals only)	Sigma-Aldrich Chemical Co.; Spectrum Chemical Co.; ICN Biomedicals, Inc.; Boehringer Mannheim Biochemicals
Cholecalciferol	Spectrum Chemical Co.
Citric acid	Univar; health food store
Cloves	San Francisco Herb & Natural Food Co. (ASK for fresh); Starwest Botanicals, Inc.
Coenzyme Q10	Spectrum Chemical Co.; Seltzer Chemicals, Inc.
Colloidal silver maker	SOTA Instruments Inc.; CTS Originals
Compass	Carolina Biological Supply Co. (#AA-75-8669); camping store
Cornstarch	Spectrum Chemical Co.
Cysteine	Spectrum Chemical Co.
Dental help in Europe	Naturheilverein
Electromagnetic field meter	Alphalab, Inc.
Empty gelatine capsules	Capsugel; health food store
Enema equipment	Medical Devices International
Epoxy coating	American Pipelining
Fat emulsion for IV use	Abbott Labs; Mexican pharmacies
Fenuthyme	Natures Way; health food store
Folic acid	Spectrum Chemical Co.
Germanium, organic	Hydrangea, coconut or other nuts
Ginger	San Francisco Herb & Natural Food Co.

Glutamine	Seltzer Chemicals, Inc.
Glutathione	Seltzer Chemicals, Inc.
Glycine	See amino acids
Goldenrod tincture	Blessed Herbs
Grain alcohol	Liquor store, get only 750 ml or 1 liter
Grains and legumes from India	Bazaar of India Imports
Gravel root (herb)	San Francisco Herb & Natural Food Co.; Starwest Botanicals, Inc.
Green Black Walnut Hull freeze-dried capsules	New Action Products; Consumer Health Organization
Green Black Walnut Hull Tincture	Nature's Meadow, New Action Products
Hair dye	Karabetian Import (black henna, red henna)
Hydrangea (herb)	San Francisco Herb & Natural Food Co.
Hydrochloric acid	Spectrum Chemical Co. (for disinfecting raw foods). You must dilute the 10% solution purchased (#HY105) to a 5% solution by adding an equal volume of water. For internal use, must be made by pharmacist.
Hydrogen peroxide 35% (food grade)	Univar
Iodine, pure	Spectrum Chemical Co.
Jade jewelry	Lapidary Art
Lecithin	Spectrum Chemical Co.
L-glutamic acid powder (this is not glutamine)	Spectrum Chemical Co.
L-lysine powder	Spectrum Chemical Co.
Lugol's iodine	Spectrum Chemical Co. or farm animal supply store (for slide staining, not internal use), for internal use must be made from scratch
Magnesium oxide	Spectrum Chemical Co.
Magnet, ceramic, high strength (e.g. 4" x 6")	BEFIT Enterprises, Ltd.
Magnetic material, low strength (thin sheet of magnetic material)	Available at fabric, art, and hobby shops.

Marshmallow root (herb)	San Francisco Herb & Natural Food Co.; Starwest Botanicals, Inc.
Methionine	See amino acids
Microscope slides and equipment	Carolina Biological Supply Company; Ward's Natural Science, Inc.; Southern Biological Supply Company
Mint oil	See peppermint oil
Niacin	Spectrum Chemical Co.
Niacinamide	Spectrum Chemical Co.
Non-alcoholic Green Black Walnut Hull capsules	See Green Black Walnut Hull freeze-dried capsules
Olive leaves for tea	San Francisco Herb & Natural Food Co.
Oregano oil	Starwest Botanicals; North American Herb & Spice, Co.
Ornithine	Spectrum Chemical Co.; Seltzer Chemicals, Inc.
Ortho-phospho-tyrosine (research chemical)	Sigma-Aldrich Chemical Co.
Ozonator	Superior Health Products
Pantothenic acid	Spectrum Chemical Co.
Peppermint oil	Starwest Botanicals
Peroxy	See Hydrogen peroxide
Plastic coated water pipes	See epoxy coating
Potassium chloride	Spectrum Chemical Co.
Potassium gluconate	Spectrum Chemical Co.
Potassium iodide, pure	Spectrum Chemical Co.
Salt (sodium chloride), pure	Spectrum Chemical Co., get USP grade
Silymarin, called "Legalon" in Mexico	Mexican pharmacies
Sodium alginate	Spectrum Chemical Co.; health food store
Sodium hypochlorite	See bleach
Stevia powder	Now Foods
Taurine	Spectrum Chemical Co.

Testing Laboratories	Aqua Tech Environmental Laboratories, Inc. (ATEL) ultra-trace thulium, other metals; Legend Technical Svcs., Inc. ultra-trace benzene, technical consultation, other analytical services; International Lab Associates (ILA); Oxford Laboratories, Inc. ultra-trace thulium, ultra-trace benzene, other metals; Braun Intertec Corp.
Thioctic acid	Spectrum Chemical Co.
Thyroid, dessicated	Your doctor
Tooth Truth	New Century Press
Uva Ursi	San Francisco Herb & Natural Food Co.
Vitamin B_1	Spectrum Chemical Co.
Vitamin B_{12}	Spectrum Chemical Co.
Vitamin B_2 (riboflavin)	Spectrum Chemical Co.
Vitamin B_6	Spectrum Chemical Co.; Seltzer Chemicals, Inc.
Vitamin C (ascorbic acid)	Hoffman-LaRoche (all other sources I tested had either toxic selenium, yttrium, or thulium pollution!)
Vitamin D	See cholecalciferol
Vitamin E capsules	Bronson Pharmaceuticals
Vitamin E Oil	Spectrum Chemical Co.
Wormwood capsules	New Action Products
Yunnan paiyao	China Healthways Institute

Abbott Laboratories
100 Abbott Park Road
Abbott Park, IL 60064
(847) 937-6100

Alphalab, Inc.
1280 South 300 West
Salt Lake City, UT 84101
(800) 769-3754
(801) 487-9492

American Pipelining
P. O. Box 5045
El Dorado Hills, CA 95762
(916) 933-4199
www.americanpiplining.com

Aqua Tech Environmental
Laboratories, Inc. (ATEL)
1776 Marion-Waldo Road
Marion, OH 43301-0436
(800) 873-2835

Bazaar of India Imports
1810 University Ave.
Berkeley, CA 94703
(800) 261-7662

BEFIT Enterprises, Ltd.
P.O. Box 5034
Southampton, NY 11969
(800) 497-9516
(516) 287-3813

Bernard Jensen Products
535 Stevens Ave.
Solana Beach, CA 92075
(800) 755-4027

Blessed Herbs
109 Barre Plaines Rd.
Oakham, MA 01068
(508) 882-3839

Boehringer-Mannheim
Biochemicals
9115 Hague Road
P.O. Box 50414
Indianapolis, IN 46250
(800) 262-1640
(317) 849-9350

Braun Intertec Corporation
6875 Washington Avenue S.
P.O. Box 39108
Minneapolis, MN 55439-0108
(612) 941-5600

Bronson Pharmaceuticals
Div. of Jones Medical Industry
1945 Craig Road
P.O. Box 46903
St. Louis, MO 63146-6903
(800) 235-3200 retail
(800) 610-4848 wholesale

Capsugel
P. O. Box 640091
Pittsburgh, PA 15264-0091
(888) 783-6361
(864) 223-2270

Carolina Biological Supply Co.
2700 York Rd.
Burlington, NC 27215
(800) 334-5551
(919) 584-0381

China Healthways Institute
115 N. El Camino Real
San Clemente, CA 92672
(949) 361-3976
(800) 743-5608

Consumer Health
Organization of Canada
1220 Sheppard Ave. E
Ste. 412
Toronto, Ontario Canada
M2K 2S5
(416) 490-0986

CTS Originals
P. O. Box 64
Lemon Grove, CA 91946
Fax (619) 644-8635

Hoffman-LaRoche
340 Kingsland St.
Nutley, NJ 07110-1199
Wholesale only
(800) 892-6510
(201) 235-5000

ICN Pharmaceuticals, Inc.
Biomedical Division
3300 Hyland Ave.
Costa Mesa, CA 92626
(714) 545-0113
(800) 854-0530

International Lab Associates
(ILA)
8 King Street E., Suite 1500
Toronto, Canada M5C1B5
(800) 291-6101
(416) 410-8314

Karabetian Import
2021 San Fernando Rd.
Los Angeles, CA 90065
(323) 224-8991

Lapidary Art
861 Sixth Ave., Suite 827
San Diego, CA 92101
(619) 234-2681
Legend Technical Services,
Inc.
775 Vandalia Street
St. Paul, MN 55114
(651) 642-1150

Mallinckrodt Baker
222 Red School Lane
Phillipsburg, NJ 08865
(800) 582-2537

Medical Devices International
3849 Swanson Ct.
Gurnee, IL 60031
(708) 336-6611

Nature's Way
1375 N. Mountain Springs
Pkwy.
Springville, UT 84663
(800) 962-8873
(801) 489-1500

Naturheilverein "Hilfe zur
Selbsthilfe" e.V.
Postfach 1238
D-65302 Bad Schwalbach
Germany
011 49 06128-41097
Tuesday and Thursday 10-12
AM Central European Time
Fax 011 49 06128-41098

New Action Products (USA)
P.O. Box 540
Orchard Park, NY 14127
(800) 455-6459 (USA only)
(716) 662-8000
New Action Products
(Canada) PO Box 141
Grimsby, Ontario Canada
L3M 4G5
(800) 541-3799
(716) 873-3738 (Canada)

New Century Press
1055 Bay Blvd., Suite C
Chula Vista, CA 91911
(800) 519-2465
(619) 476-7400

North American Herb & Spice
Co.
P.O. Box 4885
Buffalo Grove, IL 60089
(800) 243-5242

Now Foods
2000 Bloomingdale Rd.
Glendale Heights, IL 60139
(708) 545-9098

Oxford Laboratories, Inc.
1316 S. Fifth Street
Wilmington, NC 28401
(910) 763-9793

San Francisco Herb & Natural
Food Co.
47444 Kato Rd.
Fremont, CA 94538
(800) 227-2830 (wholesale)
(510) 601-0700 (retail)

Seltzer Chemicals, Inc.
5927 Geiger Ct.
Carlsbad, CA 92008-7305
(760) 438-0089

Sigma-Aldrich Chemical Co.
3500 Dekalb Street
St. Louis, MO 63118
(314) 771-5765
(800) 325-5832

SOTA Instruments Inc. (USA)
P. O. Box 1269
Revelstoke, BC Canada
V0E 2S0
(800) 224-0242
Fax (250) 814-0047

Southern Biological Supply
Co.
P.O. Box 368
McKenzie, TN 38201
(800) 748-8735
(901) 352-3337

Spectrum Chemical Co.
14422 South San Pedro St.
Gardena, CA 90248
(800) 791-3210
(310) 516-8000

Starwest Botanicals, Inc
11253 Trade Center Dr.
Rancho Cordova, CA 95742
(800) 273-4372
(916) 638-8100

Superior Health Products
13549 Ventura Blvd.
Sherman Oaks, CA 91403
(800) 700-1543
(818) 986-9456

Univar (wholesale only)
2100 Hafley Avenue
National City, CA 91950
(800) 888-4897
(619) 262-0711

Ward's Natural Science, Inc.
5100 West Henrietta Road
Rochester, NY 14692
(800) 962-2660
(716) 359-2502

Index

apoptosis, 33, 34, 39
appetite, 138, 158, 179, 190, 203,
   204, 225, 268, 300, 331, 338, 344,
   347, 373, 376, 377, 378, 390, 478,
   499, 534
Aredia, 231
arginase, 35, 164, 499
arginine, 163, 164, 191
Arichega technique, 83
arsenic, 21, 131, 252, 256, 258, 269,
   283, 294, 299, 336, 343, 377, 380,
   392, 398, 408, 417, 421, 434, 442
arterial blood, 84, 85, 574
asbestos, 21, 31, 32, 38, 43, 57, 60,
   61, 63, 97, 122, 129, 130, 131, 143,
   144, 145, 149, 166, 167, 168, 171,
   182, 184, 188, 196, 197, 202, 252,
   258, 259, 283, 285, 287, 288, 294,
   304, 325, 336, 357, 360, 363, 367,
   372, 380, 392, 434, 440, 451, 466,
   502, 505, 506, 510, 517, 518, 520,
   521, 522, 523, 524, 530, 558, 560,
   570, 574, 585, 586, 587
Ascaris, 25, 29, 32, 33, 34, 38, 53, 54,
   55, 56, 57, 61, 65, 66, 94, 126, 131,
   144, 145, 151, 153, 157, 158, 160,
   167, 172, 179, 196, 198, 204, 213,
   232, 233, 237, 239, 279, 328, 376,
   390, 421, 472, 476, 480, 481, 482,
   483, 484, 489, 492, 493, 495, 496,
   498, 499, 503, 509, 510, 511, 518,
   519, 520, 529, 531, 532, 534, 543,
   558, 578, 579, 586
aspirin, 64, 79, 85, 181, 217
AST, liver enzyme, 208, 220, 257,
   260, 263, 269, 272, 279, 282, 286,
   293, 295, 296, 298, 302, 306, 308,
   312, 317, 318, 331, 332, 335, 339,
   340, 341, 347, 353, 361, 366, 370,
   375, 378, 383, 387, 391, 396, 399,
   400, 402, 406, 409, 415, 420, 423,
   429, 433, 437, 441, 448, 456, 469,
   478, 484, 490, 493, 501, 512
autoclave, 56, 81
azo dyes, 32, 34, 57, 65, 70, 89, 114,
   115, 118, 119, 129, 130, 158, 168,
   183, 185, 212, 215, 216, 287, 420,
   435, 440, 443, 450, 458, 478, 482,
   503, 506, 523, 524, 544, 584, 585

B

bax, 20, 34, 36, 37, 39, 580, 581
benzene, 16, 17, 25, 30, 32, 53, 63,
   65, 89, 97, 121, 122, 125, 128, 129,
158, 160, 162, 166, 173, 182, 185,
194, 196, 198, 213, 214, 233, 252,
263, 283, 284, 285, 289, 290, 291,
293, 296, 297, 302, 304, 305, 306,
313, 338, 343, 357, 358, 359, 367,
368, 377, 380, 398, 415, 416, 429,
430, 434, 442, 451, 460, 485, 486,
495, 499, 500, 502, 503, 507, 510,
518, 520, 521, 523, 524, 531, 532,
545, 546, 552, 556, 559, 572, 574,
593
benzoquinone, BQ, 136, 157, 158,
   237, 256, 270, 271, 274, 276, 280,
   281, 308, 343, 571
Besnoitia, 48
beta carotene, 168, 194
betaine hydrochloride, 47, 137, 186,
   189, 191, 193, 194, 199
betapropiolactone, 32
bifidus, 44, 47
bile ducts, 52, 65, 66, 221, 241, 268,
   483, 492, 499, 510, 563, 567
bilirubin, 159, 198, 202, 208, 221, 242,
   262, 267, 268, 281, 302, 308, 309,
   311, 359, 360, 377
bioaccumulation, 90, 91
biotin, 109, 136, 154, 176, 192, 193,
   194, 199, 382, 418, 590
Black Walnut Hulls, 49
blasts, 208, 213
bleach, 56, 78, 79, 80, 81, 131, 132,
   133, 134, 182, 183, 184, 194, 238,
   295, 419, 456, 459, 547, 549, 573,
   584, 592
bleeding, 51, 64, 79, 85, 86, 87, 139,
   140, 175, 216, 217, 242, 319, 322,
   324, 332, 334, 371, 394, 422, 443,
   444, 457, 459, 470, 472, 548
bloated, bloating, 127, 139, 304, 494
blood builders, 216
blood fats, 225, 384, 386
blood iron, 142
blood osmotic force, 232
blood pressure, 228, 242, 272
blood test results, 207
blood test, perfect, 207
blood thinners, 87
blood urea nitrogen, BUN, 164, 208,
   217, 218, 219, 223, 241, 252, 256,
   257, 260, 262, 263, 268, 269, 272,
   279, 280, 282, 286, 293, 296, 297,
   298, 302, 306, 309, 310, 311, 312,
   315, 317, 318, 324, 331, 332, 335,
   339, 340, 341, 343, 347, 353, 361,
   366, 368, 370, 375, 378, 380, 383,
   386, 387, 391, 394, 396, 400, 402,

406, 409, 415, 418, 420, 423, 429, 433, 437, 441, 448, 453, 454, 455, 456, 460, 469, 472, 478, 484, 489, 493, 501, 512
body fat, 65, 114, 125, 185, 190, 195, 238
body products, 5, 9, 111, 129, 133, 134, 184, 260, 382, 429, 494
bone density, 250, 436, 501, 513
bone dissolution, 230, 231, 313, 320
bone fragment, 82, 475
bone loss, 250, 252
bone marrow, 34, 54, 78, 115, 118, 141, 144, 145, 181, 196, 212, 213, 214, 215, 216, 239, 278, 308, 313, 314, 315, 328, 348, 349, 363, 387, 390, 417, 421, 425, 427, 430, 432, 435, 458, 468, 469, 487, 488, 491, 492, 495, 496, 506, 508, 579, 584
bone marrow cancer, 118, 181
boron, 148
brace, 67, 340
bromelain, 138, 166, 185, 186, 189, 190, 191, 192, 193, 194, 195, 198, 506, 570
butter yellow, 5, 114, 116, 155, 238, 584
butyrates, 146

C

cadmium, 5, 18, 21, 69, 120, 258, 261, 283, 285, 299, 302, 319, 325, 357, 367, 372, 380, 403, 424, 434, 466
caffeine, 24
calcitonin, 230, 313, 320, 361, 370
calcium carbonate, 147, 590
calcium deposits, 22, 91, 161, 169, 171, 196, 198, 235, 502, 508, 509
calcium gluconate, 173
calcium hydroxide, 89
calories, 128, 204, 225, 226, 253, 476
Cancer Diagram, 39
canola oil, 123, 585
carbohydrate, 210
carbon dioxide, 99, 163, 208, 240, 519
carboxyethylgermanium sesquioxide, 30
carcinogenicity, 32, 70, 116
carcinogens, 5, 20, 28, 29, 33, 38, 43, 69, 70, 91, 109, 129, 195, 212, 313, 338, 413, 422, 443
caries prevention, 92
Cascara sagrada, 141, 271, 555, 590
cataract, 54, 157

cavitations, 69, 73, 75, 77, 82, 83, 84, 91, 95, 198, 270, 330, 401, 409, 453, 465
cavity, tooth, 89, 90, 92, 444
cayenne pepper, 59, 107, 334
cerium, 169, 346
cesium chloride, 147, 175, 308, 327, 368, 377
chamomile, 146
chemotherapy, 2, 9, 134, 187, 233, 260, 286, 319, 342, 371, 392, 393, 396, 397, 398, 399, 421, 438, 451, 471, 479, 502
chicken broth, 86, 165, 174, 185, 186, 514
cholanthrene, 24, 149
cholera, 55
chromosomes, 5, 19, 26, 27, 31, 36, 164, 213
chrysene, 28
citric acid, 99, 182, 545, 551, 554
clodronate, 148, 231, 255, 313, 314, 315, 320
Clostridium, 14, 15, 19, 29, 36, 37, 39, 43, 44, 45, 46, 48, 49, 50, 54, 58, 60, 69, 70, 76, 81, 82, 83, 84, 88, 92, 93, 100, 137, 144, 159, 164, 171, 217, 223, 296, 297, 304, 307, 309, 378, 399, 409, 432, 450, 459, 460, 465, 473, 474, 479, 480, 483, 485, 488, 499, 500, 501, 503, 505, 507, 548, 549, 579, 582, 583, 587, 588
clot, blood, 80, 85, 86
cloves, 49, 50, 65, 107, 108, 180, 181, 198, 199, 200, 270, 291, 299, 471, 474, 479, 481, 491, 492, 590
coal tar, 1, 25
cobalt, 21, 35, 214, 232, 313, 315, 370, 382, 427, 432, 435, 446, 492
cobalt, inorganic, 151
cobalt, organic, 151
cocoa, 126, 139, 536
codeine, 64, 289, 331
coenzyme A, 21, 105, 109, 154, 460, 472
coenzyme Q10, 104, 117, 136, 137, 154, 176, 185, 186, 189, 190, 191, 193, 194, 199, 200, 202, 204, 236, 239, 254, 256, 278, 284, 291, 297, 299, 300, 308, 309, 313, 325, 348, 354, 358, 367, 370, 373, 377, 380, 393, 398, 404, 408, 459, 471, 514, 515, 531, 590
cold packing, 88
coma, 242, 281, 471, 474, 476

X

xanthine, 142, 145, 223, 224, 431,
  445, 492, 583
xanthine oxidase, 142, 145, 223, 224,
  431, 445

Y

yeast, 100
ytterbium, 22, 169, 508
yttrium, 22, 508, 593
Yunnan paiyao, 139, 140, 176, 324,
  334, 371, 422, 443

Z

zapping, 51
zearalenone, 30, 124, 125, 129, 194,
  196, 359, 475, 502, 503, 507, 522,
  533
zinc, 78, 89, 90, 103, 168, 195, 199,
  270, 274, 308, 315, 330, 365, 447,
  455, 498
zinc oxide, 78, 89, 447, 455
zinc phosphate, 89, 90